Public Health for an Aging Society

Public Health
for an
AGING SOCIETY

Edited by

THOMAS R. PROHASKA

LYNDA A. ANDERSON

ROBERT H. BINSTOCK

The Johns Hopkins University Press
Baltimore

The Johns Hopkins University Press
2715 North Charles Street
Baltimore, Maryland 21218-4363
www.press.jhu.edu

Library of Congress Cataloging-in-Publication Data
Public health for an aging society / edited by Thomas R. Prohaska,
Lynda A. Anderson, and Robert H. Binstock.
p. ; cm.
Includes bibliographical references and index.
ISBN-13: 978-1-4214-0434-9 (hardcover : alk. paper)
ISBN-10: 1-4214-0434-6 (hardcover : alk. paper)
ISBN-13: 978-1-4214-0435-6 (pbk. : alk. paper)
ISBN-10: 1-4214-0435-4 (pbk. : alk. paper)
1. Older people—Medical care—United States.   2. Older people—Health
and hygiene—United States.   3. Health policy—United
States.   I. Prohaska, Thomas R. II. Anderson, Lynda A.   III. Binstock,
Robert H.
[DNLM: 1. Health Services for the Aged—United States.   2. Aged—
United States.   3. Health Policy—United States.   4. Public
Health—United States.   5. Social Environment—United States.   WT 31]
RA564.8.P84 2012
362.60973—dc23   2011023110

A catalog record for this book is available from the British Library.

*Special discounts are available for bulk purchases of this book. For more
information, please contact Special Sales at 410-516-6936 or
specialsales@press.jhu.edu.*

The Johns Hopkins University Press uses environmentally friendly book
materials, including recycled text paper that is composed of at least 30
percent post-consumer waste, whenever possible.

Contents

Foreword, by Kathy Greenlee   ix
Preface   xi
Acknowledgments   xv
List of Contributors   xvii

Part I   FUNDAMENTALS

1 Contemporary Perspectives on Public Health   3
TERRIE WETLE AND ANGELA SHERWIN

2 What Are the Roles of Public Health in an Aging Society?   26
LINDA P. FRIED

3 Financing and Organizing Health and Long-Term Care
Services for Older Populations   53
ROBYN I. STONE AND WILLIAM F. BENSON

4 Assessing the Health and Quality of Life of Older Populations:
Concepts, Resources, and Systems   74
SYLVIA E. FURNER AND LYNDA A. ANDERSON

Part II   SOCIAL AND BEHAVIORAL FACTORS

5 Social Determinants of Health Inequities and
Health Care in Old Age   99
STEVEN P. WALLACE

6 Disability and Functional Status   119
LAURENCE G. BRANCH, HONGDAO MENG, AND JACK M. GURALNIK

7 Behavioral Risk Factors and Evidence-Based Interventions   138
SUSAN L. HUGHES, MARCIA G. ORY, AND RACHEL B. SEYMOUR

Part III   SOCIETAL APPLICATIONS

8 Translation: Dissemination and Implementation Issues   161
THOMAS R. PROHASKA, RENAE SMITH-RAY, AND RUSSELL E. GLASGOW

9 Family Caregiving of Older Adults   181
LAURA N. GITLIN AND RICHARD SCHULZ

10 Social Engagement and a Healthy Aging Society   205
NANCY MORROW-HOWELL AND SARAH GEHLERT

11 Public Health Policy Successes   228
DAVID M. BUCHNER

Part IV   PUBLIC HEALTH INFRASTRUCTURE
FOR AN AGING SOCIETY

12 Technology and Aging   253
DAVID LINDEMAN

13 Public Health Workforce: Preparing for an Aging Society   275
JANET C. FRANK AND JOAN WEISS

14 Disaster Preparedness, Response, and Recovery   299
KATHRYN HYER AND LISA M. BROWN

Part V   EMERGING ISSUES

15 Planned and Built Environments in Public Health   327
WILLIAM A. SATARIANO, MARCIA G. ORY, AND CHANAM LEE

16 Genomics and Aging   353
STEVEN M. ALBERT AND M. MICHAEL BARMADA

17 Global Perspectives on Public Health and Aging   371
LAURENCE G. BRANCH AND HONGDAO MENG

18 Resource Allocation in an Aging U.S. Society   391
ROBERT H. BINSTOCK

Index   415

Foreword

The year 2011 marked a significant milestone for those of us in the field of aging—the nation's first baby boomers hit 65! As our baby boom generation hits retirement age, we need to be more prepared to care for our aging population, adept at managing and preventing diseases, and skilled at maintaining both physical and emotional health. As practitioners, policy makers, and researchers, we face significant challenges in promoting a healthy older population. Chronic conditions become more of a concern as we age. Older adults have the highest prevalence of multiple chronic conditions such as arthritis, asthma, chronic respiratory conditions, diabetes, heart disease, depression, and hypertension.

Public Health for an Aging Society further illustrates the many policy and practice advances that have occurred since a 1997 book on *Public Health and Aging* was published. That earlier volume explored opportunities to improve the health of the aging population and inform policy and practice in the aging services network. It is exciting to see that over the past 15 years, many of these opportunities have been realized. Tangible examples of programs that have been translated from research into community-based settings via both aging and public health networks are provided in this new volume. These are magnificent examples of how policy and practice have changed as a result of evidence-based interventions.

This book introduces many new topics relevant to public health and aging, including emergency preparedness, technology in aging, and environmental influences on health and health practices. Other pressing issues that receive significant and needed attention include workforce preparedness for the aging population, health disparities and social and behavioral determinants of health, and the role of social engagement in healthy aging.

The Aging Network, made up of State and Territorial Units on Aging, Area Agencies on Aging, and Tribal and Native Hawaiian organizations, has been working to enhance how older adults are able to access services in their communities. These services touch the lives of millions of older adults. This infrastructure, in partnership with public health and disability networks and health care providers, is rising to meet the needs of older adults with chronic conditions. The Aging Network also supports a multitude of other services for older adults such as congregate and home-delivered meals, respite care and support for caregivers, supportive services for dementia care, ombudsman support, and programs to prevent elder abuse and neglect.

The Administration on Aging supports evidence-based models of care with the translation of research to practice of programs directed toward older adults living in the community. These interventions address concerns such as chronic disease self-management, diabetes self-management, promotion of physical activity, falls management and prevention, nutrition education, and mental health support. At present, almost every U.S. state is now implementing a community-based intervention directed toward older adults living in the community and improving the health of older adults. We will continue to move in this direction and strive to touch as many lives as possible through our network of partners.

Continuity of care during transitions through the health care system is imperative to quality care. The Aging Network and their many partners in public health, academia, and the private sector are embedding evidence-based methods to minimize health complications when individuals are moving from hospitalization to rehabilitation to home or anywhere in between. For an aging population with high prevalence of multiple chronic diseases, high-quality transitions in care are critical to healthy outcomes; conversely, loss of continuity of care is wrought with risk of decline in function and health and higher health care costs. Along with care transition support, the Aging Network is also developing optimal methods for supporting care coordination and providing options counseling for older adults and those with disability.

The framework of this book will give the reader a broad lens for viewing and understanding the ecological model of how an older adult as an individual fits into a larger model of family and community, as well as exploring the larger fit within society both locally and globally. The opportunities are vast, and this context will help us to identify how to mold programs that will continue to improve the care we give to older adults in the decades to come.

I am honored to contribute to *Public Health for an Aging Society*, and I hope that it speaks to academics and students, as well as providers in health care and community-based settings who touch older adults' lives each and every day.

Kathy Greenlee
Assistant Secretary for Aging
U.S. Department of Health and Human Services

Preface

This volume advances the dialogue among researchers, practitioners, and policy makers in public health and aging which started with a previous book, *Public Health and Aging*, published by the Johns Hopkins University Press and edited by Tom Hickey, Majorie A. Speers, and Thomas R. Prohaska. That 1997 book, based on a national conference held in 1994, was designed to help create a national agenda to address scientific and public health policy issues. The book was instrumental in identifying the gaps in public health for the older population and how further public health and aging research could inform policy and practice and thereby promote the health of older adults.

Fifteen years later, the fields of public health and aging have witnessed an exponential growth and together provide important resources for improving the health and well-being of older adults. We have also entered a critical period in U.S. history, when the "baby boom" birth cohort—79 million Americans born between 1946 and 1964—is joining the ranks of the older population. By 2030, one in every five Americans will be aged 65 and older. To reflect these changes, advances, and opportunities, we titled this new book *Public Health for an Aging Society*. Given the increasing complexity of the issues posed by an aging society, we have expanded the traditional scope and treatments of public health and aging by adopting a social-ecological perspective that incorporates individual, family, community, societal, and environmental levels.

Part I, Fundamentals, presents a critical foundation for understanding public health approaches for an aging society and provides an introduction to many of the concepts examined in the sections that follow. The first chapter, by Terrie Wetle and Angela Sherwin, is an overview of public health in the second decade of this century, describing fundamental public health models, approaches, and functions and introducing many current issues that researchers, practitioners, and policy makers are facing. In the chapter that follows, Linda Fried makes a compelling case that population aging is a major successful outcome of public health interventions of the past century, that prevention matters into the oldest ages, and that public health strategies are critical and need to advance at all levels of the social-ecological model if we are to achieve our ultimate goal of optimizing healthy and successful aging. The chapter by Robyn Stone and William Benson gives an overview of the sources and mechanisms for financing medical and long-term care for older Americans. It also describes the organization of the U.S. health care system, highlighting key issues such as improving service coordination, expanding home- and community-based care services, and enhancing consumer direction in service delivery. Sylvia Furner and Lynda Anderson describe in their chapter the importance and challenges of measuring health and quality of life and then provide a number of national, state, and local data sources for doing so.

In part II, Social and Behavioral Factors, the focus is on the social determinants of health, advances in addressing disability and functional limitations, the critical role of family caregiving, and the increased knowledge of social and behavioral determinants of health, which has grown exponentially in the past decade. Steven Wallace's chapter provides an introduction to the concepts of health equity and health disparities; identifies specific populations of interest through documenting inequities by race, economic position, and gender; analyzes the impact of social determinants on the receipt of medical care in older adults; and concludes by examining how policy changes could reduce health inequities in old age. Identifying the causes and consequences of disability and functional status and strategies to prevent or delay disability is a fundamental objective in public health and aging. The chapter by Laurence Branch, Hongdao Meng, and Jack Guralnik presents advances in how disability is defined and assessed and provides epidemiological evidence on population trends in disability in older adults. Most critical to this discussion, the authors identify the mutable risk factors associated with disability and suggest strategies to change them. Susan Hughes, Marcia Ory, and Rachel Seymour's chapter contains an overview of the prevalence and associated outcomes for current major modifiable behavioral risk factors. It also provides a summary of key theories of behavior change and then discusses steps used to develop and test successful evidence-based behavior change interventions.

Part III, Societal Applications, addresses three major movements involving the translation and diffusion of evidence-based programs for older adults and the emergence of social engagement and policy successes that improve the public health of older adults. In the opening chapter of this section, Thomas Prohaska, Renae Smith-Ray, and Russell Glasgow examine the factors used to determine whether a program is evidence-based and propose approaches for enhancing the likelihood of translating research to practice. Along with examples of successful translation efforts, the authors offer recommendations to facilitate dissemination and enhance the public health impact of evidence-based programs. Using a public health lens, Laura Gitlin and Richard Schulz provide a comprehensive examination of demographic transitions shaping caregiving, the prevalence and risks of caregiving, strategies to minimize adverse outcomes among caregivers, and the global implications and needed public health responses to support family caregivers. In their chapter, Nancy Morrow-Howell and Sarah Gehlert begin with definitional issues and then undertake a comprehensive overview of current research about antecedents and outcomes of engagement. They also describe program and policy initiatives designed to increase social engagement and make recommendations for future directions. David Buchner's chapter focuses on the role of policy in the prevention of disease, chronic conditions, and disability in older adults. His discussion is particularly informative regarding the diversity and types of policies, from clinical care to housing, that have successfully impacted the health and well-being of older adults.

The most critical infrastructure concerns being discussed in the field today are the subject of part IV, Public Health Infrastructure for an Aging Society. This section delineates the increasing importance of technology, workforce preparedness, and emergency preparedness and response. David Lindeman's chapter describes the unprecedented changes in the ways technology can and will improve the health of the older population. As Lindeman makes clear, advances in technologies are reframing how health care will be delivered; how older adults, family caregivers, and service providers communicate; how the health care workforce is trained; and how older adults obtain access to care and services. A chapter by Janet Frank and Joan Weiss describes the demographics of public health personnel and their key roles in the health of older adults. It also examines the current academic preparation and needs of students and other trainees in public health and related professions. The particular vulnerability of older adults as a population that warrants special attention during all phases of disasters is the focus of a chapter by Kathryn Hyer and Lisa Brown. They analyze the structure of emergency response in the United States, the risks to and resilience of older adults in disasters, and the challenges of incorporating older people into disaster plans and responses in various types of residential settings, including nursing homes.

The final section, Emerging Issues, deals with important emerging macro-ecological factors in public health and aging. A chapter by William Satariano, Marcia Ory, and Chanam Lee focuses on the association between the built environment and healthy aging. Using the example of physical activity and walking, for instance, they illustrate how problems of neighborhood safety and "walkability" are associated with lower levels of walking and are most evident among older adults with limited mobility, which then results in a cascade of deteriorating health and well-being. In their chapter, Steven Albert and Michael Barmada address the potential of genomic information to prevent disease and promote health through the integration of genomics into public health research, policy, and practice. The authors present this emerging science clearly, conveying the importance of the association between genetics and specific behavioral risk factors—for example, the association between physical activity and telomere length. Although the authors offer examples of advances in epigenetics and aging, they also elucidate the ethical and policy challenges in this emerging field. Laurence Branch and Hongdao Meng's chapter makes clear that public health and aging are global concerns. It presents a historical perspective on increases in life expectancy in the United States and the public health factors contributing to this increase and then undertakes comparisons with recent trends in global aging. Branch and Meng also provide a convincing discussion on how the lessons learned from U.S. experiences with increasing average life expectancy can be applied globally in less developed regions. The concluding chapter, by Robert Binstock, examines the political and economic forces in the United States and other nations affecting the availability of public financial resources for health care services and other means of promoting health for older adults in the near and long term. Despite a number of contemporary pressures for cutting public resources affecting the health of the older U.S. population, he argues that effective countervailing forces to these vectors may be the political threat of bloc voting by older persons and a better rhetorical framing of the issues at stake for all generations in significant retrenchment of health care resources available for the public health of the aging population.

In preparing this book, one of our goals was to appeal to academic public health researchers and students. In addition, because of its research-to-practice perspective, the book is designed to be of value to the public health network, the aging services network, policy makers, and, to a lesser degree, clinical practitioners. Furthermore, we believe that the contents will appeal to professionals traditionally not associated with the field of public health and aging, such as those who deal with technology and health, emergency preparedness, genomics, and the role of environmental factors in health.

Finally, the high quality of this volume is due primarily to the seriousness with which the chapter authors accepted their assignments and to the goodwill with which they responded to editorial criticisms and suggestions. To these colleagues, the editors would like to express their special appreciation.

Acknowledgments

We deeply appreciate the efforts of our many colleagues who significantly contributed to the preparation of this book. We thank those who joined us — in person and by telephone—at a 2–day meeting on May 13–14, 2009, to help us outline this volume. They were Steven M. Albert, William F. Benson, Laurence G. Branch, Jacob A. Brody, David M. Buchner, Amy Eisenstein, Sylvia E. Furner, Robyn Golden, Linda Harootyan, Susan L. Hughes, Marcia G. Ory, William A. Satariano, Renae Smith-Ray, Robyn I. Stone, Steven P. Wallace, and Terrie F. Wetle. These leading individuals, drawn from various sectors of public health and aging, were well positioned to help us conceptualize this book. Many of them went on to serve as outstanding chapter authors in this volume, and we commend as well as thank them for those essential contributions. We also commend Jenny Matson Palsgrove for capturing in her notes the many ideas from the planning meeting and Carla Doan for helping with logistics. The Institute for Health Research and Policy at the University of Illinois at Chicago generously hosted the meeting.

Financial support for the meeting and for the consultants was provided by the Healthy Aging Program, Division of Adult and Community Health, National Center for Chronic Disease Prevention and Health Promotion, Centers for Disease Control and Prevention (CDC). Debra Torres and Michelle Brown provided financial oversight. Other individuals within CDC who provided critical support of this project were Wayne Giles and Kurt Greenlund. The findings and conclusions in this book are those of the authors and do not necessarily reflect the official position of CDC or the Administration on Aging.

Special thanks are due to Wendy Harris, who acquired this manuscript for the Johns Hopkins University Press, for her initial vision and encouragement to create this book, as well as her guidance in crafting and naming the volume. We are also grateful to Suzanne Flinchbaugh at the Press for her constructive suggestions and patience in moving this volume forward.

Contributors

Steven M. Albert, PhD, MSPH, MA, University of Pittsburgh

Lynda A. Anderson, PhD, Centers for Disease Control and Prevention

M. Michael Barmada, PhD, University of Pittsburgh

William F. Benson, Health Benefits ABCs

Robert H. Binstock, PhD, Case Western Reserve University

Laurence G. Branch, PhD, University of South Florida

Lisa M. Brown, PhD, University of South Florida

David M. Buchner, MD, MPH, University of Illinois at Urbana-Champaign

Janet C. Frank, DrPH, University of California at Los Angeles

Linda P. Fried, MD, MPH, Columbia University

Sylvia E. Furner, PhD, MPH, University of Illinois at Chicago

Sarah Gehlert, PhD, Washington University in St. Louis

Laura N. Gitlin, PhD, Jefferson Health System

Russell E. Glasgow, PhD, National Cancer Institute

Jack M. Guralnik, MD, PhD, National Institutes of Health

Susan L. Hughes, PhD, University of Illinois at Chicago

Kathryn Hyer, MPP, PhD, University of South Florida

Chanam Lee, PhD, MLA, Texas A&M University

David Lindeman, PhD, Center for Technology and Aging

Hongdao Meng, PhD, University of South Florida

Nancy Morrow-Howell, PhD, Washington University in St. Louis

Marcia G. Ory, PhD, MPH, Texas A&M University

Thomas R. Prohaska, PhD, University of Illinois at Chicago

William A. Satariano, PhD, MPH, University of California at Berkeley

Richard Schulz, PhD, University of Pittsburgh

Rachel B. Seymour, PhD, University of Illinois at Chicago

Angela Sherwin, MPH, Brown University

Renae Smith-Ray, University of Illinois at Chicago

Robyn I. Stone, DrPH, LeadingAge Center for Applied Research

Steven P. Wallace, PhD, University of California at Los Angeles

Joan Weiss, PhD, RN, CRNP, Health Resources and Services Administration

Terrie Wetle, MS, PhD, Brown University

PART I
Fundamentals

CHAPTER 1

Contemporary Perspectives
on Public Health

Terrie Wetle, MS, PhD
Angela Sherwin, MPH

POPULATION HEALTH

"Public health" has been characterized in a variety of ways, including as a discipline, a profession, an infrastructure, and a philosophy. At times, public health has even achieved the status of a "movement" (Raeburn and MacFarlane, 2003, p. 243). Regardless of the specific characterization of public health, maintaining and improving the health of populations is the common thread across perspectives. A 1988 report released by the Institute of Medicine (IOM) defines public health as "the fulfillment of society's interest in assuring the conditions under which people can be healthy" (IOM, 1988, p. 40). Ensuring public health requires an understanding of a population's risk factors for disease and determinants of health.

Responsibility for ensuring the public's health is dispersed among federal, state, and local branches of government. Public health surveillance is largely the responsibility of state and local governments; however, the federal government has resources, expertise, and national perspectives that inform local public health priorities and decisions. In the United States, the Department of Health and Human Services (DHHS) leads federal public health initiatives. Within DHHS, there are several key agencies that constitute the U.S. Public Health Service: the Centers for Disease Control and Prevention (CDC), the Agency for Healthcare Research and Quality, the Agency for Toxic Substances and Disease Registry, the Food and Drug Administration, the Health Resources and Services Administration, Indian Health Service, the National Institutes of Health, and the Substance Abuse and Mental Health Services Administration (IOM, 2002). Many nongovernmental organizations (NGOs) also participate in ensuring the public's health. NGOs can be involved locally, nationally, or internationally. They often focus their efforts on advocacy, fundraising, and education related to specific health concerns or on implementing interventions targeting at-risk populations.

Since the field of public health strives to improve the health of populations, understanding both the definition of health and the factors that affect health status is critical to public health practice. The World Health Organization (WHO) defines health as "a state of complete physical, mental and social well-being and not merely the absence of disease or infirmity" (Preamble to the Constitution of the WHO, 1948, p. 1). Factors that interact to affect the health of individuals and populations are called determinants of health. These factors include one's genetics, physical environment, behaviors, income, education level, relationships with friends and family, and access to and utilization of medical care (WHO, 2010b).

Several models have been developed to aid researchers and practitioners in understanding the interactions among determinants of health as they define the health of an individual or a population and dictate disease prevention pathways. Two such models are the population perspective and the social-ecological model.

The population perspective model focuses on modifying risk for the entire population rather than for specific high-risk individuals. It is possible that a preventive measure that brings substantial benefit to the population may offer little benefit to a participating individual. This phenomenon is known as the prevention paradox. Examples include public health campaigns to encourage childhood immunization or quarantining individuals with contagious diseases. A population perspective considers a continuum of risk for each determinant.

The social-ecological model assumes that health and wellness are affected by interactions among multiple determinants, including biology, behavior, social factors, and the broader environment. Upstream determinants, such as policies and societal norms, interact with downstream determinants, such as genetics and individual health behaviors, to define the health of a population. These interactions can be complex, which makes discerning any single "cause" of most health conditions impractical. An example of a multi-cause health concern is the growing obesity epidemic. Interventions can be implemented to influence determinants upstream or downstream. Interventions designed to address determinants upstream at the population level, such as reducing corn syrup in foods or removing sugary drinks from grade school vending machines, will be very different from those that intervene in individual risk factors, such as promoting individualized diet and exercise regimens.

Approaches to addressing risk factors and determinants of health often differ based on one's training. Physicians and other medical professionals are trained to diagnose and treat illnesses, making clinical decisions in the best interest of each individual patient. Clinicians generally embrace the prevention mission of public health but do so through detection of individual risk factors (Marmot, 2001). Public health professionals are trained to identify the etiology, meaning causes of disease in populations, and design appropriate interventions. A public health approach seeks to control incidence and prevalence of ill-health conditions in a population, whereas clinicians offer prevention counseling to high-risk individuals. These differing approaches are complementary. The development of health information technology, including electronic medical records, health information exchanges, geographic mapping software, and internet programs, has contributed to improvements in coordinating patient-centered medical care with population health efforts (Lurie and Fremont, 2009).

PUBLIC HEALTH FUNCTIONS

Governments play a critical role in the maintenance and improvement of the public's health. The IOM identified three core public health functions of the government in its 1988 report: public health assessment, policy development, and assurance (IOM, 1988). Ten essential services that are the responsibility of the government in addressing these three core public health functions were defined by the DHHS in 1994 (fig. 1.1). Public health *assessment* requires the government to continually monitor health status and investigate patterns of illness to identify community health problems and hazards. *Policy development* requires public health departments to inform, educate, and empower the population about health issues; mobilize community partnerships to identify and address health problems; and develop policies and plans that support individual and community health efforts. *Assurance* of the public's health requires the government to enforce laws and regulations that protect

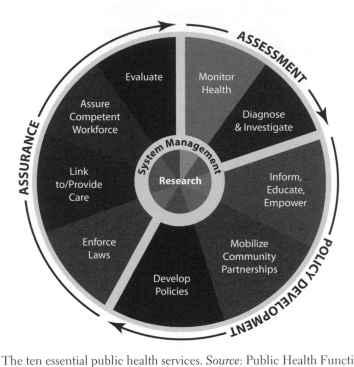

Fig. 1.1. The ten essential public health services. *Source*: Public Health Functions Project, www.health.gov/phfunctions/public.htm

health and ensure safety; link people to personal health services and assure the provision of health care; assure the competency of the public health and personal health care workforce; and evaluate effectiveness, accessibility, and quality of personal and population-based health services. As public health issues evolve, ongoing research is needed to identify and test innovative strategies that address health problems associated with each of the core functions.

More than a decade after releasing its report on the future of public health, the IOM reassessed the status of public health in the United States in a 2002 report entitled *Future of Public Health in the 21st Century* (IOM, 2002). The IOM asserted that progress had been made in aligning federal, state, and local governments to fulfill the three core public health functions but identified many areas where improved coordination and oversight were still needed. For example, strengthening local public health infrastructure is an area for continual improvement. This requires training and preparing the public health workforce, building capacity of health information systems and public health laboratories, and tightening the management and coordination of public health agencies. A strong local public health infrastructure is essential for appropriate crisis response as well as for addressing long-term public health issues, such as chronic illnesses, infectious diseases, and health promotion.

In addition to assessment, policy development, and assurance, effective communication of these core functions to the public is crucial. In many cases, the public's understanding of public health is disconnected from the reality of public health functions. Improved health status, diseases prevented, more efficient health spending, and improvements in quality of life are documented successes attributable to public health efforts. Individuals rarely link their own health successes to public health interventions and activities (Turnock, 2009).

POPULATIONS OF INTEREST

Public health research and practice depend on understanding patterns of disease and isolating determinants of health in a variety of populations, stratified by characteristics of interest. Populations may be studied at a single point in time to ascertain a snapshot of the population's health. Alternatively, population health status and characteristics may be tracked over time to assess long-term health, the impact of an intervention on a variety of populations, or to identify emerging health concerns. There may be social, geographic, ethnic, or gender differences in rates of disease occurrence. Understanding the nature of these population differences can aid public health practitioners in targeting interventions appropriately (Marmot, 2001). Common population characteristics studied in public health research include age, sex, race and ethnicity, socioeconomic status, occupational experience, and geographic location.

Children (under 18 years of age) and older adults (65 years of age and older) are two age cohorts of special interest to public health researchers and practitioners. Children encounter public health issues unique to their age group, such as the need for timely immunizations as well as minimizing exposure to lead paint and other environmental toxins detrimental to development. At the other end of the age spectrum, interest in older populations is increasing as the aging population grows. Worldwide, the percent of the population 65 years of age or older is projected to grow from 12.4% in 2000 to 19.6% in 2030 (Goulding and Rogers, 2003). This growth can be attributed to higher fertility rates in many countries immediately following World War II and to declining fertility rates more recently. A 20–year increase in the average life span between 1950 and 2000 similarly contributes to the worldwide growth of the aging population. This increased life span is a reflection, in large part, of successful public health interventions throughout the twentieth century (Goulding and Rogers, 2003).

Stratifying populations by race and ethnicity can provide insight into how these characteristics interact with other factors to produce racial disparities in health that are larger now than they were in 1950 (Krieger, 2003). These disparities are all the more important in the United States given the projected growth in the nation's racial and ethnic diversity. From 2010 to 2050, the Hispanic and Asian populations are projected to nearly double, from 16.0% to 30.2% and from 4.6% to 7.8%, respectively, while the proportion of the population that is white is projected to decrease from 64.7% to 46.3% over the same period of time (U.S. Census Bureau, 2009).

Socioeconomic status is strongly associated with health status. Approximately 1.2 billion people worldwide live in extremely impoverished conditions. Without adequate shelter, clean water, appropriate sanitation, and sufficient nutrition, poverty becomes a vehicle for chronic poor health (WHO, 2010c). A 24–year longitudinal study of British civil servants found that health behaviors, including smoking, alcohol consumption, diet, and physical activity, were associated with both lower socioeconomic status and higher mortality (Stringhini et al., 2010). In the United States, an array of health problems are associated with lower levels of education and poverty, including premature births, low birth weight, and obesity-related diseases.

Geographic location is another common population stratification used in public health. Data on local populations can shed light on environmental exposures and health risks or inform priorities of local health departments. Comparing morbidity and mortality more broadly among states and nations can identify public health issues that inform national health care investments. As global commerce and international travel become increasingly commonplace, evaluating population health with an international perspective is growing in importance. Research on aging has also begun to incorporate an international population perspective. For example, the International Network on Public Health and Aging was founded to study contextual differences that influence aging across diverse geographic locations and research disciplines to identify universal differential aspects of aging (Wahlin et al., 2008). Among developing nations, chronic diseases and other aging health concerns are a growing problem.

TRAINING PUBLIC HEALTH LEADERS

The average public health worker is 47 years old, 7 years older than the average age of the working population in the United States (Heishman, 2007). As the nation's public health workforce ages, education and training of public health professionals to replace them is critical for maintaining capacity to fulfill public health responsibilities. Approximately 20% of public health workers hold a degree specific to the field (IOM, 2003). These professionals are typically trained in the following areas: epidemiology, biostatistics, environmental health, health services administration, and social and behavioral sciences. The majority of public health professionals do not hold a public health degree but have formal education and training in a related field. These fields include medicine, nursing, dentistry, social work, allied health professions, pharmacy, law, public administration, veterinary medicine, engineering, environmental sciences, biology, microbiology, and journalism (IOM, 2003). The IOM recommends that professional training in public health must keep pace in response to evolving social, economic, technological, and demographic changes. Beyond standard training in public health, professionals may wish to achieve competency in these additional areas: informatics, genomics, communication, cultural competence, community-based participatory research, global health, policy and law, and public health ethics. A multidisciplinary approach to public health education will equip public health professionals to communicate and understand the issues, concerns, and needs of diverse populations (IOM, 2003). Educational opportunities in public health are expanding with increased interest, course work, majors, and degrees at the undergraduate, masters, and doctoral levels.

CRITICAL ISSUES IN AN EVOLVING PUBLIC HEALTH WORLD

While public health can claim many historical achievements, the field is sure to confront new challenges in the twenty-first century. An aging population will elicit many of these challenges, but also opportunities for developing effective new strategies to maximize population health. Across populations, there has been growth in both the depth and breadth of public health research, such as the inclusion of community members in the design and evaluation of new public health interventions. There has also been increased focus on public-private partnerships that address public health concerns. Critical contemporary issues in public health, discussed below, include chronic disease; infectious diseases; comorbidity and syndemics; bioterrorism and emerging diseases; health disparities; health promotion, wellness, and prevention; evidence-based health policy and action; organization of and delivery of health care services; evolving research strategies; and financing care and health reform.

Chronic Disease

The prevalence of chronic disease has steadily grown throughout the twentieth century. In 2005, 72% of the total global burden of disease among those aged 30 years and older was attributable to chronic illness (Strong et al., 2005). For example, cardiovascular disease is the leading cause of death globally. Eighty percent of all deaths due to cardiovascular disease took place in developing countries (WHO, 2010a). Contributing to this growth in chronic disease is the quickly expanding prevalence of overweight and obesity. Chronic diseases are projected to be the leading cause of death across all income groups by 2015, refuting the long-standing belief that chronic conditions are faced primarily by the affluent developed countries (Strong et al., 2005).

More than 45% of people in the United States suffer from at least one chronic condition. Common chronic conditions include arthritis, asthma, cancer, cardiovascular disease, depression, and diabetes. Arthritis is the leading cause of disability in the United States. Fifty-nine percent of Americans 65 years of age or older suffer from arthritis (Goulding and Rogers, 2003). Diabetes is one of the fastest growing epidemics, affecting approximately 10% of adults and 20% of those aged 65 years or older in the United States (Goulding and Rogers, 2003; National Diabetes Clearinghouse, 2008). Given the high percentage of the population affected by one or more chronic conditions, it is not surprising that chronic illnesses account for the majority of health care spending in the United States. More than 75 cents of every health care dollar is spent on treatment and management of chronic diseases (Partnership to Fight Chronic Disease, 2009).

Prevention and management of chronic diseases is and will continue to be a key focus of global public health efforts. Individual and population-level interventions can be implemented in tandem and complementary to each other (Strong et al., 2005). For example, interventions that target the obesity epidemic could focus on individualized coaching and counseling about appropriate nutrition and exercise habits, as well as population-level changes throughout the community, such as publishing nutritional information on menus or ensuring that neighborhoods are safe for walking. The use of patient-centered medical homes is gaining increasing popularity as a strategy for reducing the burden of chronic disease. Medical homes coordinate care for chronically ill patients through one primary care practice, thereby intersecting public health principles with medical care in an effort to decrease fragmentation in the health care delivery system, engage in appropriate health promotion, and improve quality of care.

Infectious Disease

Despite success in eradicating smallpox and minimizing the spread of other communicable diseases, infectious diseases continue to account for 51% of years of life lost. There are striking disparities across regions and nations: infectious diseases account for 68% of years of life lost in low-income countries but only 8% of years of life lost in high-income countries (WHO, 2008). Infectious diseases with high global incidence rates include tuberculosis, malaria, and HIV/AIDS, as well as diarrheal conditions in young children. Understanding determinants of health that affect the development and spread of infectious diseases can aid public health professionals in minimizing the impact of future outbreaks (McMichael and Butler, 2007).

The HIV/AIDS pandemic has dominated the landscape of infectious disease surveillance since its emergence in the early 1980s. Nearly 30 years of advocacy, harm-reduction education, and pharmaceutical advances have transformed HIV in developed countries from an acute, fatal, viral infection to a chronic infectious disease (Matic, Lazarus, and Donoghoe, 2006). Despite this progress, the early and swift evolution of HIV from an exotic infectious disease to a global pandemic provides a cautionary indication of our vulnerability to emerging diseases. Fastidious surveillance of health data to identify emerging infectious diseases continues to be a public health priority. Streamlining communication pathways throughout the public sector to disseminate analysis and interpretation of health data is a key component for infectious disease management (Binder et al., 1999). Increasing international travel and global commerce have heightened the need for international coordination of public health responses to prevent and control emerging infectious diseases. Elements of coordination include ensuring adequate supplies of safe food and drinking water, securing appropriate immunizations, improving personal hygiene, and reducing inappropriate antimicrobial use (Binder et al., 1999).

In addition to the emergence of new infectious agents, potential antimicrobial resistance may threaten public health in the future. Technological and genetic innovations may prove to be valuable tools in preventing and managing infectious disease. Possible technological advancements include biosensors and high-density DNA microarrays, which would rapidly determine the identity of an infectious agent that causes an illness and the presence of antimicrobial resistance genes in the organism. Genetic discoveries may lead to the development of individually tailored immunizations, treatments, and other infectious disease interventions (Binder et al., 1999).

Comorbidity and Syndemics

The synergistic interaction of two or more epidemics is known as a "syndemic." Syndemics contribute to excess burden of disease due to comorbidities experienced by a population (Singer and Clair, 2003). They occur when health-related problems cluster by person, place, or time. The current interaction between the global HIV pandemic and the Mycobacterium tuberculosis epidemic in the developing world is one example of a syndemic. Globally, HIV has become the greatest single risk factor for contracting tuberculosis. Approximately one-third of those infected with HIV are also positive for tuberculosis, while 10% of those infected with tuberculosis are also HIV positive (Matic et al., 2006). The comorbidity of tuberculosis in HIV-positive patients accelerates the damaging progression of HIV (Ho, 1996). To prevent a syndemic, one must not only prevent and control each disease but also control the factors linking the diseases together (Milstein, 2001). For example, coordination across tuberculosis and HIV programming for prevention and treatment is essential to maximize the impact and cost-effectiveness of these efforts.

Future directions for syndemic research include understanding the biological interactions between and among diseases, recognizing the determinants of health that exacerbate or mitigate syndemic growth, and developing interventions that target comorbidities. Assessing the role of factors such as poverty, malnutrition, stress, stigma, behaviors, and exposure to environmental toxins may shed light on the occurrence and trajectory of syndemics behavior.

Bioterrorism and Emerging Diseases

Substantial investments have been made in U.S. local, state, and federal public health infrastructure following events such as the terrorist attacks of 2001, the Gulf Coast hurricanes of 2005, and H5N1 and H1N1 influenza outbreaks in 2007 and 2009, respectively. These infrastructure investments have been almost exclusively for the purposes of upgrading the public health system's capacity for prevention of and response to large-scale public health emergencies. These investments follow years of underfunding for public infrastructure and inattention from federal policy makers. The IOM first expressed concerns with U.S. public health infrastructure in its 1988 report, but it considered the system "still in disarray" in 2002 (IOM, 2002; Lurie et al., 2006). The infrastructure investments have not come without a cost. As investments have poured into public health preparedness, health departments have identified reduction and elimination of important public health services and programs to offset the cost of preparedness, including teen pregnancy prevention, tuberculosis screening, and sexually transmitted disease (STD) contact tracing (Lurie et al., 2006).

Several changes to the public health workforce have been made as communities develop their emergency preparedness infrastructure. All states and most metropolitan areas have hired new personnel to coordinate bioterrorism responses and emergency preparedness. These new personnel are often entering the public field with experience in emergency response, law enforcement, or the military. Current public health department staffs who work in areas other than emergency preparedness have taken on new responsibilities to prepare for the event of a public health emergency. In many state and local public health departments, most employees have been trained in emergency preparedness. For many agencies, this training is the first time that all employees have collaborated to achieve a specific, common public health goal (Lurie et al., 2006). Emergency preparedness has also necessitated new partnerships between public health agencies and community agencies such as law enforcement, first responders, and other emergency personnel (Lasker, 1999). Part of this preparedness effort is recognition of the need to respond to emerging diseases, either naturally occurring or as deliberate exposure. Special considerations are required for elder populations who may have increased susceptibility to infectious or toxic agents, or who, because of mobility restrictions or other disabilities, may need additional assistance for evacuation or sheltering in place.

Health Disparities

Health disparities refer to differences in morbidity, mortality, and access to health care among populations that are defined by factors such as socioeconomic status, gender, residence, sexual orientation, race, and ethnicity. Health disparities can be costly. For example, one study estimated that from 2003 to 2006, 30.6% of direct medical care expenditures in the United States for African Americans, Asian Americans, and Hispanics were excess costs caused by health inequalities (LaViest, Gaskin, and Richard, 2009). These differences in health, when potentially avoidable, are unjust to members of these population subsets. As such, reducing health disparities is one goal of the Healthy People 2010 initiative and will likely be a priority for Healthy People 2020 (U.S. Department of Health and Human Services, 2000, p. 11).

Populations that have persistently experienced social disadvantage or discrimination often systematically experience worse health or greater health risks than more advantaged social groups (Dressler, Oths, and Gravlee, 2005; Braveman, 2006). For example, differences in health and health care have been documented across racial and ethnic divides. In fact, some have been getting worse over time, such as racial disparities in both all-cause mortality and infant mortality, which were greater in 2000 than they were in the 1950s (National Center for Health Statistics, 2001). Health disparities across sexual orientation have also been identified. Lesbian and bisexual women as compared to heterosexual women, as well as gay and bisexual men as compared to heterosexual men, have poorer overall health and mental health and higher rates of smoking and alcohol consumption (Dilley et al., 2010). One study found that men and women in same-sex relationships had significantly lower rates of health insurance coverage and higher rates of unmet medical needs than did individuals in different-sex relationships (Buchmueller and Carpenter, 2010). On a macro level, countries with greater polarization of wealth have lower life expectancies and higher mortality rates than those with more income equality. Individuals with low socioeconomic status are at higher risk for poor health because of exposure to poor working conditions, unemployment, living in disadvantaged neighborhoods, and social, economic, and environmental inequity relative to others (Wallerstein, 2002).

Racism, social inequality, and discrimination can adversely affect health through economic, environmental, psychosocial, and iatrogenic pathways (Braveman, 2006). Several conceptual models have been developed to describe health disparities. These include racial-genetic, health-behavior, socioeconomic status, psychosocial stress, and structural constructivist models (Dressler et al., 2005). The racial-genetic model explores genetic links between race and public health concerns such as high rates of low-birth-weight babies and hypertension and examines differences in genetic variance across populations. The health-behavior model accounts for health disparities via individual behaviors. The socioeconomic status model examines the confounding relationship between racial and ethnic disparities and socioeconomic status. The psychosocial stress model attempts to integrate the culture of racial and ethnic communities, stressors associated with the specific cultures, and their combined relationship with health and disease. The structural constructivist model examines the relationship between external pressures, such as social relationships, and social, psychological, and biological processes that occur in the intersection of social structure and culture. These models inform both research and intervention development.

Health care providers may intentionally or unintentionally propagate health disparities. For example, a qualitative study conducted in the Netherlands identified three patterns associated with ethnic disparities in care delivery. Disparities in care may result from language differences and resultant misunderstandings, differing perceptions of illness and or treatments, and inappropriate treatment and care because of provider prejudices against or stereotypical ideas about immigrant patients (Suurmond et al., 2010).

Despite the existing research on health disparities, many gray areas remain. For example, the lack of explicit definition of race and ethnicity is a significant barrier for research on health disparities (Dressler et al., 2005). Although long viewed as a biological factor, race has been more recently characterized as a social construct. Examining racism as a specific determinant of population health can inform public health policy and or medical decisions (Krieger, 2003). In the United States, the National Center on Minority and Health Disparities was created at the National Institutes of Health (NIH) to coordinate biomedical research and training on minority health and health disparities (Dankwa-Mullan et al., 2010). Disentangling the effects of education and socioeconomic status from race and ethnicity in analyses of disparities is an important aspect of research in this arena.

Health Promotion, Wellness, and Prevention

Health promotion involves research and interventions focused on preventing disease and promoting wellness. Studies have repeatedly linked individual behaviors with health outcomes and service use. Health promotion strategies are designed to target specific health behaviors by recognizing interactions of behaviors with social and environmental factors. Public health professionals who work in health promotion or health education encourage individuals to adopt and maintain healthy lifestyles. Engaging communities to determine wellness and prevention needs can also help to inform health promotion priorities. Health promotion messages may come through individualized counseling or may be broadly disbursed through social networks, community organizations, or public agencies (Navarro et al., 2007). Examples of health promotion efforts include programs that focus on smoking cessation, healthy diet, increasing physical activity, or safer sex practices. Other strategies include encouraging appropriate health screenings such as for cholesterol and blood pressure levels, mammography, Pap smear, and colonoscopy. Community-based health promotion initiatives have been supported by the Administration on Aging (AoA) through its Evidence-Based Prevention Program

(AoA, 2010a) in collaboration with the National Council on Aging (NCOA, 2010).

Skills required for health promotion vary widely, depending on the targeted health behavior and population. The Galway Consensus Statement, issued in 2009 after an international conference of health promotion and health education professionals, identified eight core competencies required for practicing health promotion: catalyzing change, leadership, assessment, planning, implementation, evaluation, advocacy, and building partnerships (Barry et al., 2009).

The CDC leads efforts to promote health and prevent disease in older adults in the United States. Five roles for the CDC in this endeavor include (1) providing high-quality health information and resources to public health professionals, consumers, health care providers, and experts on aging; (2) supporting health care providers and health care organizations in prevention efforts; (3) integrating public health prevention expertise with the aging services network (see chap. 3); (4) identifying and implementing effective prevention efforts; and (5) monitoring changes in the health of older adults (Goulding and Rogers, 2003).

Public health practitioners have struggled to apply evidence-based health promotion interventions to populations in real-world settings. Factors contributing to the gap between research and practice include insufficient training, lack of incentives for evidence-based practices, and inadequate infrastructures that support translation of research into practice (Glasgow, Lichtenstein, and Marcus, 2003). Bridging this gap requires adequate, timely communication and professional education about up-to-date best practices in health promotion (Cruz-Jentoft et al., 2009). Assuring funding streams for health promotion and prevention that align with these best practices and research results can also greatly affect the translation time from research to practice. Minimizing the time to bridge the gap between research and practice is a key area for improvement in health promotion. Successful efforts for evidence-based health promotion for older adults are documented at the National Council on Aging's Center for Healthy Aging website and have recently been funded by the Administration on Aging (AoA, 2010b; NCOA, 2010; see also chap. 11).

Another important direction for research in health promotion is to facilitate sustainability and long-term health benefits (McMichael and Butler, 2007). In 2006 the National Expert Panel on Community Health Promotion recommended achieving sustainability in health promotion by advancing community-based participatory research; including mental health, spirituality, and complementary and alternative medicine in the wellness paradigm;

and focusing on improving living conditions throughout the life span (Navarro et al., 2007). For older adults, compliance with recommendations for healthy behaviors can be a limiting factor in the effectiveness of health promotion and preventive interventions. Improved compliance requires sensitivity to beliefs, attitudes, preferences, expectations, limiting factors, and aspirations (Cruz-Jentoft et al., 2009).

Evidence-Based Policy and Action

Just as evidence-based medicine has become standard practice for clinicians, public health policy is grounded in evidence-based decisions. Evidence used to inform interventions, wellness programs, and health policy derives from many sources, including methodologically rigorous research studies, public opinion polls, and interviews with stakeholders. Dobrow, Goel, and Upshur (2004) propose a framework for evidence-based health policy that balances policy decisions between evidence and the broader context of all other factors taken into consideration in decision making. Their framework suggests greater emphasis on evidence than traditional political decision making, but more focused on context than evidence-based medicine. Since public health policies often impact entire populations, public scrutiny necessitates explicit justification for each decision. Grounding these decisions in data provides justification for public health decisions, improves transparency, and minimizes undue political sway.

An evidence base for health systems performance is being developed to assess and improve health care delivery and financing systems. One such effort in the United States is the work of researchers at Dartmouth who study regional differences in service use, health expenditures, and health outcomes (Dartmouth Atlas, 2010). Their work demonstrates that Medicare expenditures in the highest-cost regions are more than twice the expenditures in the lowest-cost regions, with only minor differences in health outcomes. The Commonwealth Fund compares and ranks U.S. and international health care systems based on access to care, quality of care, avoidable hospital use and costs, equity, and healthy lives (Cantor et al., 2007). The WHO developed its Health Systems Performance Assessment to establish a similar evidence base internationally (Murray and Frenk, 2001). Benchmarking health systems across nations allows policy professionals to assess various components of health care delivery systems, their influence on achieving health and social goals, system financing, and transparency and accelerates adoption of best practices across health systems.

Organization and Delivery of Health Services

Development of an evidence base for comparative health systems research, as described above, may inform future directions for organization and delivery of health services. Contemporary issues in health care organization and delivery include adoption of electronic medical records, growth of retail clinics, and establishment of accountable care organizations (ACOs).

Electronic medical records were implemented early and with much success in countries with a centralized health care delivery system, such as Sweden, Denmark, and the Netherlands (Anderson et al., 2006). Their adoption has grown much more slowly in the United States owing in part to the fragmentation of the delivery system. As adoption of electronic medical records grows throughout the United States, there will be important positive implications for the accuracy of medical information and the coordination of care, as well as an opportunity to improve tracking of disease screening and health promotion efforts for individuals. Issues of patient privacy will need to be balanced with the benefits of research using the wealth of data collected from each individual patient encounter (Binder et al., 1999).

Retail clinics provide acute medical care for simple diagnoses through nurse practitioners or physician assistants. These clinics are generally walk-in and located in retail spaces, such as pharmacies, for easy consumer access. They have grown in popularity across the nation as an alternative to primary care clinics and nonurgent emergency department visits (Laws and Scott, 2008). As retail clinics become more mainstream, it will be important to evaluate the quality of care in such clinics as compared with traditional medical settings, as well as assess the ability of these clinics to connect patients with follow-up care. Regulators will need to ensure adequate and appropriate oversight applicable to these care settings.

ACOs provide patient care to populations funded through payments for care that are tied in part to the overall performance and quality of the ACO. This model differs from earlier health maintenance organizations (HMOs) because they are built around providers rather than insurers (Gold, 2010). ACOs provide incentives for coordination of care, efficiency, and quality. ACOs may gain popularity in the United States as the Patient Protection and Affordable Care Act of 2010 (PPACA) is implemented because providers organized as ACOs will receive payments through Medicaid and Medicare for achieving cost savings. Ongoing policy issues for ACOs include establishing an adequate provider mix for each ACO and developing systems for quality and cost metrics.

Evolving Research Strategies

Conventional research methodology for evaluating public health interventions has used statistical analysis of outcome measures to assess an intervention's impact on rates of disease, disability, or death; uptake of services; or behavioral changes. Qualitative methods can be used to assess public health issues that are less easily quantifiable, such as quality of life, suffering, social justice, or equity issues. Public health research strategies are continually evolving; noteworthy advances to monitor and continually develop include community-based participatory research, geospatial mapping, and social networking.

Community-based participatory research (CBPR) is a methodology that approaches research collaboratively with community partners to "combine knowledge and action for social change to improve community health and eliminate health disparities" (Minkler and Wallerstein, 2003). CBPR methodology assumes that interventions are more effective when they incorporate both community insight and theories of etiology. Additionally, participation in the research process itself can enhance the health of participants. As a relatively new research strategy in public health, researchers using CBPR face many challenges, such as designing mechanisms to assess the effectiveness of CBPR, ensuring ethical treatment of communities as well as individual community members, and defining the researcher-community relationship (Wallerstein and Duran, 2006).

Geospatial mapping links determinants of health and health outcomes to specific geography. Mapping software can statically analyze the relationship between determinants of health and their location. Mapping can identify geographic patterns in morbidity, mortality, and health risks and can also be used to compare disease incidence with neighborhood characteristics. For example, Krieger and colleagues illustrated health disparities by socioeconomic status for sexually transmitted infections (STIs), tuberculosis, and nonfatal weapon violence, mapping the geographic prevalence and incidence of these public health issues with socioeconomic and exposure factors such as the percent of the population below poverty level (Krieger et al., 2003). Geospatial mapping technology can enhance research and development for all facets of public health through locating specific determinants of concern and more efficiently targeting interventions. This strategy can be particularly useful in identifying health risks associated with exposure to environmental toxins.

The explosion in online social networking has provided new opportunities for communication between public health professionals and the public. Social marketing campaigns that employ online social networking tools (including Facebook, Twitter, LinkedIn, YouTube, and many others) have reached their target audiences with greater speed, frequency, and ease than traditional modes of public health communication. For example, TRUTH, an anti-smoking campaign targeting adolescents, has created a variety of interactive games online for teens to play and learn about staying tobacco-free (www .thetruth.com). The CDC streams wellness and prevention videos on You-Tube (CDC, 2010). Many local health departments tweet about local health news and updates. DHHS has created a Facebook application for those who have received the H1N1 flu vaccine to share their vaccination status with their online friends. Identifying effective strategies for utilizing emerging technologies such as those described above will help to bridge generational gaps, as well as to more efficiently and effectively address population health issues.

FINANCING CARE AND HEALTH REFORM

The landscape of both public and private health care financing in the United States has changed with the passage of the PPACA (H.R. 3590, 2010). Over the next few years, Medicaid eligibility will expand to all adults under 133% of the federal poverty level. Medicare Advantage payments will be redistributed, providing higher payments to areas that currently have low fee-for-service rates. This redistribution will be coupled with quality bonuses and gradual phasing down of cost sharing for the Medicare Part D (prescription drug) "doughnut hole" coverage gap from 100% to 25%. In the private market, government regulations will implement new standards of coverage that prohibit annual and lifetime coverage limits, as well as prohibit exclusion of individuals because of preexisting conditions. All new health plans must cover a minimum set of benefits (existing plans will be "grandfathered"—that is, exempt from the minimum set). Health insurance exchanges will be created in each state to streamline purchasing for individuals and small businesses. Subsidies will be provided for those who do not qualify for Medicaid yet may not find private coverage affordable. Premium rates will be based only on age, geography, family composition, and tobacco use. These changes to both public and private health care financing systems are nuanced and complex and will require careful planning and implementation by professionals across all health care sectors.

In parallel to these financing reforms, the PPACA has the potential to directly improve the public's health. For example, PPACA requires most Americans to acquire or maintain health insurance coverage. As of 2009, 46 million people in the United States were without health insurance coverage (Statehealthfacts.org, 2010). The uninsured are less likely to receive preventive care, more likely to be hospitalized for preventable conditions, and at risk for unaffordable medical debt or bankruptcy. Access to coverage for the majority of the uninsured population may improve their health outcomes. Additionally, the minimum benefit packages required of those who have insurance may begin to close the gap for the "underinsured," facilitating access to a wider range of preventive care and treatment for those who had plans with high cost sharing or significant limitations of services covered.

The PPACA contains many provisions designed to increase the public health and primary care workforce, promote prevention, and strengthen quality measurement of health care services. PPACA expands funding for Public Health Service Act functions, including public health workforce training and development, and for student loan repayment for health care providers in rural and underserved communities. Newly established commissions will coordinate state-level and national workforce planning. Prevention efforts in PPACA include required coverage of clinical preventive services in Medicare, Medicaid, and private health insurance plans; expansion of employer wellness programs; and increased funding for prevention programs targeting public health issues including maternal and child health, oral health, and diabetes. Quality improvements include establishing a national approach to quality measurement, providing incentives for care coordination, and applying quality improvement measures across all payers—both public and private.

There is considerable controversy regarding aspects of health reform as currently legislated, and implementation at the state level, as well challenges in the courts, will play out over the next several years. Nonetheless, the debate over health care reform has raised awareness of important public health concerns, including access to health services, the importance of preventive care, and population disparities in both access and health outcomes. This increased awareness and public debate provide opportunities for improving population health, including the health of older populations.

REFERENCES

Administration on Aging (AoA). 2010a. *Evidence Based Disease and Disability Prevention Program (EBDDP)*. Department of Health and Human Services. Retrieved September 9, 2010, from www.aoa.gov/AoARoot/AoA_Programs/HPW/ Evidence_Based/index.aspx.

Administration on Aging (AoA). 2010b. *Health Prevention and Wellness Program.* U.S. Department of Health and Human Services. Retrieved September 4, 2010, from www.aoa.gov/AoARoot/AoA_Programs/HPW/index.aspx.

Anderson, G. F., B. K. Frogner, R. A. Johns., and U. E. Reinhardt. 2006. Health care spending and use of information technology in OECD countries. *Health Affairs* 25:819–31.

Barry, M. A., J. P. Allegrante, M. C. Lamarre, M. E. Auld, and A. Taub. 2009. The Galway Consensus Conference: International collaboration on the development of core competencies for health promotion and health education. *Global Health Promotion* 16(2):5–11.

Binder S., A. Levitt, J. Sacks, and J. Hughes. 1999. Emerging infectious diseases: Public health issues for the 21st century. *Science* 284:1311–13.

Braveman, P. 2006. Health disparities and health equity: Concepts and measurement. *Annual Review of Public Health* 27:167–94.

Buchmueller, T., and C. S. Carpenter. 2010. Disparities in health insurance coverage, access, and outcomes for individuals in same-sex versus different-sex relationships, 2000–2007. *American Journal of Public Health* 1003:489–95.

Cantor, J. C., D. Beloff, C. Schoen, S. K. H. How, and D. McCarthy. 2007. *Aiming Higher: Results from a State Scorecard of Health Systems Performance. The Commonwealth Fund.* Retrieved September 4, 2010, from www.commonwealthfund. org/~/media/Files/Publications/Fund%20Report/2007/Jun/Aiming%20Higher%20 %20Results%20from%20a%20State%20Scorecard%20on%20Health%20 System%20Performance/StateScorecard_EXEC_SUMM_ONLY%20pdf.pdf.

Centers for Disease Control and Prevention (CDC). 2010. CDC StreamingHealth. Retrieved September 4, 2010, from www.youtube.com/user/CDCStreamingHealth.

Cruz-Jentoft, A., A. Franco, P. Sommer, J. P. Baeyens, A. Jankowska, A. Maggi, P. Ponikoski, A. Rys, K. Szczerbinska, and A. Milewicz. 2009. European silver paper on the future of health promotion and preventive actions, basic research, and clinical aspects of age-related disease. *European Journal of Ageing* 6:51–57.

Dankwa-Mullan, I., K. B. Rhee, K. Williams, I. Sanchez, F. S. Sy, N. Stinson, and J. Ruffin. 2010. The science of eliminating health disparities: Summary analysis of the NIH summit recommendations. *American Journal of Public Health* 100:S12–18.

Dartmouth Atlas. 2010. Retrieved September 4, 2010, from www.dartmouthatlas.org/.

Dilley, J., K. W. Simmons, M. J. Boysun, B. A. Pizacani, and M. J. Stark. 2010. Demonstrating the importance and feasibility of including sexual orientation in public health surveys: Health disparities in the Pacific Northwest. *American Journal of Public Health* 100(3):460–67.

Dobrow, M. J., V. Goel, and R. E. G. Upshur. 2004. Evidence-based health policy: Context and utilization. *Social Science & Medicine* 58:207–17.

Dressler, W. W., K. S. Oths, and C. C. Gravlee 2005. Race and ethnicity in health research: Models to explain health disparities. *Annual Review of Anthropology* 34:231–52.

Glasgow, R. E., E. Lichtenstein, and A. C. Marcus. 2003. Why don't we see more translation of health promotion research to practice? Rethinking the efficacy-to-effectiveness transition. *American Journal of Public Health* 93:1261–67.

Gold, M. 2010. *Accountable Care Organizations: Will They Deliver? 2010.* Mathmatica Policy Research, Inc. Retrieved on September 4, 2010, from www.mathematica-mpr.com/publications/pdfs/health/account_care_orgs_brief.pdf.

Goulding, M. R., and M. E. Rogers. 2003. Public health and aging: Trends in aging—United States and worldwide. *Morbidity and Mortality Weekly Report* 52:101–6.

Heishman, H. 2007. Public health's aging workforce, aging leaders. *Northwest Public Health* W1–W2.

Ho, D. 1996. The influence of coinfections on HIV transmission and disease progression. *AIDS Reader* 6:114–16.

H.R. 3590. 2010. Patient Protection and Affordable Care Act. 111th Congress.

Institute of Medicine (IOM). 1988. *The Future of the Public's Health.* Washington, DC: National Academies Press.

Institute of Medicine (IOM). 2002. *The Future of the Public's Health in the 21st Century.* Washington, DC: National Academies Press.

Institute of Medicine (IOM). 2003. *Who Will Keep the Public Healthy? Educating Public Health Professionals.* Washington, DC: National Academies Press.

Krieger, N. 2003. Does racism harm health? Did child abuse exist before 1962? On explicit questions, critical science, and current controversies: An ecosocial perspective. *American Journal of Public Health* 93:194–99.

Krieger, N., P. Waterman, J. Chen, M. Soobader, and S. Subramanian. 2003. Monitoring socioeconomic inequalities in sexually transmitted infections, tuberculosis, and violence: Geocoding and choice of area-based socioeconomic measures—The Public Health Disparities Geocoding Project. *Public Health Reports* 118: 240–61.

Lasker, R. D. 1999. *Medicine and Public Health: The Power of Collaboration.* Chicago: Health Administration Press.

LaViest, T. A., D. J. Gaskin, and P. Richard. 2009. *The Economic Burden of Health Inequalities in the United States.* Washington, DC: Joint Center for Political and Economic Studies.

Laws, M., and M. K. Scott. 2008. The emergence of retail-based clinics in the United States: Early observations. *Health Affairs* 275:1293–98.

Lurie, N., and A. Fremont. 2009. Building bridges between medical care and public health. *Journal of the American Medical Association* 302:84–86.

Lurie, N., J. Wasserman, and C. Nelson. 2006. Public health preparedness: Evolution or revolution? *Health Affairs* 25:935–45.

Marmot, M. 2001. Economic and social determinants of disease. *Bulletin of the World Health Organization.* Retrieved December 26, 2010, from www.scielosp.org/scielo.php?pid=S0042–96862001001000014&script=sci_arttext&tlng=en.

Matic, S., J. Lazarus, and M. Donoghoe, eds. 2006. HIV/AIDS in Europe: Moving from death sentence to chronic disease management. Copenhagen, Denmark: World Health Organization.

McMichael, A., and C. Butler. 2007. Emerging health issues: The widening challenges for population health promotion. *Health Promotion International* 21:15–24.

Milstein, B. 2001. *Introduction to the Syndemics Prevention Network*. Atlanta: Centers for Disease Control and Prevention.

Minkler, M., and N. Wallerstein, eds. 2003. *Community-Based Participatory Research for Health*. San Francisco: Jossey-Bass.

Murray, C., and J. Frenk. 2001. World Health Report 2000: A step towards evidence-based health policy. *Lancet* 357:1698–700.

National Center for Health Statistics. 2001. *Health, United States, 2001 with Urban and Rural Health Chartbook*. Washington, DC: Centers for Disease Control and Prevention.

National Council on Aging (NCOA). 2010. Retrieved on September 4, 2010, from www.healthyagingprograms.org/.

National Diabetes Information Clearinghouse. 2008. *National Diabetes Statistics, 2007*. Retrieved on September 4, 2010, from http://diabetes.niddk.nih.gov/DM/PUBS/statistics.

Navarro, A., K. Voetsch, L. Liburd, H. W. Giles, and J. L. Collins. 2007. Charting the future of community health promotion: Recommendations from the National Expert Panel on Community Health Promotion. Preventing Chronic Disease. *Public Health Research, Practice, and Policy* 4:1–7.

Partnership to Fight Chronic Disease. 2009. *Almanac of Chronic Disease: 2009 Edition*. Retrieved on May 17, 2011, from www.fightchronicdisease.org/resources/almanac-chronic-disease-0.

Preamble to the Constitution of the World Health Organization. 1948. Adopted by the International Health Conference, New York, 19–22 June 1946; signed on 22 July 1946 by the representatives of 61 States (Official Records of the World Health Organization, no. 2, p. 100) and entered into force on 7 April 1948. Retrieved on September 4, 2010, from http://apps.who.int/gb/bd/PDF/bd47/EN/constitution-en.pdf.

Raeburn, J., and S. Macfarlane. 2003. Putting the public into public health: Towards a more people-centered approach. In *Global Public Health: A New Era*, ed. R. Beaglehole, pp. 243–52. Oxford: Oxford University Press.

Singer, M., and S. Clair. 2003. Syndemics and public health: Reconceptualizing disease in bio-social context. *Medical Anthropology Quarterly* 17:423–41.

Statehealthfacts.org. 2010. *Health Insurance Coverage of the Total Population, 2007–2008*. Kaiser Family Foundation. Retrieved on September 4, 2010, from www.statehealthfacts.org/comparetable.jsp?typ=1&ind=125&cat=3&sub=39.

Stringhini, S., S. Sabia, M. Shipley, E. Brunner, N. Hermann, M. Kivimaki, and A. Singh-Manoux. 2010. Association of socioeconomic position with health behaviors and mortality. *Journal of the American Medical Association* 303:1159–68.

Strong, K., C. Mathers, S. Leeder, and R. Beaglehole. 2005. Preventing chronic diseases: How many years can we save? *Lancet* 366:1578–82.

Suurmond, J., E. Uiters, M. C. De Bruijne, K. Stronks, and M. L. Essink-Bot. 2010. Explaining ethnic disparities in patient safety: A qualitative analysis. *American Journal of Public Health* 100:S113–17.

Turnock, B. 2009. *Public Health: What It Is and How It Works*. Sudbury, MA: Jones and Bartlett.

U.S. Census Bureau, Population Division. 2009. *Table 5. Percent Distribution of the*

Projected Population by Net International Migration Series, Race, and Hispanic Origin for the United States: 2010 to 2050 (NP2009–T5). Retrieved September 4, 2010, from www.census.gov/population/www/projections/NP2009_T5.xls.

U.S. Department of Health and Human Services. 2000. *Healthy People 2010: Understanding and Improving Health*, 2nd ed. Washington, DC: U.S. Government Printing Office. Retrieved on September 4, 2010, from www.healthypeople.gov/Document/pdf/uih/uih.pdf.

Wahlin, A., K. J. Anstey, S. W. S. McDonald, S. M. Ahmed, M. Kivipelto, K. S. S. Kunnukattil, T. T. Mai, L. G. Nilsson, P. K. Streatfield, M. P. J. van Boxtel, and Z. N. Kabir. 2008. The International Network on Public Health and Aging (INOPA): Introducing a life course perspective to the public health agenda. *Journal of Cross Cultural Gerontology* 23:97–105.

Wallerstein, N. 2002. Empowerment to reduce health disparities. *Scandinavian Journal of Public Health* 30:72–77.

Wallerstein, N., and B. Duran. 2006. Using community-based participatory research to address health disparities. *Health Promotion Practice* 7:312–23.

World Health Organization (WHO). 2008. *The Top 10 Causes of Death*. Retrieved September 4, 2010, from www.who.int/mediacentre/factsheets/fs310/en/index.html.

World Health Organization (WHO). 2010a. *Chronic Disease Risk Factors*. Retrieved May 17, 2011, from www.who.int/chp/chronic_disease_report/media/Factsheet1.pdf.

World Health Organization (WHO). 2010b. *The Determinants of Health*. Retrieved September 4, 2010, from www.who.int/hia/evidence/doh/en/index.html.

World Health Organization (WHO). 2010c. *Poverty and Health*. Retrieved September 4, 2010, from www.who.int/hdp/poverty/en/.

CHAPTER 2

What Are the Roles of Public Health in an Aging Society?

Linda P. Fried, MD, MPH

The successes of the past century in improving health and well-being have increased the life expectancy of populations around the world. These successes occurred across the full public health pyramid, from clean water, safe food, clean air, containment of spread of infectious diseases, and emergency response capability, to improved education and occupational health, supplemented by approaches elected in certain countries such as fluoridating water. Superimposed on these most basic approaches are measures to improve health at critical points in the life course: from prenatal care and prevention of infant and maternal mortality to vaccination, screening for occult infections or cancers, and effecting safe working conditions. The result has been a progressive demographic transition to longer lives worldwide. With survival to an older age comes an increased likelihood of the onset of chronic, progressive noncommunicable diseases (e.g., cardiovascular disease, diabetes, cancers, and pulmonary diseases). Public health science has now established, in many arenas, that prevention—into the oldest ages—makes a substantial difference in mortality and morbidity from these diseases. For example, as a result of evidence-based preventive interventions, mortality from cardiovascular disease has declined dramatically across all age groups in the United States. Thus, population aging is a major successful outcome of public health interventions of the past 100 years, and there is considerable evidence that morbidity can be further reduced and health enhanced during our now longer lives. Overall, prevention matters into the oldest ages, and public health approaches are critically important for an aging society. However, they will need to evolve to optimize health in aging.

POPULATIONS WORLDWIDE ARE AGING

The summary effect of these remarkable changes in population health is that all developed countries and, now, developing countries are experiencing a dramatic demographic revolution of increasing life expectancy (fig. 2.1) unprecedented in human history (Kinsella and He, 2009), and all societies are aging. There are currently more people aged 65 and older alive in the world than have previously existed in all of human history summed together. People in developed countries now live well over 30 years longer than they did 100 years ago. As a result of increased life expectancy, an increasingly large proportion of the population is older. This is visible in the day-to-day life of developed countries. In Italy and Japan, more than 21% of the population is now over 65 years of age; in the United States the proportion aged 65 and older has increased from 4% to 13% in the past 100 years, and it will increase further to 20% in the next 20 years. In developing countries, the rapidly increasing numbers of people living longer lives are often less obvious because of even greater numbers of young people. However, developing countries will see a more than 250% increase in the population aged 65 and over from 2008 to 2040, while the overall increase in older adults worldwide will be 164% during that period. China, for example, while not among the world's 25 oldest countries (2008), was home, in 2008, to 17.2% of all people aged 80 and older in the world. Overall, China expects a 206% increase in the population aged 65 and over from 2008 to 2040 (Kinsella and He, 2009). Similarly, the over-65 population will increase by 232% in Mexico, 261% in Bangladesh, and 276% in India during this period.

While longevity is increasing worldwide, there are additional dynamics affecting population aging that vary among countries. In some, the proportion that is older is greatly increased by extremely low fertility, and in others by high mortality in young and middle-aged persons such as from HIV/AIDS. For most countries, the greatest increase in older people is among the oldest

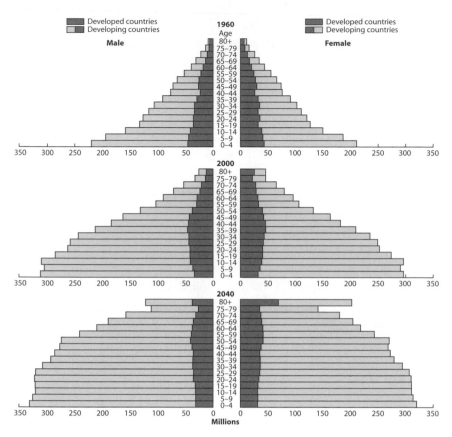

Fig. 2.1. Population in developed and developing countries by age and sex: 1960, 2000, and 2040. *Sources*: United Nations Department of Economic and Social Affairs, 2006; U.S. Census Bureau, International Data Base, accessed on December 28, 2007; Kinsella and He, 2009

old. Women's generally longer life expectancy, compared to men, increases the gender gap in survival. Thus, the population of the whole world is aging, older populations are getting older, and there are many more older women than men.

PREPARING FOR AN AGING WORLD

Notably, developing economies will experience this demographic transition to an older population more rapidly than developed countries. The latter have taken 100 years to age as a society and are continuing to go through evolutionary and sequential adjustments. Developing countries will make comparable transitions in only 40 years (Kinsella and Phillips, 2005), with the needs and opportunities of an aging society layered on top of preexisting challenges to health and productivity. Thus, developing countries will have much less time to prepare for, and transition to, an older society than developed countries have had. As stated by the Madrid International Plan of Action on Ageing in 2002, understanding the needs and necessities of an aging society must be central components of development agendas in order to foster optimal transitions to an aging society and to create the benefits that could result from this, which include increased productivity and wealth (Report of the Second World Assembly, 2002). For both developing and developed countries, it is critical that the implications, needs, and opportunities of an aging society are well understood and the roles of public health that are needed to support optimal transitions to an aging world are clear and implemented.

WHAT DO THESE CHANGES MEAN FOR SOCIETY?

Population aging affects all ages and society as a whole as much as it is about those who are older. For example, for young and middle-aged individuals anticipation of a longer life may change life expectations and offer a greater likelihood of a multigenerational family and perhaps increased cross-generational family support, connectedness, and role models. People may have four to five careers over their lifetimes, and one-third of their lives will be spent after the current retirement age. These shifts suggest needs for creating lifelong learning opportunities as well as recognition and support of many life transitions. While retirement age has dropped for some, it is being delayed by many. In the latter case, increasing age for Social Security payments in the United States and public pensions in other countries, as well as economic necessity, are significant drivers. Increased longevity may introduce new fluidity to roles and expectations along the life course. If society intentionally considers the way we have historically constructed the life course, it would be possible to redesign norms and institutions to bring new opportunities at every stage and perhaps less time famine and lower stress during child-rearing years, while extending years of productive life.

At the level of individuals, social supports and networks diminish with aging, even though they remain highly important to well-being. For society, this indicates a need for new kinds of social institutions and design of living situations to provide new social relationships and decrease social isolation with aging. Beyond continuing need for one-on-one social interactions, as people get older, many feel an increasing need to give back and contribute to the well-being and success of subsequent generations and of society as a whole. Opportunities to do this—voluntarily—have been shown to enhance health and well-being in the oldest ages and to bring substantial intergenerational benefits. New norms and social institutions for an aging society that offer opportunities for such generative contributions can both improve well-being of older adults and amplify the benefits of being an aging society. Thus, the generative desires of older adults to leave the world better, in concert with the greater number of older adults, could offer new social capital, such as for ensuring the health, success, and well-being of our children. Potentially, more older adults could mean opportunities to off-load the working generations by spreading expectations for contributions throughout the life course, as well as redistribute opportunities for lifelong learning and growth. This suggests that increasing the meaningful roles for older adults could be an important part of healthy and successful aging while addressing important unmet societal needs across the life course.

The aging of the population will affect many day-to-day experiences and needs societally. As part of that, impacts on locales may vary, for both rural and urban areas. Globally, migration of young people to cities is leaving rural areas with high concentrations of older people. In the United States, for instance, rural populations are now older than urban populations. This necessitates consideration of how to deliver services and create opportunities for older adults in rural areas. At the same time, half of the world's population now lives in cities, and that proportion is expected to increase to two-thirds by 2030 (United Nations Department of Economic and Social Affairs, 2006). According to the World Health Organization (WHO), 80% of older adults in developed countries live in cities; in developing countries, the numbers of older people in urban settings will multiply 16 times, to over 908 million, from 1998 to 2050, and one-quarter of the total urban population will be older (WHO, 2007). As stated by the WHO, "To be sustainable, cities must provide the structures and services to support their residents' wellbeing and productivity. Older people in particular require supportive and enabling living environments to compensate for physical and social changes associated with aging. Making cities more age-friendly is a necessary and logical response to promote the well-being and contributions of older urban residents and keep cities thriving" (WHO, 2007, p. 4). The built and physical environment that would be supportive for older adults would also promote well-being for all ages. The same could be said for the design of next-generation health systems.

SETTING THE STAGE FOR POPULATION HEALTH DURING LONGER
LIVES: LIFE COURSE APPROACHES TO PREVENTION

Longer lives demand understanding of the implications of exposures at one
life stage on outcomes far in the future. Knowledge from prevention science
sets the stage for taking just such a life course approach to health promotion
and prevention, optimizing key factors that affect well-being both at a given
point in the life course and for years to come. These risk factors range from
the biologic to social and structural factors, which affect health at all ages.
Key social factors are education and economic status, factors that independently predict health and well-being into the latest ages. Because of the
import of education in lifelong well-being, investments in high-quality, advanced, and lifelong education are ever-more-important parts of preparing
for an aging society and contributing to healthy aging. Access to preventive
and medical care for children and adults of all ages and the effects of social
and environmental circumstances shape health into later ages and predict
the development of health disparities.

For older adults a wide array of social factors affect outcomes, and some
are exacerbated with aging. Socioeconomic status, including education, remains an independent predictor of health outcomes, such as disability, into
the oldest ages (Szanton, Seplaki, Thorpe, Allen, and Fried, 2010). Income
declines markedly after retirement, compounded by widowhood, and rates of
poverty increase with age. Older women in the United States and globally are
more likely to be living in poverty, and alone, than older men; consequently,
gender-specific needs in income support at older ages are critical to address.

The income support and health care offered in the United States through
Social Security, Medicare, and Medicaid have made transformational differences in the well-being, security, and health of the older population while
also — intentionally — protecting working-age people from financial devasta-
tion due to the costs of caring for their parents. Thus, they are models of the
social compact across generations and cross-generational benefits in a responsible society.

Over the last 40 years, scientific evidence has shown that many people are
able to live healthy, active, and productive lives into extreme old age (Perls,
Silver, and Lauerman, 1999) and that education, prevention, and medical
care, in combination, make a substantial difference in health outcomes with
aging, for the most frail as well as those robust. One example is offered by
Hunink and colleagues, who demonstrated that half of the significant de-

clines in cardiovascular disease mortality in the United States since the 1960s are due to primary and secondary prevention, and half to improved medical care (Hunink et al., 1997). These declines occurred at every age of adulthood, including the oldest ages (Fried and Walston, 1998).

Conversely, there is clear evidence that disadvantaged groups develop health disparities across the life course, resulting in premature mortality and disability in middle and older ages. For example, a study of relatively poor African American adults living in the inner city of Saint Louis in the United States showed that disability developed at least 10 years earlier in this population compared to African American or Caucasian older adults residing in surrounding suburbs (Miller, Wolinsky, Andresen, Malmstrom, and Miller, 2008).

Evidence such as the above indicates that life course approaches to prevention are critical to improving survival to old age and the health with which people enter older ages. Such approaches are likely to decrease disparities in health status and premature mortality for populations exposed to higher levels of risk factors of all kinds, compared with those less exposed and vulnerable. Because of this and much more evidence, it has been proposed that a critical public health intervention to improve healthy aging of the U.S. population would be to ensure adequate preventive care for all. One particularly effective intervention would be to target prevention during the critical life point of the preretirement-to-postretirement transition by lowering the age of Medicare eligibility to 55 (Cassel, 2007).

Prevention of chronic, noncommunicable diseases, such as hypertension, diabetes, and cardiovascular and pulmonary diseases, and key risk states such as obesity must be a focus of public health across the full life course. It has been proposed that slowing aging in humans will also become possible (Miller, 2009; Sierra, Hadley, Suzman, and Hodes, 2009), and that this could lead to social, economic, and health benefits that have been characterized as "longevity dividends" (Olshansky, Perry, Miller, and Butler, 2006). Some have argued that this will be the most efficient approach to health promotion and disease prevention in the twenty-first century (Butler et al., 2008). Until interventions to slow aging become feasible, however, a focus on disease prevention across the life course, with modification of key risk factors, is the approach to be focused on by public health prior to reaching old age.

Preparation for healthy aging in an aging society requires a substantial shift in public health perspectives. It will require investment in sustained, multilevel, structural, all-sector approaches to optimizing health across the life course, from access to healthy foods and communities that support physical activity to improved education and other forms of building social capital. The public health system, while needing to prevent and mitigate acute events like epidemics, also has to use sustained approaches to prevention of chronic, noncommunicable diseases—across the life course—within and outside health departments. One example could be establishing distributed responsibility for access to both healthy and safe foods so as to prevent obesity and chronic diseases. Overall, numerous behavioral, social, and environmental structural factors, if modified through a public health lens, could optimize the health with which a longer-lived population enters older age and support increased health and well-being in later years.

PUBLIC HEALTH GOALS FOR AN AGING SOCIETY

Based on scientific evidence of the potential to prevent disease and optimize health during our longer lives, clear public health goals for an aging population have emerged. An overall goal is to effect a "compression of morbidity," pushing back ill health and disability to the latest possible point in a person's life so that the years of longer life are healthy years (Fries, 1980). Physical health promotion is key, but it is not the sole public health goal for an aging society. Active life expectancy is one desired outcome: not just the prevention of disease, but ability to live an active life free of disability (Katz et al., 1983). Successful aging (Rowe and Kahn, 1998), even more broadly, would additionally involve psychological and cognitive well-being and the ability to remain engaged and productive in roles meaningful to the individual and to access the creativity associated with mature minds; all of these bring benefits to family and community (Cohen, 2000; Fried, Carlson, et al., 2004). There is increasing evidence—beyond the scope of this chapter to review—that a healthy aging population brings increased productivity and economic well-being to the population at large.

With these goals in sight, there is tremendous opportunity to accomplish healthy and successful aging for older adults and bring high benefit to society from population aging. From a public health point of view, both accomplishing a compression of morbidity and supporting successful aging will require (a) supporting healthy conditions for people at each stage of the life course, as discussed above, and (b) ensuring effective public health and preventive approaches during older age itself. Public health for older adults needs to span primary, secondary, and tertiary prevention, including prevention of the onset and progression of chronic, disabling diseases and of conditions of aging (e.g., frailty, cognitive impairment, and falls) and minimizing multimorbidity, disability, and loss of independence. Also needed is the provision of community- and home-based approaches to ensuring adequate diet and physical activity, creating new opportunities for meaningful social engagement and productivity, and providing critical services to support maintaining autonomy and aging in place (Fried, Freedman, Endres, and Wasik, 1997). In addition, public health–led approaches need to be appropriately targeted, given the heterogeneity of health status and needs in older adults. Further, a public health system focused on community- and home-based health promotion and prevention needs to have gerontologic knowledge about needs and targeting as well as opportunities and be able to link to both opportunities for engagement (Fried, Ferrucci, Darer, Williamson, and Anderson, 2004) and a geriatrically knowledgeable health promotion and medical care system to be optimally effective (Fried and Hall, 2008; Institute of Medicine, 2008). Finally, an effective public health system that supports well-being of older adults needs to understand the benefits of an aging society as well as the needs, so as to set goals across multiple sectors of society that support healthy aging and do not envision older age as just the accumulation of deficits. Having this perspective would appropriately shift public perceptions toward the high return on investment for society that can come from supporting healthy aging.

With this background, the remainder of this chapter offers an overview of public health approaches for older adults within an aging society: at the individual, structural, and policy level, with an overall goal of optimizing healthy and successful aging.

PUBLIC HEALTH FOR OLDER ADULTS IN AN AGING SOCIETY: WHAT WILL IT ENTAIL?

With older age comes increased risk for emergence of chronic progressive conditions that become clinically apparent after long latency periods. These include noncommunicable chronic diseases, such as cardiovascular and pulmonary diseases, cancers, and diabetes. Their impact on older people, compared with adults under age 65, can be seen in table 2.1, which shows the prevalence of these individual diseases among people 65 and older, as well as the proportion of all adults reporting the disease who are 65 or older.

The rationale for directing prevention toward older adults themselves is demonstrated by considering that a large proportion of noncommunicable diseases develop at older ages and that the evidence shows that prevention works into these oldest ages. For most noncommunicable diseases, preven-

TABLE 2.1
*Prevalence of selected conditions reported by persons 65 years
and older, United States, 2007*

	Persons ≥65 years reporting the disease (%)	Persons ≥65 years reporting the disease, among all individuals ≥18 years reporting the disease (%)
Hypertension*	54	37
Arthritis*	48	37
Disability†	37	41
Hearing impairment†	37	40
Heart disease*	31	45
Urinary incontinence†	25	N/A
Falls†	23	N/A
Malignant neoplasm*	22	49
Obesity	21	14
Influenza*	22	N/A
Diabetes*	19	39
Visual impairment†	15	25
Alzheimer's disease*	13	96
Sinusitis*	13	18
Ulcers*	12	29
Stroke*	8	55
Asthma*	8	17
Frailty†	8	N/A
Emphysema*	5	47
Kidney disease*	4	41
Underweight	2	22
Liver disease*	2	20

Source: Fried (in press), with permission.

Note: Unless otherwise indicated, data provided by J. R. Pleis and J. W. Lucas. Summary health statistics for U.S. adults: National Health Interview Survey, 2007. National Center for Health Statistics. *Vital Health Stat* 10 (240), 2009.

* Clinical diseases

† Geriatric conditions not associated with specific diseases

tion is highly viable into the oldest ages (table 2.2), although approaches may need to vary by age group as well as health status and goals. For example, as indicated in table 2.1, over half of older adults have elevated blood pressure and 19% have diabetes, both of which put them at increased risk of cardio-vascular diseases. Secondary prevention through control of blood pressure and/or blood glucose—through exercise, diet, and medications as needed—substantially lowers risk of subsequent cardiovascular outcomes.

Evidence from the Cardiovascular Health Study (Kuller et al., 1994) indicates that one-third of older adults have clinical heart disease, stroke, or peripheral vascular disease. These individuals are also at high risk for additional cardiovascular events. At the same time, one-third of older adults have sub-

TABLE 2.2
Evidence-based prevention (primary or secondary) of chronic conditions

	Prevention effective (including exercise)	Exercise specifically effective in disease prevention
Arthritis	+	+
High blood pressure	+	+
Osteoporosis	+	+
Diabetes	+	+
Heart attack	+	+
Angina	+	+
Cancer	+	
Lung disease	+	
Stroke	+	+

clinical, but not clinical, cardiovascular diseases. Those with subclinical disease, as can be measured by decreased ankle-arm blood pressure ratio to indicate atherosclerotic narrowing of arteries in the legs, are at increased risk of incident cardiovascular disease. In contrast, older adults without subclinical disease are at low risk of developing clinical disease. Thus, evidence suggests that those with subclinical diseases are a high-risk group that would particularly benefit from targeted risk factor interventions. Thus, noninvasive screening to identify them may be a highly cost-effective approach to secondary prevention.

Another critical perspective on the importance of prevention directed to people at older ages is offered by the high proportion of all people living with these diseases who are age 65 and older: 45% of all cases of heart disease, 55% of cases of stroke, 49% of cancers, 39% of diabetes, and 96% of all Alzheimer's disease occur in older adults (table 2.1, col. b).

Population-based evidence now strongly indicates that health behaviors in older ages continue to be important to improving health. Physical activity, diet, smoking, and alcohol use remain significant modifiers of onset and progression of specific diseases and of geriatric conditions, such as frailty, falls, and disability. Physical activity has direct health benefits, as well as beneficially affecting other physiological and behavioral risk factors, including smoking cessation and sleep (Marcus et al., 1999; King, Ahn, Atienza, and Kramer, 2008). Further, social circumstances and social engagement are critical modifiers of health, well-being, and maintenance of independence with aging.

Although the likelihood of noncommunicable chronic diseases is highest with aging, they do occur in young and middle-aged adults. In contrast, some other conditions are most likely to emerge with advanced age. Prominent among these is cognitive impairment. This can be due to benign, age-related changes, or to specific disease processes, including vascular disease manifesting in strokes and/or Alzheimer's disease. At this time, life-stage-appropriate approaches to preventing strokes have the greatest evidence for potential to prevent cognitive decline. As part of this, behavioral approaches that increase cognitive activity in later ages, particularly executive function, appear to have potential to maintain cognition. Effective interventions would target older adults in early stages of cognitive impairment, to prevent further decline or actually improve cognitive function. A recent randomized trial of process-specific cognitive training, the Advanced Cognitive Training for Independent and Vital Elderly (ACTIVE) study (Jobe et al., 2001), led to improvement or maintenance of training-specific gains in memory, inductive reasoning, or speed of processing outcomes through 2- and 5-year follow-ups (Ball et al., 2002; Willis et al., 2006). The reasoning training arm also resulted in less self-reported functional decline. However, there was no transfer of training to benefits in other life activities.

In contrast, there is stronger evidence for benefits of behavioral interventions to preserve cognition via community-based programs that engage older adults in generalizable activities that can promote neurocognitive plasticity, such as the Experience Corps program (Carlson et al., 2008, 2009, submitted). The latter was intentionally designed to improve cognitive as well as physical and social activity through generative engagement in a senior volunteering program designed for high impact in improving children's success in school (Freedman and Fried, 1999; Fried, Carlson, et al., 2004). All four of the risk factors acted upon have been demonstrated, independently, to be important to healthy and successful aging. The theory of Experience Corps is that sustained improvement in multiple risk factors, through engagement in activities meaningful to the individual and the community, will result in synergistic benefits to health and well-being, while demonstrating the benefits to all of an aging society (Freedman and Fried, 1999; Fried, Carlson, et al., 2004).

With aging, physiologic function also changes, and there appears to be an increased likelihood of dysregulation of numerous physiologic systems, with resulting decreases in reserves and resilience (Fried et al., 2005). This is manifested, for example, in increased rates of elevated serum glucose and resulting increased rates of type II diabetes. This dysregulation appears to leave older adults more physiologically vulnerable to stressors, such as extremes of heat and cold, and needing longer time to recover from illness. When the dysregulation occurs in multiple physiologic systems, likely past some critical mass of systems dysregulated, older adults have a higher likelihood of becoming frail. Evidence indicates that frailty is a medical syndrome, manifesting, in a chronic, progressive manner, with a constellation of symptoms and signs of decreased strength, slowing motor functions, lower activity and energy levels, and unintentional weight loss (Fried et al., 2001; Bandeen-Roche et al., 2006). Frailty appears to also result, perhaps as a final common physiologic pathway, from wasting diseases such as severe congestive heart failure, chronic obstructive pulmonary disease, diabetes, and HIV/AIDS. Those who are frail are at high risk of disability, falls, poor outcomes, and delayed recovery after illness, hospitalization, and surgery and have high risk of institutionalization and mortality. There is potential to prevent premature frailty, particularly at earlier stages, with initial evidence suggesting that maintaining physical strength and adequate nutrition are essential.

Chronic diseases and frailty, singly and in combination, lead to geriatric conditions such as increased risk of falls, physical disability, and loss of independence with increasing age. All of the changes in health described above result in high likelihood of cumulative multimorbidity with aging, and multimorbidity increases risk of disability. These statements suggest a necessary frame shift in public health thinking, considering health outcomes like diseases as risk factors, themselves, for subsequent consequences. Prevention of chronic diseases and geriatric conditions individually is effective for many individuals and key to compressing rates of disability in the older population. Prevention of multimorbidity by attending to preventing onset of additional health problems given those already present may be a potent way to prevent disability. Prevention of distal outcomes of falls, frailty, and disability can have significant benefit. For example, multi-risk factor interventions, both in community and in patient-focused interventions, led to a 33% decrease in fall risk (Tinetti et al., 1994). Early data indicate that increased strength and walking programs can maintain mobility and potentially prevent frailty and disability onset and progression (Fiatarone et al., 1994; LIFE Study Investigators, 2006); this success is amplified by adequate nutrition.

Overall, gerontologically sophisticated public health and medical care must recognize that there is great heterogeneity in the older population in terms of health status (fig. 2.2; Fried and Hall, 2008), related prognosis, and the appropriate preventive and clinical approaches. Level of overall health status and the presence of multiple, concurrent health problems must modify both preventive and clinical care goals and approaches. This is exemplified by the need to intervene on one issue in a way that does not exacerbate or

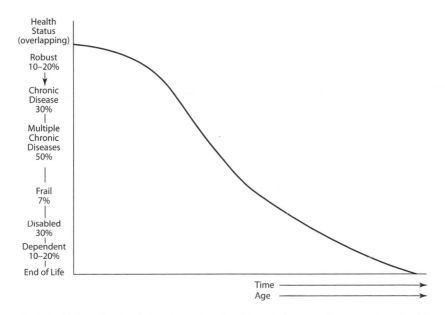

Fig. 2.2. Roles of geriatricians in caring for older adults according to patient health status.

precipitate another (Fried, Ferrucci, et al., 2004; Boyd et al., 2005) and, in many instances, to define person-appropriate preventive screening and interventions based on prognosis and individual goals (Walter and Covinsky, 2001; Durso, 2006). For example, a 70–year-old with few or no health problems, who is robust and has a life expectancy of another 15–20 years, would likely benefit from screening for conditions where prevention would affect outcomes in more than 5 years, while an individual with severe congestive heart failure, frailty, or cancer with life expectancy of less than 5 years would have low likelihood of benefit from such screening or related interventions. Goals for health may change over time, and interventions need to be directed to the individual's goals and be sensitive to life expectancy. This marked heterogeneity of health status and goals with aging requires more targeting of public health and preventive approaches than is usual in young and middle-aged populations, based on health and functional status of the individual.

Both clinical care and public health approaches for older adults are confronted by the complexity of highly multifactorial risk factors and outcomes with aging and dynamic health states that can change significantly over short periods of time. As people age, chronic health concerns are often a result of multiple causes, and the outcomes themselves are sometimes complex. For example, disability is often a product of multiple physical and cognitive changes and can span limitations on roles and productive abilities, e.g., mobility, ability to manage a household and live independently, and ability to perform basic self-care tasks, such as bathing and dressing. Individuals compensate for impairments so as to preserve function (Fried, Bandeen-Roche, Chaves, and Johnson, 2000). As people become frail or seriously disabled, such compensations must be increasingly provided extrinsically by community- and home-based supports and services (Baltes, Freund, and Li, 2005). Further, one condition can precipitate another; for example, psychological issues such as anxiety and depression can be precipitants of outcomes and also result, understandably, from intrinsic and extrinsic losses with aging. Finally, body, mind, purpose, context, and resources affect each other significantly in older age; enhancement in one area can improve others (Baltes, Freund, and Li, 2005). All of these issues can be supported and benefit from preventive approaches at the level of clinic, community, and home. Notably, because of the complexity of precipitants and outcomes, successful interventions for older adults are often multifactorial and require effective targeting.

FUTURE PUBLIC HEALTH APPROACHES FOR OLDER ADULTS

Many of the preventive, public health approaches to support health and well-being with aging must occur at the level of communities and policies and, optimally, be aligned with clinical prevention for the individual to meet the needs of longer life expectancy and an aging society. The range of these structural approaches is broad, including design of housing to decrease social isolation and increase intergenerational mutual supports, ensuring access to transportation that can help older adults utilize their community's opportunities and services, and new public health approaches for older adults in emergency situations—whether extremes of heat or cold that may disproportionately affect frail older adults or emergencies where frail older adults must be quickly identified and supported. Further, current institutions need to be modified to decrease risk. This is exemplified by the high risk of hospitalization for vulnerable older adults, who may acquire infections difficult to treat when in hospital or become confused while ill in an unfamiliar setting. These risks suggest a need to develop alternatives to hospitalization when possible. Thus, the aging of the population brings new needs and challenges that can best be addressed by gerontologically sophisticated public health approaches.

Approaches designed to enhance physical activity and optimize other health behaviors through structural interventions are also key. Multilevel approaches for older adults, as for all age groups, are key to improving physical activity, through designing environments to become more activity-friendly (Sallis, Story, and Lou, 2009) and addressing policies that thwart activity (King and Sallis, 2009). Further, design of new social institutions that facilitate engagement will foster increased activity levels (Fried et al., 1997). Overall, the aging of the population brings new needs and challenges that can best be addressed by gerontologically sophisticated public health approaches.

HEALTHY AGING SUPPORTS SOCIETAL WELL-BEING

At the same time that risks for older adults need to be mitigated by public health approaches, opportunities can be created so that the benefits of being an aging society can be fully experienced. The current population of older adults is better educated and healthier than ever before: 39% report being in excellent, very good, or good health. At the same time, the health of older adults appears to be critical to strengthening the economic well-being of society. Further, those who are not disabled report ability and goals of ongoing contributions to society. In fact, many individual elders report goals of increased societal engagement and seeking opportunities to give back to society and ensure the well-being of future generations. The increased numbers and proportion of older adults can offer substantial benefits to society along many dimensions. Optimizing healthy aging through primary, secondary, and tertiary prevention and along social, cognitive, and physical dimensions is critical to amplifying these benefits.

TWENTY-FIRST-CENTURY PUBLIC HEALTH APPROACHES FOR OLDER ADULTS

Public health for an aging society needs to implement life-stage-appropriate approaches for older adults with interventions at the levels of health systems, communities, the environment (both built and physical), and policies. New, multilevel, public health approaches and social institutions are needed to create the opportunities for as well as to meet the needs of longer life expectancy and an aging society. This section summarizes those perspectives.

An organizing structure for these approaches would recognize that older adults are heterogeneous and that opportunities and needs vary by health status and goals. Broadly, the continuum of health status among older adults can be categorized as in figure 2.2, along a continuum of robust, usual functioning, low functioning but independent community-dwelling older adults, and then the subset who are dependent (whether in home-based, assisted living, or institutional care) and those at the end of life.

A schema for the breadth of public health and clinical prevention for heterogeneous older adults, according to the health, functional status, and life expectancy of the individual, can be seen in table 2.3. While most issues are appropriate to older adults of any health status, the particular approaches will need to vary by the individual's status and goals. For example, intensity, type, and location of exercise would obviously vary by health and function, while remaining physically active to the degree possible is relevant for all older adults. Screening for cholesterol level would have more saliency for a healthy older adult than one who is terminally ill. Additionally, the responsibilities for prevention would best be integrated among clinical, public health, and community services.

Community-Based Approaches

New social institutions will be needed that can bring community-based prevention to all older adults. These can range from swimming programs, providing exercise to those who have arthritis without the stress from weight-bearing exercise, to programs of social engagement that are also designed to enhance health (Fried, Carlson, et al., 2004). For the latter, one community-based approach to increasing activity was mentioned above: new roles for social engagement that lead to enhanced physical activity, as well as cognitive and social activity. Experience Corps, designed to do just this through 15 or more hours per week of service in public elementary schools in roles designed to benefit children's academic success—with evidence-based health promotion embedded in the design—has been shown to increase physical activity by older adults who were previously inactive to levels sought in formal exercise trials. Further, older adults who volunteer for Experience Corps serve a full school year, and 80% return for a second year (Fried, Carlson, et al., 2004). This suggests that designing new roles for older adults that meet their needs for generative, meaningful engagement can also deliver significant and sustained doses of prevention and engage all older adults—including those who have least access to formal prevention programs. These programs offer evidence of the win-wins of an aging society, where multiple sectors benefit by investing in older adults.

New, multilevel, public health approaches and social institutions are needed to create the opportunities for as well as to meet the needs of longer life expectancy and an aging society. The aging of populations raises many

Public health: Broad approaches to targeting and optimizing health in aging

Functional status spectrum

Topics/issues	Community			Dependent home-based or institutionalized care 10%–15%		End-of-life/hospice
	High functioning/robust 30%	Usual functioning—at risk 30%	Low functioning 30%	Assisted living	Long-term care	
A. Financial security						
B. Mobility						

C. Health behaviors
  Physical activity
  Healthy foods
  Smoking
  Alcohol
  Sleep						

D. Housing						
E. Social engagement						
F. Mental health						
G. Issues of isolated older adults						
H. Transportation and safety, including emergency preparedness/monitoring						
I. Access to geriatrically knowledgeable clinical screening, prevention, and care						
J. Community-based self-management of chronic diseases and prevention						
K. Community-based supportive services						

Note: Each square includes primary, secondary, tertiary, and quaternary levels of actions/interventions. To address health status heterogeneity, actions or interventions will need to be tailored, in multilevel interventions according to (1) delivery setting (e.g., clinical office by physician vs. home visit by nurse vs. community by health professionals and policy and regulatory approaches) and (2) stratum-specific actions or interventions that will comprehensively address complementary domains, for example, medical (e.g., screening for diseases, diagnosis, prescription; access to care and prevention); health behaviors (e.g., physical activity, nutrition, smoking, drinking, sexual activity, vaccination); social (e.g., leisure activities, volunteerism); environmental (e.g., home, neighborhood); education, information (e.g., dissemination of public health messages, programs, appropriate to physical and cognitive status and education); access (e.g., referral systems); financial (e.g., acquisition of medications); and legal issues.

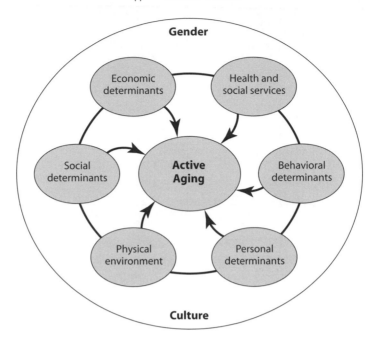

Fig. 2.3. Determinants of active aging. *Source*: WHO, 2007

needs in terms of design of the built environment and the availability and selection of appropriate services. Such services and institutions are critical to well-being and independence with aging. One aspect of this is the question of housing design, with evidence that multigenerational housing supports social needs of isolated older adults while potentially offering support for the needs of young and middle-aged generations.

More broadly, WHO has recommended that cities, 50% of which will be rebuilt in the coming 30 years, should become age-friendly. WHO recommends that cities focus on the determinants of active aging (figs. 2.3 and 2.4) (from WHO Global Age-Friendly Cities, 2007 pp. 5–6), so that "policies, services, settings and structures support and enable people to age actively," while protecting those who are most vulnerable. This WHO report recommends that cities optimize their approaches in eight key areas, listed in table 2.4 (WHO, 2007).

WHO also calls for integrated and mutually enhancing urban features, suggesting the need for a systems approach to design. An example would be a design in which transportation and infrastructure support linking to opportunities for social, civic, and economic participation, as well as to essential health services.

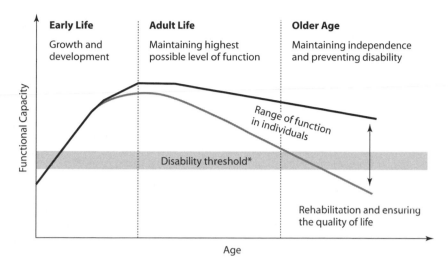

Fig. 2.4. Maintaining functional capacity over the life course. *Sources*: WHO, 2007; Kalache and Kickbusch, 1997

New Metrics to Guide Public Health for an Aging Society

Becoming an aging society requires not only the application of new evidence to effective prevention for older adults but also new formulations of goals and outcomes. To accomplish this, public health will require new measures to frame our vision for successful aging and characterize success. While a wide variety of approaches are needed, many of which are discussed above, this section will focus on three types of measures as examples.

First, setting goals for health for older adults has been shown to need positive aspirations as well as measures of limitations. For the former, a watershed was accomplished for public health by the concept of successful aging (Rowe and Kahn, 1998) and the public health goal of compressing morbidity (see fig. 2.3; WHO, 2007). Then, the ability to apply this in actual measurement was initiated through the development of the measure of active life expectancy, or remaining years of life lived without disability (Katz et al., 1983). Ongoing refinements will be needed to represent the multidimensional components of successful aging and set goals and outcomes for public health interventions.

Second, aspirations and objectives for health in an aging society are significantly constrained by current metrics such as the support-dependency ratio. This measure portrays older adults as a uniformly dependent population, when that is far from the case. More valid measures that represent the

TABLE 2.4
Eight key areas for age-friendly cities to optimize approaches

1. *Outdoor spaces and buildings*
   Environment, green spaces and walkways, outdoor seating, pavements, roads, traffic, cycle paths, safety, services, buildings accessible and with special features, public toilets

2. *Transportation*
   Availability, affordability, reliability and frequency, travel destinations, age-friendly vehicles, specialized services for older people, priority seating and passenger courtesy, transport drivers, safety and comfort of public transport, transport stations and stops, taxis, community free transport, information on transport options, driving conditions, courtesy toward older drivers, parking

3. *Housing*
   Affordability, essential services, design, modifications, home maintenance service and cost, access to services in one's home, aging in place offers community and family connections in familiar environment, range of housing options in familiar environment, living environment with sufficient space, privacy and safety

4. *Social participation*
   Accessible opportunities, affordable activities, range of opportunities, awareness of activities and events, encouraging participation and addressing isolation, integrating generations, cultures and communities

5. *Respect and social inclusion*
   Respectful and disrespectful behavior, ageism and ignorance, intergenerational and family interactions, public education, community inclusion, helpfulness of the community, economic inclusion

6. *Civic participation and employment*
   Volunteering options for older people, better employment options and more opportunities, flexibility to accommodate older workers and volunteers, encouraging civic participation, training, entrepreneurial opportunities, valuing older peoples' contributions, pay

7. *Communication and information*
   Widespread distribution, right information at the right time, oral communication, printed information, plain language, automated communication and equipment meet older peoples' needs, computers and the Internet: access and assistance as needed

8. *Community support and health services*
   Accessible care, wider range of health services, aging well services: disease prevention and health promotion services and programs, home care, residential facilities for people unable to live at home, network of community services, volunteers to support older adults, emergency planning and care

Source: WHO, 2007

benefits and contributions as well as costs, needs, and dependencies of different age groups would foster recognition of value of all age groups and mutual benefits from different generations. They would also strengthen our social compact toward optimizing successful aging.

Third, community indicators are needed that offer measures of the components necessary to support health and well-being. Building on the WHO recommendations for age-friendly cities, the AdvantAge Initiative, a project

TABLE 2.5
Components of an elder-friendly community

Addresses basic needs
    affordable housing that is safe and facilitates independence
    sufficient food
    financial security
    neighborhood
    transportation and safety
    information and how to access it readily available

Optimizes physical and mental health and well-being
    promotes healthy behaviors
    access to preventive health services
    access to medical, social, and palliative services with minimal obstacles
    supports community activities that enhance well-being

Promotes social and civic engagement
    fosters meaningful connections
    promotes active engagement
    provides opportunities for meaningful paid and voluntary work
    makes aging issues a community-wide priority
    social capital—community residents help and trust each other

Maximizes independence for the frail and disabled
    mobilizes resources to facilitate "living at home"
    provides accessible transportation
    supports family and other caregivers
    service-system navigable

Source: Feldman and Oberlink, 2003

of the Center for Home Care Policy and Research, conducted focus groups with older adults in diverse communities and formal needs assessment. This work led to identification of community indicators to assess the progress of communities in becoming age-friendly and in promoting the health and well-being of older adults. These measures (Feldman and Oberlink, 2003) synthesize many of the elements recommended by the WHO into measurable outcomes in four areas (table 2.5).

Needs for Health System, and Services for Older Adults

Gerontologically informed public health and clinical geriatrics approaches make substantial differences in accomplishing healthy aging. These should be incorporated into the next-generation public health system, which must take responsibility for older adults in an aging society. To do so in the United States will require both new contents and better linking of public health and aging services networks (Palombo et al., 2005), ensuring that the public health system is committed to accomplishing healthy aging, and clarifying

authority and responsibility for both prevention and the provision of supportive services. Further, geriatric medicine has demonstrated that systems of
care designed and based on geriatric principles are necessary to support provision of geriatrically expert contents of care—and prevention. These lessons
and practices should be linked to public health system approaches as well.

CONCLUSION

There is compelling evidence that public health and health care system approaches designed to benefit the health of older adults will likely benefit all
ages. One reason is that communities and systems that can support the needs
of the more vulnerable can be beneficial to all. For example, structural approaches like designing parks and public spaces so that older adults can be
active and safe and ensuring availability and affordability of healthy foods
within walking distance of older adults would benefit people of all ages. At
the same time, these plans require design features specific to the needs of
older adults, such as pleasant places to sit in parks designed for the abilities
and socializing of older adults, while also designing playgrounds for the children. In a parallel way, designing a health system of public health and medical/
geriatric care based on geriatric knowledge and needs of the most vulnerable
subsets of older adults will ensure the ability to take optimal care of older adults;
this would include expertise and systems designed for people with high risk for
multiple incident problems and rapid changes in health status, while offering
the design of a coordinated, continuous system of care that is holistic and cost-
effective. It would likely be beneficial if extended to adults of all ages.

Increased longevity and the aging of society require new public health approaches specific to the prevention and health promotion needs of older
adults, but potentially beneficial to people of all ages. They also require reframing public health approaches at all ages and stages to ensure a life course
approach to prevention so that people living longer lives will be healthy into
the oldest ages. All of these issues suggest a need for fresh approaches and
evaluating whether new or redesigned social and health institutions and systems are needed to prepare for the needs, as well as harness the benefits and
opportunities, of an aging society.

REFERENCES

Ball, K., D. B. Berch, K. F. Helmers, J. B. Jobe, M. D. Leveck, M. Marsiske, J. N. Morris, G. W. Rebok, D. M. Smith, S. L. Tennstedt, F. W. Unverzagt, and S. L. Willis,
for the ACTIVE Study Group. 2002. Effects of cognitive training interventions

with older adults. A randomized controlled trial. *Journal of the American Medical Association* 288:2271–81.

Baltes, P. B., A. M. Freund, and S. C. Li. 2005. The psychological science of human ageing. In *The Cambridge Handbook of Age and Ageing*, ed. M. L. Johnson, V. L. Bengston, P. G. Coleman, and T. B. L. Kirkwood, pp. 47–71. Cambridge: Cambridge University Press.

Bandeen-Roche, K.,Q. L. Xue, L. Ferrucci, J. Walston, J. M. Guralnik, P. Chaves, S. L. Zeger, and L. P. Fried. 2006. Phenotype of frailty: Characterization in the Women's Health and Aging Studies. *Journals of Gerontology Series A: Biological Sciences and Medical Sciences* 61A:262–66.

Boyd, C. M., Q. L. Xue, C. F. Simpson, J. M. Guralnik, and L. P. Fried. 2005. Frailty, hospitalization, and progression of disability in a cohort of disabled older women. *American Journal of Medicine* 118(11):1225–31. PMID: 16271906.

Butler, R. N., R. A. Miller, D. Perry, B. A. Carnes, T. F. Williams, C. Cassel, J. Brody, M. A. Bernard, L. Partridge, T. Kirkwood, G. M. Martin, and S. J. Olshansky. 2008. New model of health promotion and disease prevention for the 21st century. *British Medical Journal* 337:a399.

Carlson, M. C., K. I. Erickson, A. F. Kramer, M. W. Voss, N. Bolea, M. Mielke, S. McGill, G. W. Rebok, T. Seeman, and L. P. Fried. 2009. Evidence for neurocognitive plasticity in at-risk older adults: The Experience Corps program. *Journals of Gerontology Series A: Biological Sciences and Medical Sciences* 57(9):1604–11.

Carlson, M. C., J. M. Parisi, J. Xia, Q. L. Xue, G. W. Rebok, K. Bandeen-Roche, and L. P. Fried. Submitted. Lifestyle activities and aging: Variety may be the spice of life. The Women's Health and Aging Study II.

Carlson, M. C., J. S. Saczynski, G. W. Rebok, T. Seeman, T. A. Glass, S. McGill, J. Tielsch, K. D. Frick, J. Hill, and L. P. Fried. 2008. Exploring the effects of an "everyday" activity program on executive function and memory in older adults: Experience Corps. *Gerontologist* 48(6):793–801. PMID: 19139252.

Cassel, C.K. 2007. *Medicare Matters: What Geriatric Medicine Can Teach American Health Care*. Berkeley: University of California Press.

Cohen, G. D. 2000. *The Creative Age: Awakening the Human Potential in the Second Half of Life*. New York: Avon Books.

Durso, S. C. 2006. Using clinical guidelines designed for older adults with diabetes mellitus and complex health status. *Journal of the American Medical Association* 295:1935–40.

Feldman, P. H., and M. R. Oberlink. 2003. Developing community indicators to promote the health and well-being of older people. *Family and Community Health* 26:268–74.

Fiatarone, M. A., E. F. O'Neill, N. D. Ryan, K. M. Clements, G. R. Solares, M. E. Nelson, S. B. Roberts, J. J. Kehayias, L. A. Lipsitz, and W. J. Evans. 1994. Exercise training and nutritional supplementation for physical frailty in very elderly people. *New England Journal of Medicine* 330:1769–75.

Freedman, M., and L. P. Fried. 1999. *Launching Experience Corps: Findings from a 2-Year Pilot Project Mobilizing Older Americans to Help Inner-City Elementary Schools*. Oakland, CA: Civic Ventures.

Fried, L. P. In press. Epidemiology of aging: Implications of the aging of society. In *Cecil Textbook of Medicine*, ed. L. Goldman and D. Ausiello. Philadelphia: Saunders.

Fried, L. P., K. Bandeen-Roche, P. M. Chaves, and B. Johnson. 2000. Preclinical mobility disability predicts incident mobility disability in older women. *Journal of Gerontology: Medical Sciences* 55A:M43–52.

Fried, L. P., M. C. Carlson, M. Freedman, K. D. Frick, T. A. Glass, J. Hill, S. McGill, G. W. Rebok, T. Seeman, J. M. Tielsch, B. Wasik, and S. Zeger. 2004. A social model for health promotion for an aging population: Initial evidence on the Experience Corps® model. *Journal of Urban Health* 81(1):64–78.

Fried, L. P., L. Ferrucci, J. Darer, J. D. Williamson, and G. Anderson. 2004. Untangling the concepts of disability, frailty, and comorbidity: Implications for improved targeting and care. *Journals of Gerontology Series A: Biological Sciences and Medical Sciences* 59:M255–63. http://sageke.sciencemag.org/content/vol2005/issue31/.

Fried, L. P., M. Freedman, T. E. Endres, and B. Wasik. 1997. Building communities that promote successful aging. *Western Journal of Medicine* 167:216–19.

Fried, L. P., E. C. Hadley, J. D. Walston, A. Newman, J. M. Guralnik, S. Studenski, T. B. Harris, W. B. Ershler, and L. Ferrucci. 2005. From bedside to bench: Research agenda for frailty. 2005. *Science of Aging Knowledge Environment* 2005(31): pe24. Retrieved December 9, 2010, from http://sageke.sciencemag.org/content/vol2005/issue31/.

Fried, L. P., and W. J. Hall. 2008. Editorial: Leading on behalf of an aging society. *Journal of the American Geriatrics Society* 56:1791–95.

Fried, L. P., C. M. Tangen, J. Walston, A. B. Newman, D. Hirsch, J. Gottdiener, T. Seeman, R. Tracey, W. Kop, G. Burke, and M. A. McBurnie. 2001. Frailty in older adults: Evidence for a phenotype. *Journal of Gerontology: Medical Sciences* 56: M146–56.

Fried, L. P., and J. Walston. 1998. Frailty and failure to thrive. In *Principles of Geriatric Medicine and Gerontology*, 4th ed., ed. W. R. Hazzard, J. P. Blass, W. H. Ettinger, Jr., J. B. Halter, and J. Ouslander, pp. 1387–1402. New York: McGraw-Hill.

Fries, J. F. 1980. Aging, natural death, and the compression of morbidity. *New England Journal of Medicine* 303:130–35.

Hunink, M. G., L. Goldman, A. N. Tosteson, M. A. Mittleman, P. A. Goldman, L. W. Williams, J. Tsevat, and M. C. Weinstein. 1997. The recent decline in mortality from coronary heart disease, 1980–1990. The effects of secular trends in risk factors and treatment. *Journal of American Medical Association* 277:535–42.

Institute of Medicine. 2008. *Retooling for an Aging America: Building the Health Care Workforce*. Washington, DC: National Academies Press.

Jobe, J. B., D. M. Smith, K. Ball, S. L. Tennstedt, M. Marsiske, S. L. Willis, G. W. Rebok, J. N. Morris, K. F. Helmers, M. D. Leveck, and K. Kleinman. 2001. ACTIVE: A cognitive intervention trial to promote independence in older adults. *Controlled Clinical Trials* 22:453–79.

Kalache, A., and I. Kickbusch. 1997. A global strategy for healthy ageing. *World Health* 50(4):4–5.

Katz, S., L. G. Branch, M. H. Branson, J. A. Papsidero, J. C. Beck, and D. S. Greer. 1983. Active life expectancy. *New England Journal of Medicine* 309:1218–24.

King, A. C., D. F. Ahn, A. A. Atienza, and H. C. Kraemer. 2008. Exploring refinements in targeted behavioral medicine intervention to advance public health. *Annals of Behavioral Medicine* 35:251–60.

King, A. C., and J. F. Sallis. 2009. Why and how to improve physical activity promotion: Lessons from behavioral science and related fields. *Preventive Medicine* 49:286–88.

Kinsella, K., and W. He. 2009. U.S. Census Bureau, International Population Reports, P95/09–1, *An Aging World*. Washington, DC: U.S. Government Printing Office.

Kinsella, K., and D. R. Phillips. 2005. Global aging: The challenge of success. *Population Bulletin* 60(1). Washington, DC: Population Reference Bureau.

Kuller, L., N. Borhani, C. Furberg, J. Gardin, T. Manolio, D. O'Leary, B. Psaty, and J. Robbins. 1994. Prevalence of subclinical atherosclerosis and cardiovascular disease and association with risk factors in the Cardiovascular Health Study. *American Journal of Epidemiology* 139:1164–79.

LIFE Study Investigators. 2006. Effects of a physical activity intervention on measures of physical performance: Results of the lifestyle interventions and independence for Elders Pilot (LIFE-P) study. *Journals of Gerontology Series A: Biological Sciences and Medical Sciences* 61:1157–65.

Marcus, B. H., A. E. Albrecht, T. K. King, A. F. Parisi, B. M. Pinnto, M. Roberts, R. S. Niaura, and D. B. Abrams. 1999. The efficacy of exercise and an aid for smoking cessation in women: A randomized controlled trial. *Archives of Internal Medicine* 159:1229–34.

Miller, D. K., F. D. Wolinsky, E. M. Andresen, T. K. Malmstrom, and J. P. Miller. 2008. Adverse outcomes and correlates of change in the Short Physical Performance Battery over 36 months in the African American health project. *Journals of Gerontology Series A: Biological Sciences and Medical Sciences* 63:487–94.

Miller, R. A. 2009. "Dividends" from research on aging—can biogerontologists, at long last, find something useful to do? *Journal of Gerontology: Biological Science* 64A:157–60.

Olshansky, S. J., D. Perry, R. A. Miller, and R. N. Butler. 2006. In pursuit of the longevity dividend. *Scientist* 20:28–36.

Palombo, R., J. Alongi, A. Goldman, R. Greene, T. Lambert, and S. Smith. 2005. Opportunities for collaboration: Linking public health and aging services networks. *Generations* 29(2):48–53.

Perls, T. T., M. H. Silver, and J. F. Lauerman. 1999. *Living to 100: Lessons in Living to Your Maximum Potential at Any age*. New York: Basic Books.

Report of the Second World Assembly on Ageing. 2002. Madrid, 8–12 April 2002. New York: United Nations. Retrieved December 7, 2010, from www.un.org/ageing/madrid_declaration02.html.

Rowe, J. W., and R. L. Kahn. 1998. Successful aging. *Aging. Milano* 10:142–44.

Sallis, J. F., M. Story, and D. Lou. 2009. Study designs and analytic strategies for environmental and policy research on obesity, physical activity, and diet: Recommendations from a meeting of experts. *American Journal of Preventive Medicine* 26(Suppl. 2):S72–77.

Sierra, F., E. Hadley, R. Suzman, and R. Hodes. 2009. Prospects for life span extension. *Annual Review of Medicine* 60:457–69.

Szanton, S. L., C. L. Seplaki, R. J. Thorpe, J. K. Allen, and L. P. Fried. 2010. Socioeconomic status is associated with frailty: The Women's Health and Aging Studies. *Journal of Epidemiology and Community Health* 64(1):63–67.

Tinetti, M. E., D. I. Baker, G. McAvay, E. B. Claus, P. Garrett, M. Gottschalk, M. L. Koch, K. Trainor, and R. I. Horwitz. 1994. A multifactorial intervention to reduce the risk of falling among elderly people living in the community. *New England Journal of Medicine* 331:821–27.

United Nations Department of Economic and Social Affairs. 2006. *World Urbanization Prospects: The 2005 Revision.* Retrieved December 7, 2010, from www.un.org/esa/population/publications/WUP2005/2005wup.htm.

Walter, L. C., and K. E. Covinsky. 2001. Cancer screening in elderly patients: A framework for individualized decision making. *Journal of the American Medical Association* 285:2750–56.

WHO. 2007. *Global Age-Friendly Cities: A Guide.* Retrieved December 7, 2010, from http://whqlibdoc.who.int/publications/2007/9789241547307_eng.pdf.

Willis, S. L., S. L. Tennstedt, M. Marsiske, K. Ball, J. Elias, K. M. Koepke, J. N. Morris, G. W. Rebok, F. W. Unverzagt, A. M. Stoddard, and E. Wright, for the ACTIVE Study Group. 2006. Long-term effects of cognitive training on everyday functional outcomes in older adults. *Journal of the American Medical Association* 296:2805–14.

CHAPTER 3

Financing and Organizing Health and Long-Term Care Services for Older Populations

Robyn I. Stone, DrPH
William F. Benson

For the elderly population medical and long-term care (LTC) services represent a key component of the public health landscape. Older adults are more likely than younger people to have multiple chronic diseases and functional disabilities, leading them to consume a proportion of health services that is larger than their percentage of the population. Data from the 2007 Medical Expenditure Panel Survey indicate that the noninstitutionalized elderly (data are not available for nursing home residents) were 13% of the population but accounted for 34% of all personal health care expenditures (AHRQ, 2010). The median per capita health care spending for the elderly population in 2007 was $4,447, five times higher than the median spending per person under age 65. Older adults, furthermore, spent much more out of pocket than their younger counterparts, averaging $1,357 in 2007 compared with $623 for the under-65 population. It is estimated that in 2008 older Americans spent 12.5% of their total expenditures on health care, more than twice spent by all consumers (AoA, 2009). The distribution of these older persons' expenditures included 62% for insurance, 17% for needed services, 18% for drugs, and 3% for supplies.

The elderly need and consume an array of medical services that include acute care, post-acute care and rehabilitation, specialty and primary care, chronic care, and palliative/end-of-life care. Services are provided in a range of settings including hospitals (inpatient and outpatient), skilled nursing facilities, physician offices, clinics, and individual homes. Older persons also consume both prescription and over-the-counter drugs and durable medical equipment (e.g., wheelchairs, canes, walkers). Chronically disabled older adults also need a range of LTC services that address their physical and cognitive functional limitations and that are designed primarily to enhance independence as much as possible and to ensure quality of life. Services are provided in a range of settings, including nursing facilities, assisted living and other residential environments, adult day care centers, and individual homes.

To understand the role that health care for older persons plays in the larger public health arena, it is important to understand how care for older adults is financed and delivered in the United States. In the following section, sources and mechanisms for financing medical care and LTC are described. This is followed by a brief review of the organization of the health care system with an emphasis on current and proposed initiatives for (1) improving service coordination and integration, (2) expanding home- and community-based care services, and (3) including more consumer direction in service delivery. The chapter concludes with the identification of key factors that must be considered in light of a rapidly aging society and increasing financial constraints at all governmental levels.

FINANCING OF CARE FOR THE ELDERLY POPULATION

Financing of health care (medical care and LTC) for older adults in the United States is both a public and private sector responsibility. Public programs play a dominant role in financing the spectrum of services. Medicare (which provides national health insurance for most older persons) pays a large proportion of the medical care bill, and Medicaid, the federal-state health insurance program for specific categories of poor persons, covers a large portion of the LTC expenditures. The various sources of funding for health care spending on the elderly in 2004 (CMS, 2010b)—the most recent date for which published data on spending are available for both the nursing home– and community-dwelling elderly population—are displayed in figure

Payment Source

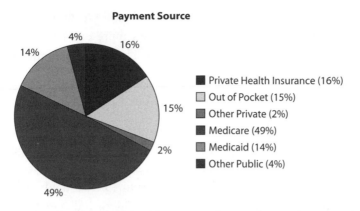

Fig. 3.1. Distribution of personal health care spending on the population aged 65+ in the United States by payment source, 2004. *Source*: Centers for Medicare and Medicaid Services Office of the Actuary, National Health Statistics Group

Type of Service

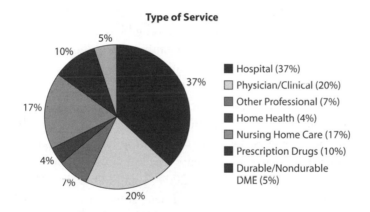

Fig. 3.2. Distribution of personal health care spending on the population aged 65+ in the United States by type of service, 2004. Source: Centers for Medicare and Medicaid Services Office of the Actuary, National Health Statistics Group.

3.1; the distribution of spending by type of service is displayed in figure 3.2. This patchwork system of funding streams is summarized below.

Medical Care

Public financing of medical care—including acute, post-acute (post-hospital), primary, and chronic care—is primarily a Medicare responsibility, with Medicaid and other public programs (such as those of the Department of Veterans Affairs and the Indian Health Service) providing additional support for special populations. As noted in the introductory section, despite significant public financing, out-of-pocket expenses represent a large part of the health care expenditures pie for older adults. The range of financing mechanisms is described below.

Medicare

Established in 1965, Medicare is a social insurance program that finances the health care of most individuals ages 65 and older (and for younger people who are receiving federal disability insurance, or have end-state renal disease, or have Alateral Myotrophic Sclerosis). Prior to 1965, roughly half of older adults lacked medical insurance; today 98% of elderly individuals have health insurance under Medicare. The program helps to pay for many important health care services, including hospitalizations, physician services, prescription drugs, post-acute care in skilled nursing facilities and in the home, and hospice care. Individuals contribute payroll taxes to Medicare throughout their working lives and generally become eligible for Medicare when they reach age 65, regardless of income or health status. Medicare expenditures were an estimated 12% of the federal budget and more than one-fifth of total national health expenditures in 2010 (KFF, 2010b).

Medicare has four parts, each structured differently and financing a different set of benefits. Part A—the Hospital Insurance (HI) program that covers inpatient hospital services, subacute or post-hospital care in skilled nursing facilities and at home, and hospice care—accounted for approximately 36% of total Medicare benefit spending in 2009 (Topoleski, 2009). Although Part A has no monthly premiums, beneficiaries are subject to various deductibles (such as $1,060 for each hospital stay in 2010) before Medicare payments begin. Part B—the Supplementary Medical Insurance (SMI) program—helps pay for outpatient services such as outpatient hospital care, physician visits, and preventive services, as well as ambulance services, clinical laboratory services, durable medical equipment (e.g., wheelchairs and oxygen), and diagnostic tests. Part B is funded by a combination of general revenues and beneficiary premiums (a minimum of $110.50 per month in 2010), with wealthier beneficiaries paying a higher income-related monthly premium. Part B is voluntary, but about 95% of Part B beneficiaries enroll in it when they enroll in Part A.

Part C—the Medicare Advantage (MA) program—allows beneficiaries to enroll in a private plan, such as a health maintenance organization, preferred provider organization, or private fee-for-service plan, as an alternative to the traditional Parts A and B fee-for-service programs. These plans receive prospective payments from Medicare to provide covered benefits, including hospital, physician, and, in most cases, prescription drugs. According to the Medicare Payment Advisory Commission (MedPAC, 2009), Medicare payments to private plans in 2010 are higher, on average, than Medicare fee-for-service costs. This difference in costs (sometimes referred to as "overpayments") will be gradually eliminated by the Patient Protection and Affordable Care Act (referred to as the Affordable Care Act), the new national health care reform law enacted in 2010 (CMS, 2010a).

Part D—the outpatient drug benefit—was established by the Medicare Modernization Act of 2003 and launched in 2006. The benefit is delivered through private plans that contract with Medicare. Individuals who sign up for a Part D plan generally pay a monthly premium along with cost-sharing amounts for each prescription; those with modest income and assets are eligible for government assistance with premiums and cost-sharing amounts. Plans are required to provide a "standard" benefit, or one that is actuarially equivalent, and may offer more generous benefits. More than 27 million Medicare beneficiaries are enrolled in a Part D plan as of April 2010.

Since its inception, many Medicare beneficiaries have experienced a serious gap in their drug coverage—referred to as the "doughnut hole." With passage of the Affordable Care Act, any beneficiary in that situation will receive a $250 rebate in 2010. The following year, this subset of beneficiaries will receive a 50% discount when buying Part D–covered brand-name prescription drugs. They will receive additional savings over the next 8 years until the gap is closed in 2020 (CMS, 2010a).

Supplemental Insurance for Medical and Long-Term Care

A majority of Medicare beneficiaries have some type of supplemental insurance coverage to help fill in the gaps in Medicare's benefit package and help with the program's cost-sharing requirements. In 2007, 59% of noninstitutionalized older adults had some type of private health insurance (AoA, 2009). One in three Medicare beneficiaries receives supplemental coverage through an employer- or union-sponsored plan (KFF, 2010b). Access to retiree health benefits, however, is on the decline. The share of large firms offering this coverage has dropped by more than half over the past two decades, from 66% in 1988 to 29% in 2009 (KFF, 2009).

So-called "Medigap" policies are also sold in the private market to help cover the cost-sharing requirements and fill benefit package gaps. Twelve standard plans are available, each offering a different menu of benefits. As of June 2010, four of these plans will no longer be for sale and two new plans

will be available (CMS, 2010a). In 2007, about one in five Medicare beneficiaries had an individually purchased supplemental insurance policy, with
premiums varying by plan type, insurer, age of the enrollee, and state of residence. Another segment of elderly individuals receives supplemental coverage for benefits such as vision and dental care by enrolling in Medicare Advantage plans.

Medicaid, the federal-state program that covers health care (as well as
LTC) expenses for specific categories of low-income Americans of all ages (see
more detail later in this chapter), is a source of supplemental insurance for
close to 9 million Medicare enrollees with low incomes and modest assets—
referred to as the "dual eligibles" (Coughlin, Waidmann, and O'Malley
Watts, 2009). Most of these individuals—6.3 million in 2009—qualify for full
Medicaid benefits, including LTC and dental services, as well as having their
Medicare premiums, benefit co-pays, and drug costs subsidized by Medicaid.
In 2009, approximately 1.8 million dual eligibles did not qualify for full Medicaid benefits, but the program did assist with Medicare premiums and some
required cost-sharing through the Medicare Savings Program (MSP) admin-
istered under Medicaid.

Other Financing Sources

There are a number of other public programs that help to finance older
adults' medical bills. Almost 4 million elderly veterans (out of a veteran population of 8.5 million) received some type of services from the Department of
Veteran Affairs in 2008, including coverage to supplement Medicare payments (DVA, 2010). The Indian Health Service also provides benefits and
services to elderly Native Americans.

A significant amount of out-of-pocket expenses also finance health care for
elderly individuals with both chronic conditions and functional disabilities
that live in the community (The Lewin Group, 2010). Those with Medicare
and private insurance coverage spend, on average, $1,808 annually. Even
with Medicaid coverage, dual eligibles spend an average of $808 annually.
This estimate, furthermore, would be much higher if the elderly nursing
home population were included.

Long-Term Care

American families today are struggling to pay for LTC. For those needing
LTC services—particularly individuals with extensive LTC needs—services
can be costly. In 2010, the average annual cost of nursing home care was

$72,270 for a semiprivate room and $79,935 for a private room (Mature Market Institute and LifePlans, Inc., 2009). The national average annual cost for assisted living was $37,572. Care purchased outside of an institution typically is purchased in smaller increments. Charges for home health aides average $21 per hour; homemaker services average $19 per hour. LTC might be needed for 3 months, 2 years, 10 years, or more, with varying amounts, types, and hours of care required. The estimated median annual out-of-pocket expenditures on nursing home care in 2009 were $12,680; the comparable estimate for home- and community-based care was $6,648 (Kaye, Harrington, and LaPlante, 2010).

The financing of LTC services is currently a patchwork of funds from the federal, state, and local levels and private dollars, primarily paid from the consumer's own pocket. It is difficult to assess the exact amount of dollars spent on the elderly because most of the existing estimates include funding for the nonelderly population that represents almost one half of LTC recipients. One recent analysis using 2004 and 2005 national survey data indicates that in 2009 dollars, Americans spent $119 billion on LTC services for the elderly (Kaye, Harrington, and LaPlante, 2010). Another analysis using projections from the Long-Term Care Financing Model suggests that this estimate could be as high as $182 billion (The Lewin Group, 2010). The majority of LTC spending is for nursing home care, although the proportion of expenditures for home- and community-based alternatives has increased substantially over the past 25 years.

Public funds, primarily Medicaid and Medicare (if post-acute skilled nursing and home health care are included in the LTC definition), accounted for approximately 71% of national LTC spending on the elderly and nonelderly population in 2008 (The Lewin Group, 2010). Out-of-pocket spending accounted for 18%, private LTC insurance for 7%, and various other federal, state, and local agencies for most of the rest. These estimates do not include the dollar value of the vast amount of unpaid care, including the value of wages forgone by informal caregivers. AARP estimated the economic value of this care (including family care provided to the nonelderly LTC population) at approximately $375 billion in 2007 (Gibson & Houser, 2008). About half of family caregivers contribute financially, with an average of $200 per month.

Medicaid

Medicaid is the nation's largest source of financing for LTC, paying for 49% of all LTC expenditures (for elderly and nonelderly recipients) in 2008 (The Lewin Group, 2010). This jointly federal-state-funded, state-administered health insurance program for the poor is required to provide coverage for nursing home care for elderly and disabled people who meet certain financial eligibility requirements (because they are low income and have negligible assets). In 2007, nursing home care accounted for 73% of total Medicaid spending on LTC for elderly individuals and younger people with physical disabilities (Houser, Fox-Grage, and Gibson, 2009).

Since 1970, states have been required to cover home health services (though not personal care services) for those who are eligible for Medicaid-covered nursing home care. Since the mid-1970s, states have had the option to offer personal care services under their Medicaid state plans (Ng, Harrington, and O'Malley Watts, 2009). In 1981, Congress authorized the waiver of certain federal requirements to enable a state to provide home and community services (other than room and board) to individuals who would otherwise require skilled nursing facility (nursing home) services reimbursable by Medicaid. Waiver services include case management, homemaker, home health aide, personal care, adult day health, habilitation, and respite care. As noted above, by 2007, 27% of Medicaid LTC expenditures for elderly and younger people with physical disabilities covered personal care and home- and community-based services (HCBS; Houser, Fox-Grage, and Gibson, 2009). Medicaid policies toward HCBS, however, vary tremendously by state. In 2006, only seven states spent 40% or more of their Medicaid LTC dollars on home- and community-based care (Kassner, Reinhard, Fox-Grage, Houser, and Accius, 2008).

Medicare

The extent to which Medicare finances LTC depends on one's definition of the term. If post-acute care delivered in skilled nursing facilities and in individual homes is considered an LTC service, then the Medicare program financed 20% of overall national LTC expenditures in 2005 — 16% of nursing home care and 27% of home health care (Komisar & Thompson, 2007). Although Medicare was enacted primarily to pay for acute and primary care, the program pays for the first 20 days, and in part for an additional 80 days, of care in a skilled nursing facility for individuals requiring post-acute services, including intensive rehabilitation, following a hospital stay of at least 3 days. Medicare also pays for home health care—skilled nursing, therapy, and social work and aide services—for individuals who are not able to leave their homes because of their health condition and who require intermittent skilled care. In 2005, approximately 3 million Medicare beneficiaries received services from home health agencies, most for relatively short periods of time.

Other Public Financing

In addition to Medicaid, several other federal programs provide modest support for LTC delivered to older adults. Title III of the Older Americans Act (OAA), initially legislated in 1965, supports a network of aging services providers in every state—administered by state units on aging (SUAs) and local Area Agencies on Aging (AAAs)—and authorized funding for meals programs and other community-based services. Title VI of the OAA established a comparable service system for Native Americans in the United States. Unlike the Medicaid program, OAA funds are not means-tested; all elders aged 60 and over are eligible for benefits, although most programs use a variety of strategies to target services to those most in need. On average, 30% of the SUA budget comes from the OAA; one in four SUAs report that OAA funding is 10% or less of their budget (NASUA, 2009). Other sources of funding include state appropriations, foundations and private grants, targeted taxes that include a tobacco tax, income tax checkoff or other targeted tax assessments, and state lotteries in New Jersey, Pennsylvania, and West Virginia.

The Department of Veterans Affairs also funds a range of LTC services for elderly and nonelderly disabled veterans. The Indian Health Service issued a Letter of Intent in May 2010 to award 8–10 Elder Care Initiative LTC grants to help the tribes meet the needs of their elderly populations.

Private Insurance

As noted above, private LTC insurance financed only about 7% of the elderly population's LTC in 2008. An LTC insurance market has existed since the 1960s, but it is only since the mid-1980s that national insurance companies began developing and marketing policies nationwide. About 1.2 million policies were in force in 1990, compared with 8 million in 2009 (Stevenson, Cohen, Tell, and Burwell, 2010). The majority of LTC insurance purchasers buy their policies directly through individual insurance sales agents. On average, purchasers select daily benefit amounts of about $145, a benefit period between 3 and 5 years, and policies that offer a comprehensive set of benefits (Tumlinson, Aguiar, and O'Malley Watts, 2009). About half of individual policies sold in 2006 included 5% compound inflation protection. A policy purchased in 2008 priced to reflect the most typical coverage decisions cost between $2,140 and $2,460 per year for a single 60–year-old. The comparable policy for a married couple ranged between $2,952 and $3,340.

Insurers are selling a growing number of policies through employers and other groups. Purchasers in this market tend to earn less and be younger than individual policy holders—age 41 on average. Unlike employer-sponsored health plans, individuals who purchase LTC insurance through an employer usually pay 100% of the premium and, as long as they continue to pay premiums, remain covered under the policy regardless of where they are employed. Employers can also permit employees to purchase separate LTC insurance policies for spouses or parents. In 2005, 29% of LTC insurance policies in force were held through employer-based programs (Kassner, 2007). In 2002, the federal Office of Personnel Management (OPM) began to offer access to LTC insurance (with no employer contribution) to all federal employees and their parents, as well as to federal retirees. Despite the fact that the federal program's features have produced considerably lower premiums than are available in the current individual market, the take-up rate for this product has been similar to the experience of other employers offering LTC insurance.

In the Deficit Reduction Act of 2005, Congress promoted the "Long-Term Care Partnership"—state programs that allow people who purchase approved private insurance policies to qualify for Medicaid while retaining a higher level of assets than would otherwise be allowed for program eligibility. As of July 2010, 36 states had adopted a Partnership program (Stevenson et al., 2010). The experience in four states that have had this program since the 1990s shows that this Partnership program has influenced the design of higher-quality products. But improved policies have not meant an increased volume of purchases, particularly among people of modest means to whom the program is targeted (Ahlstrom, Clements, Tumlinson, and Lambrew, 2004). Most purchasers of Partnership policies have substantial assets—the majority of purchasers in California, Connecticut, and Indiana had more than $350,000 in assets. These individuals would never previously have qualified for Medicaid, resulting in greater expenditures for the states in which these claimants lived. The Government Accountability Office (2007) has estimated that on balance, enabling all states to offer Partnership arrangements would result in a small increase in Medicaid costs—$86 million nationwide over 10 years.

The New Federal CLASS Long-Term Care Program

A number of factors have influenced the lack of expansion of the private LTC insurance market (Tumlinson, Aguiar, and O'Malley Watts, 2009). Cost to policy purchasers remains a key perceived barrier to expanding the private insurance role in LTC financing. Since most potential consumers must undergo a detailed health screening to determine their insurability and risk rating, health risk also is a limitation for many would-be consumers. Buyers, furthermore, face complex product design issues and decisions that discourage many individuals from purchasing policies. Since it can be 20 to 30 years before the purchased insurance is used, the time lag between purchase and receipt of benefits is a deterrent for many potential buyers. A lack of consumer confidence in insurers to pay benefits when the care is needed and to maintain stable premiums is another limiting factor.

The Community Living Assistance Services and Supports (CLASS) program, included in the Affordable Care Act of 2010, establishes a new federally administered, voluntary program for LTC designed to address many of the private insurance limitations (Justice, 2010). Program premiums are to be fully paid for by individual workers through payroll deductions. In an attempt to increase participation, individuals whose employers agree to offer the program will automatically be enrolled, retaining the right to "opt out" at any point. Premium amounts are to be set by the secretary of the Department of Health and Human Services (DHHS) at a level to maintain program solvency. Unlike most private policies, no underwriting based on preexisting conditions can be used to prevent enrollment or to determine monthly premiums. To qualify for benefits, individuals must have paid premiums for at least 5 years, have a disability expected to last at least 90 days, and meet the functional eligibility criteria established by the secretary. To ensure maximum flexibility and consumer choice, a cash benefit is provided, with the amount varying by level of disability. (The architects of the program expect the benefit to average $50 per day.) There are no lifetime or aggregate limits.

At the time of this writing, staffs from DHHS and the U.S. Department of Treasury are working on the implementation of the CLASS provisions. A number of concerns have been raised that have important implications for the long-term solvency of this program. The lack of underwriting and the voluntary nature of the program suggest the likelihood of substantial adverse selection, that is, the potential that high-risk individuals (those with disabilities or at risk of becoming disabled) are most likely to enroll. These program elements, in turn, are key factors in determining the premium levels that need to be set to ensure a sustainable program. If the premium levels are too high, there will be little incentive for younger, healthier working-age individuals to enroll in the program. There are also substantial implementation issues, including the relationship between CLASS and Medicaid and who will assume responsibility for legibility determination and benefit administration. Finally, program benefits are limited. The average daily benefit may be adequate to cover the costs of HCBS for elderly persons with moderate LTC needs, but it would not be sufficient to cover the costs of nursing home care.

The current health care delivery system is primarily shaped by two key factors: the public funding streams (Medicare and Medicaid) and the knowledge, skills, and competence of the health care workforce. Because the formal (paid) care sector is dominated by public finding, the nature and scope of Medicare and Medicaid have shaped, in large part, the organization and delivery of services to the elderly population. Each program has different eligibility and coverage rules, benefit structures, and regulatory environments that frequently conflict with each other (Grabowski, 2007). These programs, furthermore, have created silos of service primarily tied to settings (e.g., hospital, physicians' offices and clinics, nursing homes, home care) that fail to support a person-centered system for elderly consumers and their families (who often make most of the care decisions). In addition, most of the physicians, nurses, social workers, therapists, allied health professionals, and direct care workers are not trained to address, in a comprehensive fashion, the range of medical care, LTC, and other prevention and supportive services for older adults (IOM, 2008).

Consequently, the "system" is really a nonsystem of fragmented services that fail to address the twin goals of quality of care and quality of life, particularly for chronically disabled elderly individuals who require services from all segments of the health care sector. Within the LTC sub-sector, family and other unpaid friends and neighbors constitute the major part of the delivery system. Data from the 1999 National Long-Term Care Survey—the most recent published estimates—indicate that nearly two-thirds of disabled elderly individuals relied entirely on informal caregivers (primarily spouses and adult children) for LTC assistance (Spillman and Black, 2005). For those elderly consumers receiving care from the formal sector, public financing continues to have an institutional bias, despite the fact that most individuals prefer to receive their services in the community. Moreover, even many of the HCBS programs do not provide the level of choice and discretion that today's and particularly tomorrow's older adults prefer. The following section presents a brief summary of existing and proposed models of service integration and coordination, efforts to rebalance the LTC system toward more home- and community-based care, and the evolution of consumer-directed care.

Models of Service Integration/Coordination

Over the past 25 years, a number of model programs have been developed at the federal, state, and local levels to improve care coordination and to achieve better service integration. The recently enacted Affordable Care Act builds on past experience and establishes a number of demonstration programs that provide financial incentives for further development of such programs. While there is no consensus on the definition of "integration," key elements being sought typically include (1) broad and flexible benefits, (2) far-reaching delivery systems that include care management in the community and linkage of medical and LTC providers, (3) adoption of specific processes and tools to facilitate integration (e.g., care planning protocols, interdisciplinary care teams, integrated electronically based information systems), (4) overarching quality-control systems with a single point of accountability, and (5) flexible funding streams with incentives to integrate dollars and minimize cost shifting. The models described below reflect past and current efforts in the public and private sectors to achieve better service coordination and integration.

Federal Initiatives

Perhaps the most well-known program designed to integrate the full range of medical care, LTC, and other supportive services for very disabled older adults is the Program of All-Inclusive Care for the Elderly (PACE). The PACE model is centered on the belief that it is better for the well-being of seniors with chronic care needs and their families to be served in the community whenever possible. PACE serves individuals who are aged 55 or older, are certified by their state to need nursing home care, are able to live safely in the community at the time of enrollment, and live in a PACE service area. Most of the enrollees are low-income, chronically disabled elderly dual eligibles. Through an intensive care management approach conducted by interdisciplinary care teams, PACE programs strive to keep individuals in community care and out of nursing homes and hospitals. Providers receive a combined Medicare/Medicaid capitation payment per client and rely on the adult day care setting as the focal point for service coordination. PACE organizations gained permanent Medicare and Medicaid provider status in 1997, and as of 2010 74 PACE programs were operating in 30 states. Another five programs were operating as Pre-PACE—receiving a Medicaid capitation payment and fee-for-service payment from Medicare.

Using Medicare and Medicaid waivers, the EverCare program—developed by United Healthcare (a private health insurance company) in 1986—is a model of integrated primary care and LTC in nursing homes. The program enrolls nursing home residents in a risk-based HMO, with the nursing home costs covered by Medicaid or private insurance. Teams of geriatric physicians and nurse practitioners provide intensive primary care services to the residents and coordinate this care with the LTC services provided by the facility's nursing staff. Because EverCare pays for all medical services incurred by the resident, there is no incentive for the nursing home provider to shift costs to Medicare by hospitalizing a resident.

The U.S. Department of Veterans Affairs' Home-Based Primary Care (HBPC) program provides care through a multidisciplinary team in the individual's home after discharge from a hospital or nursing home (Beales and Edes, 2009). The program screens patients to identify those at highest risk and targets care to them, designates a care manager within the multidisciplinary team, provides 24–hour contact, requires prior approval for hospitalizations, and involves the team in any hospital admission planning. Services include management and administration of medication; wound, pain, and medical management; laboratory draws; tele-home care; and care coordination between DVA and community-based LTC providers.

The Affordable Care Act includes several payment and health delivery reforms to encourage better care coordination and service integration, delivered more efficiently and at less cost (KFF, 2010a). The law establishes a pilot program to bundle payments to hospitals, physician groups, and post-acute care providers (skilled nursing facilities and home health agencies) with the goal of reducing rehospitalization rates and improving the quality of care delivered in the community. Another 3-year demonstration provides an additional Medicare payment to accountable care organizations—groups of hospitals, physician groups, health plans, and other community-based providers that are successful in achieving better care coordination and care outcomes. Several demonstrations focus specifically on improving the transitions from the hospital to other residential and home-based settings, targeting high-risk Medicare beneficiaries. The Independence at Home Demonstration provides a payment based on a spending target for interdisciplinary teams of physicians, nurse practitioners, and other providers who deliver home-based primary care and intensive care coordination to chronically disabled older adults not able to get to physician offices and other ambulatory care settings.

The law also creates a new CMS Office of Innovation to test new payment and service delivery models and establishes a Federal Coordinated Health Care Office to improve the integration of care delivered to the dual eligibles.

State Initiatives

States have also experimented with the integration of services for their chronically disabled elderly populations. Arizona's LTC system is part of a mandatory Medicaid managed care program begun in the late 1980s. Medicaid acute, long-term, and behavioral health services are included in the package, but Medicare funding is not integrated. The program implicitly achieves a degree of integration at the contractor level, because Medicare services are usually delivered through the organization that receives the Medicaid capitation to provide the LTC services (Grabowski and Bramson, 2008).

Minnesota was the first state to receive Medicare and Medicaid waivers to integrate acute care and LTC services for elders in seven counties. The Minnesota Senior Health Options (MSHO) program, developed in 1995, offers a package of acute care and LTC services on a voluntary basis; plans pay for community-based care, case management for high-risk patients, up to 180 days of nursing home costs, and financial incentives to minimize nursing home use and to encourage early nursing home discharges (Kane, Homyak, Bershadsky, Lum, and Siadaty, 2003). Other states (Massachusetts, Maine, Florida, Texas, Wisconsin) have established integrated initiatives combining Medicaid Home and Community-Based Waiver programs with fee-for-service Medicare through various coordination mechanisms (Grabowski and Bramson, 2008). Despite the theoretical underpinnings of this model, there is little evidence to support the hypothesis that these programs have been cost-effective. MSHO—the only integrated state program to be thoroughly studied to date—saw stable quality of care but higher Medicare and Medicaid costs, though this cost rise may be partially attributable to higher-than-anticipated levels of enrollment (Kane et al., 2003).

The Medicare Modernization Act of 2003 provided a catalyst for states wishing to coordinate Medicare and Medicaid programs through the creation of the Special Needs Plans (SNPs). Under Medicare Advantage (Part C described above), SNPs receive a capitated rate for each Medicare enrollee and are also capable of enrolling Medicaid beneficiaries under a single capitation, without the burden of seeking any Medicaid waivers. Three states—Minnesota, Texas, and Arizona—took full advantage of the SNP program, enrolling 23,000, 18,000, and 8,000 individuals, respectively (Milligan and Woodstock, 2008). Additional states (e.g., New York, Massachusetts, and Washington) have also begun to take advantage of the SNP option. Grabowski and Bramson (2008) note, however, that there is no consensus on the cost-effectiveness of these new efforts. Since the initial spurt of enrollment following the rollout of the SNP program, growth has been much more modest. The Affordable Care Act extends the SNP demonstration through 2014. Payments to SNPs for individuals with chronic conditions will be risk adjusted based on the costs of enrollees with the same health conditions, beginning in 2011 (KFF, 2010a).

Rebalancing the LTC Delivery System

As noted above, public financing for LTC services is heavily biased in favor of nursing home coverage. Beginning in the early 1980s, the federal and state governments began to experiment with various initiatives to (1) serve greater numbers of people in their homes or community-based residential settings (e.g., assisted living, adult foster homes, personal care homes) and (2) shift more resources toward HCBS to balance Medicaid spending between institutional care and HCBS (Kassner et al., 2008). The U.S. Supreme Court ruling in *Olmstead v. L.C.* (119 S. Ct. 2176, 1999)—requiring states to provide services to people with disabilities in the "least restrictive setting"—provided additional incentives for states to offer Medicaid beneficiaries more alternatives to institutional care.

The federal government's 2001 New Freedom Initiative provided grants to states to encourage a "rebalancing" of the system from nursing homes to HCBS. These include (1) Real Choice Systems Change Grants ($270 million since 2001) to help states expand HCBS options, (2) Nursing Facility Transition Grants to help move residents into HCBS settings, (3) Money Follows the Person Grants ($1.4 billion over a 5–year period) to accelerate nursing home diversion and transition programs, and (4) funds to develop Aging and Disability Resource Centers (ADRCs) in each state to serve as a single point of entry and one-stop shopping for elderly and younger disabled people receiving LTC services.

To date, the impact of these efforts has been mixed. As noted above, there is great interstate variation in the shift of dollars. In 2006, the percentage spent on HCBS ranged from 5% to 50% (Kassner et al., 2008). The spending increase for waiver programs serving the nonelderly population with intellectual/developmental disabilities was four times greater than spending for institutional programs; spending for HCBS and nursing homes for elderly people was roughly equivalent. Therefore, the rebalancing attributed to waiver expansion has been much more likely to benefit the younger disabled population than the elderly population.

The Affordable Care Act includes several policy changes and initiatives to encourage state rebalancing efforts (Justice, 2010). The federal government will provide financial incentives (up to $3 billion) to states that are interested in expanding their waiver programs and home health and personal assistance benefits under their Medicaid state plans. Participating states with less than 25% of their FY 2009 Medicaid LTC spending allocated to noninstitutional services will receive a five-percentage-point increase in the Federal Medicaid Assistance Percentage (FMAP) during FY 2010–15. All other states in which less than 50% of Medicaid LTC spending was for HCBS will receive FMAP incentive payments of two percentage points.

The Affordable Care Act also provides more flexibility for states through their various waiver programs and creates a Community First Choice Option that enables states to adopt for Medicaid HCBS the more generous existing eligibility criteria for Medicaid institutional care of up to 300% of the income threshold for Supplemental Security Income (SSI) benefits. The aim is to equalize access to personal care services and institutional care based on financial criteria. Beginning in 2014, this law also equalizes the spousal protection from impoverishment between those whose spouse enters a nursing home and those who choose to receive Medicaid HCBS. Allowing the non-disabled spouse to retain some joint income and assets without jeopardizing the ability for the disabled spouse to qualify for home- and community-based care will undoubtedly help to expand noninstitutional options.

Developing a More Consumer-Directed Long-Term Care System

Catalyzed by younger people with disabilities who strongly oppose institutionalization and demand a range of community-based options controlled by consumers, a trend toward more consumer involvement and direction in HCBS has evolved among the elderly and their families (Doty, Mahoney, and Sciegaj, 2010). Consumer direction supports individuals with LTC needs in actively choosing the care and setting that fit their needs and preferences. This approach emphasizes privacy, autonomy, and the right to "negotiate and manage one's own risk."

Historically, there has been controversy about the degree of discretion publicly subsidized consumers should have in making their service and setting choices and, in particular, the extent to which elderly people needing LTC prefer and are capable of making their own decisions about care. Over the past decade, however, there has been a growing recognition among policy makers, researchers, and advocates for the elderly LTC population that consumer direction is a viable option for at least a subset of older adults. In addition to recognizing the preferences of many consumers and their families, many policy makers see consumer direction as a potential way to save money through more efficient allocation of resources, fewer administrative costs, and more tailored care delivery.

Policy and program options range from active participation in care planning and decision making to the ultimate in consumer direction—providing cash benefits to beneficiaries and letting them purchase their own services and supports. Most consumer direction has occurred at the state level, through Medicaid waivers and state-funded personal assistance service programs. Programs generally reimburse providers through a fiscal intermediary or directly rather than providing vouchers or direct payments to clients. The recently enacted CLASS program within the Affordable Care Act—which provides a cash benefit to enrollees—is the first national initiative to embrace consumer direction.

One of the most controversial aspects of consumer direction has been the option to pay family caregivers as formal providers. All but six states currently allow payments to family members (excluding spouses) to provide care through one or more of their consumer-directed programs (Houser, Fox-Grage, and Gibson, 2009). There is great variation, however, in the nature and scope of these programs.

CONCLUSION

As the aging of the baby boomers becomes a reality, policy makers, providers, elderly consumers, and other stakeholders are grappling with several health care–related issues. The first is how to control the growth in national spending on Medicare and federal and state spending on Medicaid. The second issue is how to develop a quality delivery system that is person centered and that produces better health, functional, and quality-of-life outcomes for the elderly individual. These are not mutually exclusive goals; in fact, many argue that a more integrated financing and delivery system that focuses attention on prevention, early intervention, and self-care management and the avoidance of high-cost procedures and settings will help to lower costs and achieve better quality as well.

It is clear that the system is fragmented; some say it is broken. The payment and delivery reform initiatives highlighted in this chapter offer some promising opportunities to improve quality while at the same time bending the cost curve. The implementation of the new voluntary LTC insurance program (CLASS) is now underway, although questions remain as to the future solvency of the program, the implications for the Medicaid program, and the impact on further development of the private LTC insurance market. A quality system will also require a quality workforce that is trained to understand the comprehensive needs of elderly consumers (and their families) and that knows how to deliver care in a holistic way (Stone and Harahan, 2010). New technologies, including interoperable electronic health records across settings and assistive devices to maximize elder independence, have the potential to mitigate some of the demands on the workforce. But technology should be seen as a tool, rather than the magical panacea to the nation's health care challenges in the face of an aging society. While many issues remain unresolved, one thing is clear: the financing and organization of health care for America's elderly is and will become an even greater public health challenge with the graying of our society.

REFERENCES

Administration on Aging (AoA). 2009. *Aging Statistics Profile.* Retrieved May 24, 2010, from www.aoa.gov/AoARoot/Aging_Statistics/Profile/2009/14.aspx.

Agency for Healthcare Research and Quality (AHRQ). 2010. Total health services mean and median expenses per person with expense and distribution of expenses by source of payment: United States, 2007. *Medical Expenditure Panel Survey Household Component Data.* Retrieved September 24, 2010, from www.meps.ahrq.gov/mepsweb/data_stats/quick_tables_results.jsp?component=1&subcomponent=0&year=-1&tableSeries=1&searchText=&searchMethod=1&Action=Search.

Ahlstrom, A., E. Clements, A. Tumlinson, and J. Lambrew. 2004. *The Long-Term Care Partnership Program: Issues and Options.* Report prepared for the Retirement Security Project. Washington, DC: Brookings Institution.

Beales, J. L., and T. Edes. 2009. Veterans Affairs home based primary care. *Clinical Geriatric Medicine* 25(1):149–54.

Centers for Medicare and Medicaid Services (CMS). 2010a. *Medicare and the New Health Care Law: What It Means to You.* CMS Prodsuct No. 11467. Washington, DC: CMS.

Centers for Medicare and Medicaid Services (CMS). 2010b. *Total Personal Health Care Spending by Age Group, Calendar Year 2004.* Retrieved September 23, 2010, from www.cms.gov/NationalHealthExpendData/downloads/2004–age-tables.pdf.

Coughlin, T., T. Waidmann, and M. O'Malley Watts. 2009. *Where Does the Burden Lie: Medicaid and Medicare Spending for Dual Eligible Populations?* Issue Brief #7895. Washington, DC: Kaiser Family Foundation. Retrieved June 5, 2010, from www.kff.org/medicaid/upload/7895–2.pdf.

Department of Veterans Affairs (DVA). 2010. *Analysis of Unique Veterans Utilization of VA Benefits and Services.* Retrieved May 24, 2010, from www1.va.gov/VETDATA/docs/SpecialReports/uniqueveteransMay.pdf.

Doty, P., K. J. Mahoney, and M. Sciegaj. 2010. New state strategies to meet long-term care needs. *Health Affairs* 29:49–56.

Gibson, M. J., and A. Houser. 2008. *Valuing the Invaluable: The Economic Value of Family Caregiving.* Washington, DC: AARP. Retrieved January 6, 2010, from http://assets.aarp.org/rgcenter/il/i13_caregiving.pdf.

Government Accountability Office. 2007. *Long-Term Care Insurance: Partnership Programs Include Benefits That Protect Policyholders and Are Unlikely to Result in Medicaid Savings.* GAO-07–2010. Retrieved September 24, 2010, from www.gao.gov/new.items/d07231.pdf.

Grabowski, D. C. 2007. Medicare and Medicaid: Conflicting incentives for long-term care. *Milbank Quarterly* 85:579–610.

Grabowski, D. C., and J. Bramson. 2008. State initiatives to integrate the Medicare and Medicaid programs for dually eligible beneficiaries. *Generations* 32(3):54–60.

Houser, A., W. Fox-Grage, and M. J. Gibson. 2009. *Across the States: Profiles of Long-Term Care and Independent Living.* Washington, DC: AARP.

Institute of Medicine (IOM). 2008. *Retooling for an Aging America: Building the Health Care Workforce.* Washington, DC: National Academies Press.

Justice, D. 2010. *Long-Term Services and Supports and Chronic Care Coordination: Policy Advances Enacted by the Patient Protection and Affordable Care Act.* Portland, ME: National Academy for State Health Policy.

Kaiser Family Foundation (KFF). 2009. *KFF/HRET Employer Health Benefits 2009 Survey.* Retrieved March 6, 2010, from http://ehbs.kff.org/.

Kaiser Family Foundation (KFF). 2010a. *Focus on Health Care Reform: Summary of Key Changes to Medicare in 2010 Health Reform Law.* Issue Brief #7948–02. Washington, DC: Kaiser Family Foundation.

Kaiser Family Foundation (KFF). 2010b. *Medicare: A Primer.* Washington, DC: Kaiser Family Foundation.

Kane, R. L., P. Homyak, B. Bersahdsky, Y. S. Lum, and M. S. Siadaty. 2003. Outcomes of managed care of dually eligible older persons. *Gerontologist* 43:165–74.

Kassner, E. 2007. *Long-Term Care Insurance: Fact Sheet.* Washington, DC: AARP Public Policy Institute.

Kassner, E., S. Reinhard, W. Fox-Grage, A. Houser, and J. Accius. 2008. *A Balancing Act: State Long-Term Care Reform.* Washington, DC: AARP.

Kaye, S. H., C. Harrington, and M. P. LaPlante. 2010. Long-term care: Who gets it, who provides it, who pays and how much? *Health Affairs* 29:11–21.

Komisar, H. L., and L. S. Thompson. 2007. *National Spending for Long-Term Care.* Fact Sheet (February). Washington, DC: Georgetown University Long-Term Care Financing Project.

The Lewin Group. 2010. *Individuals Living in the Community with Chronic Conditions and Functional Limitations: A Closer Look.* Report prepared under contract #HHS-100–95–0046 for the U.S. Department of Health and Human Services,

Office of the Assistant Secretary for Planning and Evaluation. Retrieved March 10, 2010, from www.lewin.com/content/publications/ChartbookChronicConditions.pdf.

Mature Market Institute and LifePlans, Inc. 2010. *Market Survey of Long-Term Care Costs: The 2010 Market Survey of Nursing Home, Assisted Living, Adult Day Services and Home Care Costs*. Westport, CT: Metlife Mature Market Institute.

Medicare Payment Advisory Commission (MedPAC). 2009. *Report to the Congress: Medicare Payment Policy*. March, 2009. Washington, DC: Author.

Milligan, J., and C. H. Woodstock. 2008. *Medicaid Advantage Special Needs Plans for Dual Eligibles: A Primer*. Report prepared for the Commonwealth Fund. New York: Commonwealth Fund.

National Association of State Units on Aging (NASUA). 2009. *State of Aging: 2009 State Perspectives on the State Units on Aging Policies and Practices*. Washington, DC: National Association of State Units on Aging and Disabilities.

Ng, T., C. Harrington, and M. O'Malley Watts. 2009. *Medicaid Home and Community-Based Services Programs: Data Update*. Report prepared for the Kaiser Commission on Medicaid and the Uninsured. Washington, DC: Kaiser Family Foundation.

Spillman, C., and K. J. Black. 2005. *Staying the Course: Trends in Family Caregiving*. Report prepared for the AARP/Public Policy Institute. Washington, DC: AARP.

Stevenson, D. G., M. A. Cohen, E. J. Tell, and B. Burwell. 2010. The complementarity of public and private long-term care insurance. *Health Affairs* 291:96–101.

Stone, R. I., and M. F. Harahan. 2010. Improving the long-term care workforce serving older adults. *Health Affairs* 29(1):109–15.

Topoleski, J. 2009. The long-term outlook for Medicare, Medicaid and national health. In *The Long-Term Budget Outlook*. Washington, DC: Congressional Budget Office, 21–35.

Tumlinson, A., C. Aguiar, and M. O'Malley Watts. 2009. *Closing the Long-Term Care Funding Gap: The Challenge of Private Long-Term Care Insurance*. Report #7879. Washington, DC: Kaiser Family Foundation.

CHAPTER 4

Assessing the Health and Quality of Life of Older Populations

Concepts, Resources, and Systems

Sylvia E. Furner, PhD, MPH
Lynda A. Anderson, PhD

How health is defined, and consequently measured and tracked, is fundamental to understanding and designing strategies that can promote or maintain health. By tradition, the field of public health focuses on the health of populations, whereas the aging services network concentrates on delivering services to improve the health of individuals (Kane, 1997). In recent years, however, both of these disciplines increasingly recognize that their differing approaches are complementary and equally integral to improving the health of an aging society. Professionals working in this important arena must be able to assess and interpret factors that affect the health and well-being of older adults, as individuals and as a group, and to examine the effects of environments in which they live.

Data, when appropriately assembled and analyzed, yield valuable information for practitioners, providers, planners, researchers, and policy makers. Potential uses of data are vast and include identifying and tracking changes in the age distributions of populations, identifying and monitoring health events in a population, understanding the process and outcomes of various diseases and conditions, and determining factors in causation (Tulchinsky and Varavikova, 2000). Such information is pivotal at local, state, regional, national, and global levels in providing direction for the design of programs and policies, as well as monitoring their impact on health outcomes.

Although their potential uses are numerous and diverse, data are generally derived from six major sources: through surveys and surveillance systems, medical records, and vital records such as birth and death certificates; during the course of a research study; and unobtrusively through documents related to social and environmental policies or events such as tobacco sales or motor vehicle accidents. Surveys, in particular longitudinal studies of aging, have been critical in conceptualizing the aging process and are essential to understanding the relationship between risk factors and aging and quantifying age-related changes over time.

A complete discussion of this field is beyond the scope of this chapter; however, some general concepts about surveys and surveillance systems are provided. In addition, it is important to note the various ways that data are featured throughout all of the chapters in this text—from introducing the scope of a problem to reporting on the efficacy of an intervention. In this chapter the concepts of health and quality of life and several models for understanding their assessment and determinants are introduced. The challenges to measuring and interpreting findings related to aging are examined. A number of sources of data at national and state levels and tools are provided. Finally, future directions and opportunities are described.

DEFINING HEALTH

More than 60 years ago, the World Health Organization (WHO) definition of health emerged: "Health is a state of complete physical, mental and social well-being and not merely the absence of disease or infirmity" (World Health Organization, 1946). Over time, multiple definitions of health have emerged. The most cogent of these recognize the multidimensionality of health (Patrick and Erickson, 1993; Crimmins, 2004).

The determinants of health are both complex and interrelated—making measurement challenging, subject to individual interpretation, and potentially imprecise. As McDowell states, "For more than 100 years, Western nations have collected statistical data characterizing social conditions. Measurements of health have always formed a central component in such public accounting; they are used to indicate major health problems confronting society, to contribute to the process of setting policy goals, and to monitor the effectiveness of medical and health care" (McDowell, 2006, p. 10).

Because of this complexity, monitoring trends using just one dimension of health (e.g., mortality) is simply not sufficient to describe the full spectrum of population health. Trends in healthy life, as Crimmins (2004) articulates, are a combination of mortality and morbidity dimensions affected by many different dynamic processes including the age-specific incidence of disease, the rapidity with which people with these diseases deteriorate, and the likelihood that people with and without the disease will die. Further, as proposed by Crimmins, the different dimensions of health include risk factors, diseases, conditions or impairments, loss of functioning, disability, and death. Evaluation of trends in any one of these dimensions has been used as evidence of health trends overall, but in fact they may each represent unique aspects of health and be affected differently by separate processes. Relying on unidimensional trends may lead to flawed public health policy and inappropriate investments in preventive community-based interventions and programs.

Further, the definitions of health may vary depending on the segment of the population for which the definition is being developed (e.g., select age groupings, select socioeconomic groupings, or different countries), the purposes for which the constructs are being used (e.g., research or practice), or, perhaps most importantly, the breadth of the perspective on aging. Major shifts in perceptions about aging in the United States began around 50 years ago as a result of longitudinal studies showing the variability in the health of older persons and subsequent research sponsored by the MacArthur Foundation and others that changed the focus from predictors of poor health to predictors of successful aging (Satariano, 2006). The MacArthur studies were designed to examine successful aging and the factors associated with differences in health and functioning in an aging cohort. Based on these studies, Rowe and Kahn coined the term "successful aging" and defined three broad domains related to (1) an individual's health, the absence of disease, and the risk factors for disease; (2) high physical and cognitive abilities; and (3) active engagement with life (Rowe and Kahn, 1998). Recent reviews of the literature have explored this concept further and found numerous definitions of successful aging—but with commonalities (Phelan and Larson, 2002; Depp and Jeste, 2006). According to Phelan and Larson, these commonalities revolve around high functioning (both physical and cognitive), active engagement with life (including strong social support networks), physical activity, and freedom from chronic illnesses.

The WHO definition has also been embraced by the Patient-Reported Outcomes Measurement Information System (PROMIS) initiative. The Steering Committee of the PROMIS initiative adopted the WHO definitional framework of physical, mental, and social domains because it is sufficiently broad and inclusive and will support examination of social dimensions of health (Cella et al., 2007).

Understanding population aging within the United States and across the world requires a broad-based approach such as that provided by the social-ecological model of aging. This model considers the complex interplay among individual, relationship, community, and societal factors that unfold throughout the life course of individuals, families, and communities (Smedley and Syme, 2000; Satariano, 2006). It theorizes that determinants of health such as age, sex, and socioeconomic status influence the context in which individuals function and therefore can directly or indirectly affect risk factors and health outcomes. The model allows for a broad perspective to define and assess health for the aging population, including measuring the various elements related to health risks and outcomes, and has been used to describe and explain the effects of multilevel factors on the causes of health conditions and the consequence or trajectories of those conditions. An example of the application of the social-ecological model can be seen in how public health approaches disability in older adults. The likelihood of disability in populations has received special attention and has been examined within the "disablement process" (Verbrugge and Jette, 1994). This model considers a broad range of factors contributing to disability, including the functional status of the individual and the environmental challenge faced by persons with functional limitations. Further, this model has served as an important frame of reference for research in the epidemiology of aging and disability and is explored more fully in chapter 6.

The definition of "healthy aging," proposed by the Centers for Disease Control and Prevention's (CDC) Healthy Aging Research Network, reflects both the WHO definition and the social-ecological framework first developed by McLeroy, Bibeau, Steckler, and Glanz (1988) and later refined by Sallis, Bauman, and Pratt (1998): "Healthy aging as the development and maintenance of optimal physical, mental, and social well-being and function in older adults. It is most easily achieved when physical environments and communities are safe and support the adoption and maintenance of attitudes and behaviors known to promote health and well-being and when health services and community programs are used effectively to prevent or minimize the impact of acute and chronic disease on function." This definition reinforces a social-ecological view of the determinants of health and recognizes the interactions among individuals, groups, and communities while also considering the broader environmental and policy arenas.

DEFINING QUALITY OF LIFE

Like health, defining quality of life requires a multidimensional approach. CDC defines quality of life as "an overall sense of well-being including aspects of happiness and satisfaction with life as a whole" (CDC, 2000). This is a broad concept with inherent measurement challenges, since the meaning of quality of life is deeply personal and rooted in an individual's culture and beliefs.

Albert and Teresi (2002) posit two distinct domains of quality of life: health-related quality of life and non-health-related quality of life (or environment-based quality of life). With regard to the former, Erickson, Wilson, and Shannon (1995) state that "when subjective complaints and symptoms (e.g., mental, physical, and social functioning; general health assessment; and social opportunity) are combined to describe health, the resulting multidimensional concept is generally referred to as health-related quality of life." Non-health-related quality of life encompasses material and security necessities (access to shelter, food, medical care, social support, safety, and economic resources that are fundamental to a healthy life) and life activities (purposeful activity to maintain identity and health, including engagement in both formal paid or unpaid activities and leisure activities) (Rowe and Kahn, 1998; Hawkins, 2005).

Table 4.1 provides various single-item measures of health-related quality of life (HRQOL). HRQOL measures can vary considerably in scope, complexity, and objectives. Although not an exhaustive list, the measures presented are those most commonly used to describe HRQOL. Each of these measures can be used by themselves or, in the case of the healthy days measure, in combination to describe individuals or populations. In contrast to table 4.1, which describes individual items, table 4.2 presents select survey instruments often used to assess an individual's health and quality of life. These instruments incorporate several dimensions or components of health.

DATA RESOURCES AND TOOLS

Much of the data available to assess the health and quality of life of older adults come from cross-sectional analyses (e.g., survey data). In practice, how-

TABLE 4.1
Commonly used measures of health-related quality of life

Measure	Description
Self-reported health status	This is a global assessment asking respondents to rate their overall health with categories ranging from excellent to poor. It is widely used in population-level surveys nationally and globally (Idler and Benyamini, 1997).
Physically un-healthy days	Respondents are asked, "Now thinking about your physical health, which includes physical illness and injury, for how many days during the past 30 days was your physical health not good?" This variable is sometimes reported as mean days but more often categorized into 0, 1-13, and 14+ days (CDC, 2000).
Mentally un-healthy days	Respondents are asked, "Now thinking about your mental health, which includes stress, depression, and problems with emotions, for how many days during the past 30 days was your mental health not good?" Responses are reported in the same way as physically unhealthy days (CDC, 2000).
Overall unhealthy days	This measure is calculated from the sum of physically and mentally unhealthy days (not to exceed 30 days). Responses are reported in the same way as physically unhealthy days (CDC, 2000).
Recent activity limitation days	Respondents are asked, "During the past 30 days, for about how many days did poor physical or mental health keep you from doing your usual activities, such as self-care, work, or recreation?" Responses are reported in the same way as physically unhealthy days (CDC, 2000).
Active life expectancy	This measure is defined as the expected remaining years of functional well-being in terms of the activities of daily living (Katz et al., 1983).
Healthy life expectancy	This index of a population's state of health is derived from mortality and disability estimates introduced by the World Health Organization (2000). It is intended to answer the question of whether the increases seen in life expectancy are also accompanied by decreases in morbidity (Robine and Ritchie, 1991).
Disability-free life expectancy	This measure is the average number of years an individual is expected to live free of disability if current patterns of mortality and disability continue to apply (Colvez, 1996).
Healthy People 2020 measures	Includes a number of measures of general health status that "provide information on the health of a population" and are considered as foundational measures in Healthy People 2020 (http://healthypeople.gov/2020/about/Gen HealthAbout.aspx).
Life expectancy	This refers to the "average number of healthy years a person can expect to live if age-specific death rates and age-specific morbidity rates remain the same throughout his or her lifetime." It is assessed through three measures, which are defined below (http://healthypeople.gov/2020/about/GenHealthAbout.aspx).
Years of healthy life without activity limi-tation	This measure is defined as the average number of years a person can expect to live free from limitation in activities, the need for assistance in personal or routine care needs (www.healthypeople.gov/Data/midcourse/html/execsummary/Goal1.htm).
Years of life without spec-ified diseases	This measure is defined as the average number of years a person can expect to live without developing one or more of the following selected conditions for which nationally representative data are available: arthritis, asthma, cancer, diabetes, heart disease, hypertension, kidney disease, or stroke (www.healthy people.gov/Data/midcourse/html/execsummary/Goal1.htm).
Years of life in good or bet-ter health	This measure is defined as the average number of years a person can expect to live in good or better health (based on self-reported health) (www.healthy people.gov/Data/midcourse/html/execsummary/Goal1.htm).

TABLE 4.2
Survey instruments used to measure an individual's health and quality of life

Instrument	Description
HUI (Health Utilities Index) Mark 3	This instrument defines health in terms of physical, role, and social and emotional function, as well as health problems (Feeny, Furlong, Torrance, and Barr, 2002; Horsman, Furlong, Feeny, and Torrance, 2003; Feeny, Huguet, McFarland, and Kaplan, 2009). It includes a health status classification system and a "multi-attribute utility function" that uses community data (e.g., Orpana et al., 2009). There are eight dimensions: vision, hearing, speech, ambulation, dexterity, emotion, cognition, and pain and discomfort; each ranges from severely impaired to no impairment (Feeny et al., 2005; Orpana et al., 2009). Overall scores range from 1.00 (considered perfect health) to –0.36 (health status considered worse than death) (Kaplan et al., 2008).
SF-36 (Medical Outcome Study)	The 36 items in this instrument address eight domains (physical functioning, role limitations due to physical problems, bodily pain, general health perceptions, vitality, social functioning, role limitations due to emotional problems, and mental health). Two summary scores are also produced: physical component score and mental component score (Ware and Sherbourne, 1992; Ware, 1997).
RAND-12	This uses the same health status assessment questionnaire as the SF-12 (a shorter alternative to the SF-36), but the scoring differs in two ways (Feeny et al., 2005): the Rand-12 (Hays, 1998) allows for "correlation between physical and mental health and scores are based on weights derived from item response theory." Two summary scores are generated: the physical health composite and the mental health composite.
SIP (Sickness Impact Profile)	This instrument was developed to include 12 domains that are self-rated: ambulation, mobility, body care and movement, communication, alertness behavior, emotional behavior, social interaction, sleep and rest, eating, work, home management, and recreation (Bergner, Bobbit, Pollard, Martin, and Gilson, 1976).
QWB-SA (Quality of Well-Being Scale—Self-Administered)	This instrument assesses health over the past 3 days and combines domains of functioning (mobility, physical activity, and social activity) with a list of symptoms and health issues. A summary score is created for each of the last 3 days, and the final score is an average of the 3 days' scores (Andresen, Rothenberg, and Kaplan, 1998).
HALex (Health and Activities Limitations index)	This instrument consists of two domains, six levels of activity limitation, and five levels of self-reported health and is used to track years of healthy life in HP2000 and HP2010 (Erickson, 1998).

ever, changes that occur over time are often of greater interest. Three causal factors frequently described in demographic research are age, period, and cohort effects.

1. *Age*. The consequences of growing older exemplify an age effect. Examining age effects is central to a number of disciplines, such as gerontology and life course, in which questions about the consequences of aging are key. For example, it is believed that voting and other forms of political participation typically increase as young adults take on greater work and family responsibilities (Glenn, 2007). However, estimating age effects is not easy because these effects may be confounded with cohort or period effects. For example, when assessing the relationship between depression and aging, cross-sectional studies frequently report a positive association between depression and aging; Yang (2007), however, using data from a four-wave panel study, documented that aging per se was not associated with increases in depression and that different birth cohorts experienced different patterns of increases or decreases in depression with age. The author concluded that there was substantial cohort variation in depression, as well as age and cohort interactions.

2. *Period*. Period effects are the consequences of influences that vary through time and can be thought of as extrinsic factors (Glenn, 2007). One example of this is the fluoridation of the water supply, which greatly reduced the incidence of dental caries. Comparing the incidence of dental caries over time without consideration of the addition of fluoride is likely to lead to misinterpretation. A similar example is the change in policy to include annual mammography in the services covered by Medicare Part B. Over time a comparison of the incidence of breast cancer in older women would need to take into consideration the effects of this policy change.

3. *Cohort*. Finally, in addition to age and period effects, there are also cohort effects. Cohort effects are the consequences of being born within a certain time frame or come into existence by entry into a group such as a graduating class. Cohort effects pertain to the differences across age cohorts in life experiences, attitudes, education, environment, and the nature of available health care. All of these effects may affect health and quality of life; thus, evaluating such outcomes cross-sectionally over time may lead to incorrect interpretation—especially when disease or disability rates are changing over that same period.

Much information on the health of older adults in the United States comes from secondary analysis of data that have been gathered for other purposes. The main providers of health-related information are (1) individuals (and/or their proxies) through community needs assessment, surveys, or surveillance systems; (2) care providers and related documentation through medical records; and (3) entities (governmental and nongovernmental) that collect data about a variety of issues (Parrish and McDonnell, 2000). This chapter focuses on the first source and briefly describes the major features, strengths, and limitations of community assessment, surveys, and surveillance systems.

Community assessment. A community assessment gathers information on various current conditions of persons, systems, and resources in the community. The information comes from many sources and can be obtained through interviews, focus groups, and review of demographic data collected by local agencies, including local health departments. Often there are a variety of people from different disciplines and perspectives involved in the assessment, and thus the information obtained tends to reflect a broad view of the community. Because the focus is local, the assessment provides an understanding of the context in which community members live, the health priorities and other issues they feel are important, the resources that are available or need to be developed, and the strategic challenges that should be addressed. The strengths of community assessment include the local focus, the community "buy-in," and the potential for relatively fast policy change. Its limitations include the lack of ability to compare one community's results to other communities; the oftentimes limited resources for such assessments, which in turn limit their scope; and the potential lack of representativeness of the respondents. When undertaking a community assessment, practitioners and researchers are encouraged to examine some of the existing tools available for this purpose to not only ease the cost of creating a new tool but also build on the experience and lessons learned by others. Should existing tools not elicit information about some issue of interest, an existing tool can certainly be augmented or adapted and the reliability and validity reestablished. The following are a few resources or tools available for community assessment:

- Community Health Status Indicators: This instrument originated in 2000 and provides county-level health profiles for all U.S. counties (http://communityhealth.hhs.gov/AboutTheData.aspx?GeogCD=&Peer Strat=&state=&county=). Programs addressing community health can readily access pertinent health indicators for their respective counties on over 300 items related to disease prevalence, birth characteristics and outcomes, causes of death, environmental health, availability of health services, behavioral risk factors, HRQOL, vulnerable populations, health disparities, summary health measures, and population measures (Metzler et al., 2008).

- The AdvantAge Initiative: This set of indicators is designed to "encourage and facilitate community action for the benefit of older adults" (www.vnsny.org/advantage/survey.html). There are 33 essential elements of an elder-friendly community across four major components: addressing basic needs, optimizing physical and mental health and well-being, promoting social and civic engagement, and maximizing independence for frail and disabled adults (Feldman and Oberlink, 2003).
- Administration on Aging (AoA) Performance Outcomes Measures Project: This initiative helps states and Area Agencies on Aging address their own planning and performance reporting needs, while assisting the AoA to meet the accountability provisions of the Government Performance and Results Act and the Office of Management and Budget's (OMB) program assessment requirements. OMB uses its Program Assessment Rating Tool to evaluate program performance (www.aoapomp .net/default.asp). Measurement surveys have evaluated caregivers, case management, senior centers, transportation services, service recipients, and providers among other areas.
- Chronic Disease Indicators: This initiative allows states, territories, and large metropolitan areas to uniformly define, collect, and report chronic disease data that are important to public health practice (http://apps .nccd.cdc.gov/cdi/). At the time of review, the database included 97 indicators organized around seven chronic conditions. Of particular interest here is that the database includes the Healthy Days measures.

Surveys. Surveys are data collection tools to gather information about individuals. The information sought can be collected via a questionnaire that individuals complete themselves, a structured interview where participants are asked questions by an interviewer, or a combination of these two approaches. Surveys are generally standardized to ensure that they have reliability (consistency of responses) and validity (questions measure what they are intended to measure) and that they can be generalized to the larger population. Surveys have several strengths: (1) a large amount of data can be collected in a relatively short time period; (2) a wide array of topics can be included; (3) surveys are often less expensive than other data collection techniques, although the cost rises if part of the data collection includes interviews; and (4) surveys can be developed quickly and administered easily. There are important limitations to surveys that must also be considered: (1) the data collected from a survey are only good if the survey is constructed and administered well; (2) question-answer choices need to allow for an accurate reflection of the participant's feelings; and (3) low response rates can lead to biased results, severely limiting the usefulness of the data.

Surveillance. Public health surveillance is another important source of data. As defined by CDC, surveillance is "the ongoing systematic collection, analysis, and interpretation of health data, essential to the planning, implementation, and evaluation of public health practice, closely integrated with the timely dissemination of these data to those who need to know" (Teutsch and Churchill, 2000). In contrast to surveys, surveillance involves the *continuous gathering* of health data to monitor a population's health status so that needed services can be provided or unnecessary services can be eliminated or revised. The main purposes of surveillance are to (1) follow trends in the health status of a population over time, (2) establish public health and health care priorities, (3) detect and respond to epidemics, (4) ensure that priorities are set that address those with greatest need, and (5) evaluate the effectiveness of programs and services. Examples of surveillance data include communicable disease surveillance (seasonal influenza surveillance), surveillance of hospital-acquired infections, and monitoring of behavioral risk factors (Parrish and McDonnell, 2000).

Public health surveillance is critical to states because it provides timely information to identify cases of disease, initiate control and prevention activities, and help ensure efficient use of resources by documenting the impact of interventions. As indicated by Birkhead and Maylahn (2000), there are a number of challenges to carrying out surveillance at state and local levels. Challenges faced by states include a lack of dedicated funds to support surveillance systems, lack of trained staff to access and use data in the most efficient and effective way, and fragmentation and inefficiencies in different surveillance systems developed to track different issues and conditions (for in-depth information about surveillance see Teutsch and Churchill, 2000).

As stated previously, there are many sources of data for assessing health and quality of life of the older population. A recent publication from the Federal Interagency Forum on Aging-Related Statistics, *Data Sources on Older Americans (DSOA)*, highlights the contents of government-sponsored surveys and products containing statistical information about the older population (www.agingstats.gov/agingstatsdotnet/Main_Site/Data/2009_Documents/Final_DSOA2009_508.pdf). Table 4.3 presents a select number of resources that are readily accessible in the public domain and categorizes them by source (government or nongovernment) and unit of observation. Also offered are example questions the practitioner or researcher could answer from the relevant data source.

TABLE 4.3
Data sources for assessing quality of life in older populations

Source	Description	Example question
Government resources: national level		
Vital Statistics (mortality data)	Mortality data are a fundamental source of demographic, geographic, and cause-of-death information. Vital Statistics is one of the few sources of health-related data in the United States that are comparable for small geographic areas and available for a long time period. The data can also be used to examine characteristics of those who have died, determine life expectancy, and compare mortality trends with other countries. www.cdc.gov/nchs/nvss/about_nvss.htm	What are the 10 leading causes of death for those over 65 years of age, and how have they changed over time?
Vital Statistics (National Mortality Followback Survey)	This survey uses a sample of United States residents who die in a given year to supplement the death certificate with information from the next of kin or another person familiar with the decedent's life history. Data provide a unique opportunity to study the etiology of disease, demographic trends in mortality, and other health issues. www.cdc.gov/nchs/nvss/nmfs.htm	What were the access and utilization rates of health care facilities in the last year of life for persons 65 years of age and over? Did these vary by race and ethnicity?
National Health Interview Survey (NHIS)	NHIS has monitored the health of the nation since 1957 using data on a broad range of health topics collected through personal household interviews. Survey results have been instrumental in providing data to track health status, health care access, and progress toward achieving national health objectives. www.cdc.gov/nchs/nhis.htm	Are there different patterns of participation in exercise and sports activities and self-perceptions of their physical activity levels in men 65 years of age and over compared with women 65 years of age and over? Do activities of daily living (ADL) and/or instrumental activities of daily living (IADL) vary by age, gender, and race/ethnicity?
National Health and Nutrition Examination Survey (NHANES)	NHANES is a program of studies designed to assess the health and nutritional status of adults and children in the United States. The survey is unique in that it combines interviews and physical examinations. www.cdc.gov/nchs/nhanes.htm	What is the prevalence of obesity in the population 65 years of age and over? What percentage of persons 65 years of age and older have radiographic knee osteoarthritis?

continued

TABLE 4.3 *continued*

Source	Description	Example question
National Health Care Surveys	The National Ambulatory Medical Care Survey provides information on the provision and use of ambulatory medical care services based on a sample of visits to nonfederally employed office-based physicians. The unit of observation is visits, not persons; however, person characteristics for each visit are also available. www.cdc.gov/nchs/ahcd.htm	What are the patient and provider characteristics for ambulatory care visits to physician offices and hospital outpatient and emergency departments? What are the top five diagnoses at visits to office-based physicians and hospital outpatient departments by patient age and sex?
	The National Hospital Ambulatory Medical Care Survey provides information on ambulatory care services in hospital emergency and outpatient departments, not including federal, military, or VA facilities. The unit of observation is visits, not persons; however, person characteristics for each visit are also available. www.cdc.gov/nchs/nhcs.htm	
National Survey of Ambulatory Surgery	This survey is a nationally representative sample of ambulatory surgery visits. The unit of observation is visits, not persons; however, person characteristics for each visit are also available. www.cdc.gov/nchs/nsas.htm	What are the number, percent distribution, and rate of ambulatory surgery visits, by sex, age, and region in the United States?
National Hospital Discharge Survey	This is a nationally representative survey on inpatients discharged from nonfederal short-stay hospitals. www.cdc.gov/nchs/nhds.htm	What are the number and rate of discharges from short-stay hospitals with a diagnosis of hip fracture, by selected characteristics and selected years?
National Nursing Home Survey	This is a national sample survey of nursing homes residents and staff. www.cdc.gov/nchs/nnhs.htm	Are there racial differences in functioning among nursing home residents?
National Home and Hospice Care Survey	This survey provides information about the agencies that provide home health and hospice care, including their patients and discharges. www.cdc.gov/nchs/nhhcs.htm	What are the characteristics of home health or hospice care users over 65 years of age?

Resource	Description	Research questions
National Long-Term Care Surveys	This is a longitudinal survey designed to study changes in the health and functional status of Americans aged 65 and older. It also tracks health expenditures, Medicare service use, and the availability of personal, family, and community resources for caregiving. Both elderly in the community (including those not impaired) and those residing in institutions are represented in the samples. www.nltcs.aas.duke.edu/index.htm	What is the prevalence of chronic disability among the population 65 years of age and older? Has this prevalence changed over time?
Government resources: state level		
Behavioral Risk Factor Surveillance System (BRFSS)	BRFSS is an annual telephone survey conducted by all state health departments, the District of Columbia, Puerto Rico, the Virgin Islands, and Guam. It monitors preventable chronic disease, injuries, and infectious disease and helps states monitor and track health problems and evaluate public health programs. www.cdc.gov/BRFSS	What is the health-related quality of life among persons with arthritis? What is the prevalence rate of diabetes in the population 65 years of age and older? What percentage of the older population uses preventive care services (e.g., mammography and immunizations)?
Cancer registries	Virtually all states and the District of Columbia have cancer registries that collect information on the incidence of cancer, types of cancers, location of cancers, and staging of cancers. Registry example: www.idph.state.il.us/cancer/statistics.htm	What counties in Illinois have the highest incidence of breast cancer? Does the incidence of prostate cancer vary by race/ethnicity and county?
The Long-Term Care Minimum Data Set	This data resource contains physical, psychological, and psychosocial functioning of residents in long-term care facilities that are certified to participate in Medicare or Medicaid. The University of Minnesota Research Data Assistance Center can assist the researcher to obtain access to these data. www.resdac.umn.edu/MDS/data_available.asp	Summarize the percentage of nursing home residents within your state who have low levels of physical functioning (based on activities of daily living).

continued

TABLE 4.3 *continued*

Source	Description	Example question
Healthcare Effectiveness Data and Information Set (HEDIS)	HEDIS is a widely used set of performance measures in the managed care industry, developed and maintained by the National Committee on Quality Assurance (NCQA). HEDIS was designed to allow consumers to compare health plan performance to other plans and to national or regional benchmarks. An incentive for many health plans to collect HEDIS data is a (CMS) requirement that HMOs submit Medicare HEDIS data in order to provide HMO services for Medicare enrollees under the program called Medicare Advantage. www.advantageplan.com/pdfs/HEDIS2010MeasurementGuide.pdf	*Compare health plans on the coverage of select preventive care procedures for the older population.*
Nongovernment resources		
Community health status indicators	Sponsored by the Public Health Foundation, these indicators provide an overview of key health indicators for local communities. There are over 200 measures (see text under head Data Resources and Tools). www.communityhealth.hhs.gov	*What are the leading causes of death associated with alcohol consumption within a particular community?*
National Health Measurement Survey	Coordinated by the University of Wisconsin, this survey examines older adults' perceptions of HRQOL using multiple indexes to compare across measures. The design oversampled African Americans and older individuals to allow subgroup analyses. www.disc.wisc.edu/NHMS/nhms_study.html	*How well does an HRQOL index assess health status in African American older adults as compared with Caucasian older adults?*

FUTURE DIRECTIONS AND EXPANDING OPPORTUNITIES

New and emerging issues and developments are anticipated to impact the study of aging. In addition to embracing the social-ecological model, the study of aging should incorporate a life course approach to enhance knowledge of patterns of health, quality of life, and aging. As indicated by Satariano (2006), the life course approach needs to include research on the interplay between age, period, and cohort effects at the population and individual levels. Further, more attention should be paid to the socioeconomic factors and health (Herd, Goesling, and House, 2007).

As racial and ethnic minority groups continue to make up an increasingly larger percentage of the U.S. population, the reality of health disparities continues to severely impact the nation's health. Of particular concern is the growing problem of health disparities in older adults. Many racial and ethnic minority groups have persistently higher rates of illness and death than the U.S. population as a whole (CDC, 2007). In particular, more attention is needed regarding the causes and consequences of disparities in aging populations and public health strategies to reduce these disparities (National Research Council, 2004). Every 10 years, the U.S. Department of Health and Human Services leverages scientific insights and lessons learned from the past decade, along with new data and knowledge on trends and innovations. Healthy People 2020 will reflect assessments of major risks to health and wellness, changing public health priorities, and emerging issues related to the nation's health preparedness and prevention. As with Healthy People 2010, a major emphasis of Healthy People 2020 will be to achieve increased quality and years of healthy life and to eliminate health disparities (Koh, 2010). Racial and Ethnic Approaches to Community Health across the U.S. (REACH U.S.) is an important cornerstone of CDC's efforts to eliminate health disparities in the United States. Its fundamental objective is to address the Healthy People 2010 goal of eliminating health disparities among segments of the population, including differences that occur by race, ethnicity, education, income, or geographic location. By developing, implementing, and evaluating a broad range of innovative strategies, REACH communities have been able to make measureable and sustainable improvements to community systems and infrastructures (www.cdc.gov/reach/about.htm). The REACH U.S. Risk Factor Survey gathers health-related information annually from selected communities across the nation where REACH interventions have been launched. The survey contains questions about health, chronic diseases, diet, exercise, preventive services, and adult immunizations. The results of the survey are used in many ways, including improving REACH U.S. programs (www.cdc.gov/reach/risk_factor_survey.htm).

Healthy People and the definitions of successful and healthy aging also acknowledge that improving social, economic, and physical environments are essential to increasing years of quality life and eliminating health disparities. Additionally, there are increased calls for the development of relevant indicators (Birkhead and Maylahn, 2000; Metzler et al., 2008; CDC, AARP, AMA, 2009). Questions assessing financial security, access to housing, mobility options, and social participation should be collected in concert with other monitoring tools, such as geographic information systems.

Although there is increasing recognition of the importance of addressing conditions that have an impact on health across public health and aging arenas, current surveillance systems have limited coverage of positive aspects of health, as well as few questions covering social and environmental factors that affect health. Increased availability of social and environmental measures in major surveys can support the inclusion of such measures in tools used by states and communities to identify priorities and appropriate interventions for local programs and policies. Having social and environmental indicators will allow researchers and practitioners to refine conceptual frameworks that identify relationships between context and health, examine the intersection across multiple levels from the individual to the environment (Satariano, 2006), and support the development of intervention studies in this area.

Work on indicators and measures is occurring on many fronts. As an example, CDC developed a social context module within the Behavioral Risk Factor Surveillance System (BRFSS) that is based on the work of the WHO Commission on Social Determinants of Health (Marmot and Bell, 2009). This module consists of six questions that explore day-to-day concerns about access to housing and nutritious food, financial security, time at work, and participation in civic activities. In 2009, it was used in 12 states and the District of Columbia.

Efforts are also underway to develop new tools that can reliably and validly measure outcomes important to the study of aging. An example is the PROMIS initiative. PROMIS is a collaboration between the National Institutes of Health and a network of primary research sites to develop and test a large bank of items measuring patient-reported outcomes, create a publicly available system that can be added to and modified periodically, and allow researchers access to a common repository of items and computerized adaptive tests. The PROMIS network will develop and test a large bank of items measuring patient-reported outcomes, create a computerized adaptive testing system, and develop a publicly available system that can be added to and modified periodically and allow researchers to access a common repository of items and computerized adaptive tests. The questions cover a broad range of topics about different aspects of health-related quality of life such as depression, social functioning, physical functioning, and quality of sleep. The measures are being subjected to a multistage development and testing program to ensure that the information meets scientific standards of reliability, with the goal of enabling researchers and clinicians to have access to efficient, precise, valid, and responsive indicators of a person's health status. These measures will be available for use across a wide variety of chronic diseases and conditions and in the general population (www.nihpromis.org/default.aspx).

Finally, special efforts are being pursued to make data more understandable. Over the past decade, the display of geospatial data has become more routinely incorporated into public health projects and reports. This approach adds to our understanding of the broader social-ecological environmental factors contributing to the health of our populations. As indicated by Heitgerd et al. (2008), much has evolved in the area of geospatial mapping because of the decreased costs and increased accessibility of geographic information systems. Through mapping of public health and other statistical data, practitioners and researchers have new ways to assist audiences in viewing, examining, and exploring data. Mapping of data can help users understand complex data or data sets, allow them to find patterns and relationships among the mapped data, and even facilitate further inquiries (Heitgerd et al., 2008). For example, the second version of the Community Health Status Indicators (CHSI) includes an Internet mapping application to highlight spatial relationships between peer and contiguous counties, promote spatial data exploration, produce maps and graphs of sufficient quality to be included in presentations and reports, and be simple to navigate (Heitgerd et al., 2008; Metzler et al., 2008). Additionally, CDC's BRFSS website allows users to map BRFSS data for numerous variables and years (http://apps.nccd.cdc.gov/gisbrfss).

SUMMARY

Research has contributed significantly to understanding health and quality of life and their determinants. The use of a social-ecological model is essential for the study of aging. Information gathered from surveys and other methods can help identify and track health and quality of life and form the basis for planning, organizing, and tracking numerous prevention efforts at local, state, and national levels. As demonstrated in this chapter, data on older populations are widely available in health statistics and published reports of all kinds. Use of these data by researchers, professionals, providers, and policy makers requires seeking out the appropriate data sources, asking the right questions, conducting appropriate analysis, interpreting new or published data, and communicating findings to appropriate audiences.

DISCLAIMER

The findings and conclusions in this report are those of the authors and do not necessarily represent the official position of the Centers for Disease Control and Prevention.

REFERENCES

Albert, S. M., and J. A. Teresi. 2002. *Quality of Life, Definition and Measurement. Encyclopedia of Aging.* Retrieved July 29, 2010, from www.encyclopedia.com/doc/1G2–3402200344.html.

Andresen, E. M., B. M. Rothenberg, and R. M. Kaplan. 1998. Performance of a self-administered mailed version of the Quality of Well-Being (QWB-SA) questionnaire among older adults. *Medical Care* 36:1349–60.

Bergner, M., R. A. Bobbit, W. E. Pollard, D. P. Martin, and B. S. Gilson. 1976. The sickness impact profile: Validation of a health status measure. *Medical Care* 14: 57–67.

Birkhead, G. S., and C. M. Maylahn. 2000. State and local public health surveillance. In *Principles and Practices of Public Health Surveillance,* 2nd ed., ed. S. M. Teutsch and R. Elliott Churchill, pp. 253–86. New York: Oxford University Press.

Cella, D., S. Yount, N. Rothrock, R. Gershon, K. Cook, B. Reeve, D. Ader, J. F. Fries, B. Bruce, and R. Matthias, on behalf of the PROMIS cooperative group. 2007. The Patient Reported Outcomes Measurement Information System (PROMIS): Progress of an NIH Roadmap Cooperative Group during its first two years. *Medical Care* 45(5):S3–11.

Centers for Disease Control and Prevention (CDC). 2000. *Measuring Healthy Days: Population Assessment of Health Related Quality of Life.* Atlanta: Author.

Centers for Disease Control and Prevention (CDC). 2007. *The Power to Reduce Health Disparities: Voices from REACH Communities.* Atlanta: Author.

Centers for Disease Control and Prevention, AARP, American Medical Association (CDC, AARP, AMA). 2009. *Promoting Preventive Services for Adults 50–64: Community and Clinical Partnerships.* Atlanta: National Association of Chronic Disease Directors.

Colvez, A. 1996. Disability free life expectancy. In *Epidemiology in Old Age,* ed. S. Ebrahim and A. Kalache, pp. 41–48. London: BMJ Books, World Health Organization.

Crimmins, E. M. 2004. Trends in the health of the elderly. *Annual Review of Public Health* 25:79–98.

Depp, C., and D. Jeste. 2006. Definitions and predictors of successful aging: A comprehensive review of larger quantitative studies. *American Journal of Geriatric Psychiatry* 14(1):6–20.

Erickson, P. 1998. Evaluation of a population-based measure of quality of life: The Health and Activity Limitation Index (HALex). *Quality of Life Research* 7:101–14.

Erickson, P., R. Wilson, and I. Shannon. 1995. *Healthy People 2000. Statistical Notes. Years of Healthy Life*. Hyattsville, MD: National Center for Health Statistics.

Feeny, D., K. Farris, I. Cote, J. A. Johnson, R. T. Tsuyuki, and K. Eng. 2005. A cohort study found the RAND-12 and Health Utilities Index Mark 3 demonstrated construct validity in high-risk primary care patients. *Journal of Clinical Epidemiology* 58(2):138–41.

Feeny, D., W. Furlong, G. W. Torrance, and R. D. Barr. 2002. Multi-attribute and single-attribute utility functions for the Health Utilities Index Mark 3 System. *Medical Care* 40(2):113–28.

Feeny, D., N. Huguet, B. H. McFarland, and M. S. Kaplan. 2009. The construct validity of the Health Utilities Index Mark 3 in assessing mental health in population health surveys. *Quality of Life Research* 18:519–26.

Feldman, P. H., and M. R. Oberlink. 2003. The AdvantAge Initiative: Developing community indicators to promote the health and well-being of older people. *Family and Community Health* 26(4):268–74.

Glenn, N. D. 2007. Age, period, and cohort effects. In *Blackwell Encyclopedia of Sociology*, ed. G. Ritzer, *Blackwell Reference Online*. Retrieved December 27, 2010, from www.blackwellreference.com/public/book?id=g9781405124331_9781 405124331.

Hawkins, B. A. 2005. Aging well: Toward a way of life for all people. *Preventing Chronic Disease* [serial online]. Retrieved July 29, 2010, from www.cdc.gov/pcd/issues/2005/jul/05_0018.htm.

Hays, R. D. 1998. *RAND 36 Health Status Inventory (R36 H.S.I.)*. Orlando: Psychological Corporation / Harcourt Brace.

Heitgerd, J. L., A. L. Dent, J. B. Holt, K. A. Elmore, K. Melfi, J. M. Stanley, K. Highsmith, N. Kanarek, K. Frederickson Comer, M. M. Metzler, and B. Kaplan. 2008. Community health status indicators: Adding a geospatial component. *Preventing Chronic Disease* 5(3). Retrieved July 20, 2010, from www.cdc.gov/pcd/issues/2008/jul/07_0077.htm.

Herd, P., B. Goesling, and J. S. House. 2007. Socioeconomic position and health: The differential effects of education versus income on the onset versus progression of health problems. *Journal of Health and Social Behavior* 48:223–38.

Horsman, J., W. Furlong, D. Feeny, and G. Torrance. 2003 The Health Utilities Index (HUI): Concepts, measurement, properties and applications. *Health and Quality of Life Outcomes* 1:54.

Idler, E., and Y. Benyamini. 1997. Self-rated health and mortality: A review of twenty-seven community studies. *Journal of Health and Social Behavior* 38(1):21–37.

Kane, R. L. 1997. The public health paradigm. In *Public Health and Aging*, ed. T. Hickey, M. A. Speers, and T. R. Prohaska, pp. 3–16. Baltimore: Johns Hopkins University Press.

Kaplan, M. S., N. Huguet, H. Orpana, D. Feeny, B. H. McFarland, and N. Ross.

2008. Prevalence and factors associated with thriving in older adulthood: A 10–year population-based study. *Journal of Gerontology: Medical Sciences* 63A:1097–104.

Katz, S., L. G. Branch, M. H. Branson, J. A. Papsidero, J. Beck, and D. S. Greer. 1983. Active life expectancy. *New England Journal of Medicine* 309:1218–24.

Koh, H. K. 2010. A 2020 vision for healthy people. *New England Journal of Medicine* 362: 1653–56.

Marmot, M. G., and R. Bell. 2009. Action on health disparities in the United States: Commission on social determinants of health. *Journal of the American Medical Association* 301:1169–71.

McDowell, I. 2006. *Measuring Health: A Guide to Rating Scales and Questionnaires*, 3rd ed. New York: Oxford University Press.

McLeroy, K. R., D. Bibeau, A. Steckler, and K. Glanz. 1988. An ecological perspective on health promotion programs. *Health Education and Behavior* 15:351–77.

Metzler, M., N. Kanarek, K. Highsmith, R. Bialek, R. Straw, I. Auston, J. Stanley, and R. Klein. 2008. Community health status indicators project: The development of a national approach to community health. *Preventing Chronic Disease* 5(3). Retrieved July 29, 2010, from www.cdc.gov/pcd/issues/2008/jul/07_0225.htm.

National Research Council. 2004. *Critical Perspectives on Racial and Ethnic Differences in Health in Late Life.* Edited by N. B. Anderson, R. A. Bulatao, and B. Cohen. Panel on Race, Ethnicity, and Health in Later Life. Committee on Population Health, Division of Behavioral and Social Sciences and Education. Washington, DC: National Academies Press.

Orpana, H. M., N. Ross, D. Veeyn, B. McFarland, J. Bernier, and M. Kaplan. 2009. The natural history of health-related quality of life: A 10–year cohort study. *Health Reports* (Statistics Canada, Catalogue 82–003–XPE) 20(1):29–35.

Parrish, R. G., II, and S. M. McDonnell. 2000. Sources of health-related information. In *Principles and Practice of Public Health Surveillance*, 2nd ed., ed. S. M. Teutsch and R. Elliott Churchill, pp. 30–57. New York: Oxford University Press.

Patrick, D. L., and P. Erickson. 1993. Health status and health policy: Quality of life in health care evaluation and resource allocation. New York: Oxford University Press.

Phelan, E., and E. Larson. 2002. "Successful aging"—where next? *Journal of the American Geriatrics Society* 50:1306.

Robine, J. M., and K. Ritchie. 1991. Healthy life expectancy: Evaluation of global indicator of change in population health. *British Medical Journal* 32:457–60.

Rowe, J. W., and R. L. Kahn. 1998. *Successful Aging.* New York: Random House, Pantheon Books.

Sallis, J. F., A. Bauman, and M. Pratt. 1998. Environmental and policy interventions to promote physical activity. *American Journal of Preventive Medicine* 15:379–97.

Satariano, W. 2006. *Epidemiology of Aging: An Ecological Approach.* Sudbury, MA: Jones and Bartlett.

Smedley, B. D., and S. L. Syme, eds. 2000. *Promoting Health: Intervention Strategies from Social and Behavioral Research.* Washington, DC: National Academies Press.

Teutsch, S. M., and R. Elliot Churchill. 2000. *Principles and Practice of Public Health Surveillance*, 2nd ed. New York: Oxford University Press.

Tulchinsky, T. H., and E. A. Varavikova. 2000. *The New Public Health. An Introduction for the 21st Century*. San Diego: Academic Press.

Verbrugge, L. M., and A. M. Jette. 1994. The disablement process. *Social Science & Medicine* 38(1):1–14.

Ware, J., and C. Sherbourne. 1992. The MOS 36–item Short Form Health Survey (SF-36): Conceptual framework and item selection. *Medical Care* 30:473–83.

Ware, J. E., Jr. 1997. *SF-36 Physical and Mental Health Summary Scales: A User's Manual*. Boston: Quality Metric.

World Health Organization. 1946. Preamble to the Constitution of the World Health Organization as adopted by the International Health Conference, New York, 19–22 June, 1946; signed on 22 July 1946 by the representatives of 61 States (Official Records of the World Health Organization, no. 2, p. 100) and entered into force on 7 April 1948.

World Health Organization. 2000. *World Health Report 2000. Health Systems: Improving Performance*. Geneva: World Health Organization.

Yang, Y. 2007. Is old age depressing? Growth trajectories and cohort variations in late-life depression. *Journal of Health and Social Behavior* 48:16–32.

PART II
Social and Behavioral Factors

Social Determinants of Health Inequities and Health Care in Old Age

Steven P. Wallace, PhD

Public health is grounded in an understanding of the social and environmental determinants of health. It grew out of the sanitary movement in the nineteenth century that focused on population health risks in the physical environment, such as contaminated water, and in the social environment, such as poverty and overcrowded housing. The discovery of germs as a cause of disease began a shift toward more individual-level prevention and treatment. When chronic diseases replaced infectious diseases as the leading cause of death in the mid-twentieth century, individual-level health risk factors, such as smoking and sedentary lifestyles, gained attention while social and environmental factors that shape those individual risks received little attention (Lindheim and Syme, 1983). Recent methodological innovations allow a more accurate measurement of neighborhood effects on health, and together with increased attention to the social determinants of health differences between population groups, public health is reemphasizing its hallmark strategy of addressing population-level health.

Social determinants, the conditions in which people are born, live, work, and age, are largely responsible for health inequities between populations. These circumstances are shaped by the distribution of resources at global, national, and local levels and are influenced by policy choices (Estes and Wallace, 2010). For older adults, the inequities apparent in old age are a function of both current and lifelong social inequities.

This chapter starts with an overview of the definitions and distinctions between the concepts of health equity and health disparities. It then documents key social determinants that are grounded in systematic inequities in race, economic position, and gender. The role of economic position and other social determinants on health status is documented, with particular attention to the role of education. Social determinants are then shown to impact medical care in old age. The underlying mechanisms that explain how social determinants lead to those outcomes, including the different ways that the life course interacts with social determinants, are reviewed. It concludes with perspectives for the future and by providing suggestions of how policy changes could reduce health inequities in old age.

HEALTH EQUITY AND PUBLIC HEALTH

Almost 40 years ago, Beauchamp (1976) described "public health as social justice." He argued that health and disease were the result of social arrangements that privilege some groups at the expense of others, and that treating health and its determinants as a "market good" that depended on individuals' purchasing power and preferences prevented many from achieving the universal right to decent health. Instead, he saw public health as orienting collective action to meet "social goods" outside of market dynamics, goods that had an inherent value independently of their ability to generate profits. More recently, Sen has written about health within a "capacities" approach that similarly argues that health is a basic right independent of market forces. He argues that health is fundamental to the exercise of other rights, making health equity central to the broader issue of social justice (Sen, 1998).

The United States is unique in discussing avoidable and/or inequitable differences in health status and health care use between populations as "health disparities." For example, in 2010 the National Institutes of Health (NIH) established the National Institute on Minority Health and Health Disparities (Williams, 2010), the Centers for Disease Control and Prevention (CDC) has an office of Minority Health and Health Disparities (www.cdc.gov/omhd/), and the federal government annually publishes a National Healthcare Disparities Report (www.ahrq.gov/qual/measurix.htm) that examines indicators of differences in medical care by race, income, age, gender, rural, and disability.

Other countries and the World Health Organization use the concept of health inequity instead of health disparities. The term "disparity" tends to draw attention to the group with the worse health, establishing categories of them versus us. Health equity, on the other hand, draws attention to a more collective context where health and health care are distributed in a fair manner across all groups. The CDC defines health inequities as those that result from the social determinants of health, in particular the unjust distribution of resources, while disparities are any observed health differences between social groups that are defined by characteristics such as race or income (Brennan Ramirez, Baker, and Metzler, 2008). This definition allows CDC's "social determinants of health" workgroup to emphasize health equity within a larger federal framework that continues to focus on health disparities.

Braveman (2006) defines inequities as systematic and unjust differences grounded in social positions of privilege and exclusion. Thus, the finding of a particular health indicator where non-Latino whites are worse than African Americans, such as breast cancer diagnosis rates (Horner et al., 2009), is not a health inequity because whites are privileged in the overall position of power in American society. A difference must be part of a pattern and associated with broader social inequities to rise to the level of a health inequity. In this chapter, health inequities are defined as avoidable differences between populations that are part of a pattern of health determinants, outcomes, and resources that are associated with broader social inequities. This definition focuses on patterns of outcomes rather than any specific health outcome, as well as on patterns of social injustice.

The major axes of inequity in American society are formed across race, gender, class, and age. In this chapter, race is used to denote groups defined in society by parentage and physiological characteristics that are socially and politically created as significant, that lead to differential power in society, and that are the basis for social, economic, and political conflict (Omi and Winant, 1994). This structural definition of race includes Latinos, who have historically been treated as a separate group in the U.S. racial order. Class denotes a group sharing a common economic position. It is not the continuous variable of income, but rather a categorical set of relationships related to life chances and resources that are not easily crossed. Finally, age serves as a social category that affects individuals' status and treatment by social institutions (Estes and Wallace, 2006), in addition to being a measure of the length of exposure to the inequities caused by race, gender, and class.

SOCIAL INEQUITY BY RACE, CLASS, AND GENDER IN LATER YEARS

In American society, one of the key means to social and economic success is through education. A child born to a family with limited economic resources in a community with poor schools is much more likely than one born into better circumstances to have a low educational attainment, poor working conditions, and an insecure old age (Rouse and Barrow, 2006). Relatively low levels of economic mobility among the wealthiest and poorest segments of American society can be explained in part by differential access to and quality of education for the rich and poor, combined with economic returns to educational attainment (Beller and Hout, 2006). Educational attainment and the return on education are also affected by gender and race, which establish lifelong patterns of access to employment, knowledge about health and access to healthy environments, and related life chances.

The relationship between education and occupation is critical because the resources that older people depend on are largely linked to their lifetime occupation and related earnings. Although Medicare and Social Security are near-universal, employment-linked pensions and supplemental health insurance are not. Just over one-quarter of older adults in the United States have Medicare supplemental insurance paid for by their former employer, while just under one-quarter pay for similar coverage privately (Employee Benefit Research Institute, 2010). While 89% of those aged 65 and over are collecting Social Security benefits, only 31% are collecting benefits from a private pension or annuity. For the poorest 40% of older adults, Social Security accounts for over 80% of their total incomes, with pensions and assets accounting for less than 10%. In contrast, the 20% of older adults at the top of the income distribution rely on Social Security for only 18% of their total income and receive 37% of their current income from pensions and assets (Forum, 2010, table 9b).

Social norms and ideologies can also create inequities. For example, women on average marry men who are older than they are. Given current morbidity patterns that are reinforced by gender roles, women are more likely than men to provide care for their spouses in later life, which has labor force and economic consequences (for additional information on caregiving see chap. 9). Women are also more likely to live for a number of years as widows with a reduced income. Among those between the ages of 75 and 84, over half (52.5%) of women are widows, compared with less than one-fifth (18.7%) of men (Forum, 2010, table 3).

Among adults aged 65 years and older, income inequalities are evident in

TABLE 5.1
Poverty (FPL) by race/ethnicity and gender, persons aged 65 and over, 2008
(by population and percentages)

	0%–99% FPL	100%–199% FPL	200%+ FPL	Total
Men				
Non-Latino white	1,074,092 (8.0%)	2,202,682 (16.5%)	10,102,507 (75.5%)	13,379,281 (100%)
Non-Latino black	244,255 (19.5%)	310,968 (24.9%)	695,077 (55.6%)	1,250,300 (100%)
Non-Latino Asian/Pacific Islander	69,274 (12.0%)	107,906 (18.7%)	399,718 (69.3%)	576,898 (100%)
American Indian/ AK Native	24,595 (16.1%)	40,663 (26.7%)	87,167 (57.2%)	152,425 (100%)
Latino	204,107 (18.1%)	320,474 (28.4%)	605,532 (53.6%)	1,130,113 (100%)
Total	1,606,712 (9.8%)	2,965,182 (18.1%)	11,848,269 (72.2%)	16,420,163 (100%)
Women				
Non-Latino white	2,624,221 (14.6%)	4,042,452 (22.5%)	11,324,696 (62.9%)	17,991,369 (100%)
Non-Latino black	556,759 (27.8%)	543,293 (27.1%)	903,088 (45.1%)	2,003,140 (100%)
Non-Latino Asian/Pacific Islander	105,773 (13.8%)	147,918 (19.3%)	513,150 (66.9%)	766,841 (100%)
American Indian/ AK Native	47,936 (22.5%)	62,000 (29.1%)	102,895 (48.3%)	212,831 (100%)
Latino	351,298 (23.4%)	435,478 (29.0%)	713,665 (47.6%)	1,500,441 (100%)
Total	3,666,521 (16.4%)	5,200,569 (23.2%)	13,509,664 (60.4%)	22,376,754 (100%)

Source: U.S. Census, 2010
Note: Total includes "other" race not shown separately. As a result of rounding, not all totals equal 100%. FPL = Federal Poverty Threshold levels.

the poverty rates by race and gender (table 5.1). Older women are more likely to live in poverty than older men of the same racial group, and within each gender, racial and ethnic minorities usually have higher rates than non-Latino whites. The official Federal Poverty Guideline levels (FPL) significantly understate the income needed by older adults, especially in higher-cost states like California (Wallace, Padilla-Frausto, and Smith, 2010). In many states, renters need about 200% of the FPL to pay for basic expenses (WOW, 2010). For those under 200% FPL, the basic pattern of inequities is similar, but the rates of those without enough money to make ends meet grow dramatically. For men and women combined, about half of non-Latino black and Latino older adults have incomes under 200% of FPL, compared with just under one-third of non-Latino white older adults.

HEALTH STATUS OF OLDER ADULTS BY SOCIAL AND ECONOMIC POSITION

Social determinants of health involve the intersection of race, gender, and class dynamics, each of which has an independent role in determining health status, as well as interacting with each other. Race has long been known to be a social determinant of health status. Older African Americans consistently show higher rates than non-Latino whites of major health problems, including hypertension, diseases of the circulatory system, and diabetes. They also have the highest rates of functional limitations. Although the gap in disease and disability rates diminishes when black-white population differences in wealth and other socioeconomic characteristics are controlled, most studies continue to find that race has an independent effect on poor health. This may be the result of multiple factors, including stress and social exclusion associated with race that exists across all socioeconomic statuses (Zarit and Pearlin, 2005).

The disease and disability pattern of Latino older adults does not reflect their low economic position as clearly as does that of African Americans. Most evidence suggests that Latino men have a lower prevalence of heart disease and major cancers than whites, but it is not clear why. With the exception of Cuban Americans, Latinos are clearly disadvantaged socioeconomically, have very high rates of diabetes and obesity, and engage less in exercise. In addition, hypertension is at least as prevalent among Mexican American older adults as it is among the general elderly population. Smoking and alcohol consumption rates among Latino males are also high. Any advantages in diseases of the heart and cancer among Latino males cannot be explained by known risk factors and may be related to selective immigration (Markides, Rudkin, and Wallace, 2007).

There is extensive research on economic resources as a social determinant of health (Hajat, Kaufman, Rose, Siddiqi, and Thomas, 2010). Mortality rates increase as poverty increases, with the effect most dramatic in the age groups 25 to 44 and 45 to 64 (table 5.2). A similar, but smaller, increase in mortality rates occurs for older adults living in neighborhoods with high poverty rates (Rehkopf et al., 2006). Longitudinal studies examining the incomes

TABLE 5.2

Rate ratio (confidence intervals) for all-cause mortality, by percentage of census tract residents below poverty (FPL), Massachusetts, 1999–2001

	0%–4.9%	5.0%–9.0%	10%–19.9%	≥20%
Ages 25–44	1 (reference)	1.34 (1.26, 1.43)	1.85 (1.73, 1.98)	2.52 (2.36, 2.70)
Ages 45–64	1 (reference)	1.31 (1.27, 1.36)	1.74 (1.68, 1.81)	2.29 (2.20, 2.38)
Ages 65+	1 (reference)	1.11 (1.10, 1.13)	1.19 (1.17, 1.21)	1.14 (1.11, 1.17)

Source: Adapted from Rehkopf et al., 2006
Note: FPL = Federal Poverty Threshold levels.

of individuals find a similar effect of income on mortality risk, with the effect declining with age (Bassuk, Berkman, and Amick, 2002). It is likely, therefore, that the higher total mortality in older ages washes out some of the income effects, in addition to those most vulnerable to the disadvantages of low incomes having died in younger ages.

Disability rates also vary among older adults by income. Overall disability rates for those aged 70 and over are declining, but the poorest quartile of older adults has experienced the least overall decline and has increasing rates of activities of daily living (ADL), while higher-income groups experienced declines in ADL rates. The disadvantages of the lowest-income group exist even after controlling for age, gender, education, and race (Schoeni, Martin, Andreski, and Freedman, 2005).

Self-reported health is also related to income. Table 5.3 shows that as income levels increase, the proportion of older adults rating their health as fair or poor decreases. In addition, those with low incomes experience health declines at earlier ages than wealthier individuals (Crimmins, Kim, and Seeman, 2009). The association between poverty and poor health in old age is reciprocal—poverty causes poor health (social causation) and poor health causes low incomes (social selection)—but social causation is the dominant direction. This suggests that poverty reduction is an effective way to reduce health declines and improve health equity in old age.

Sen (1998) notes that improvements in life expectancy at the national level are driven by broad-based economic growth when growth works to reduce poverty (e.g., in South Korea) or by the expansion of "supports" even without economic growth when basic health-enhancing services reach all residents (e.g., in Costa Rica). In contrast, when economic growth goes largely to those already well-off, and where public services for those with low incomes are inadequate, economic growth has a marginal impact on national health outcomes. Studies at the subnational level show that inequality influences both mortality and self-assessed health after a threshold level of income

TABLE 5.3
Self-assessed health fair/poor, age 65 and over, by household income as percentage of poverty (FPL), age adjusted, 2006–8

	<100% FPL	100%–199% FPL	≥200% FPL
Non-Latino white	39.7%	31.5%	19.1%
Non-Latino black	49.3	35.6	28.0
Latino	41.9	40.5	29.1

Source: National Center for Health Statistics, 2010
Note: FPL = Federal Poverty Threshold levels.

is reached, especially at the highest levels of inequality (Kondo et al., 2009). The inequality effect for mortality is most apparent for persons under age 65, where the leading causes of death include unintentional injury, suicide, homicide, and HIV, all conditions that are particularly sensitive to social conditions (Backlund et al., 2007).

Education is a powerful indicator of social and economic position. People with higher education have longer life expectancies, lower rates of most health conditions, and lower levels of disability, independently of their income and health insurance. The health status gap between those with the highest and lowest educational levels has been increasing for the past several years, indicating that the advantages of more education (and disadvantages of less education) are of growing importance in health inequities.

The educational gap in mortality rates increased between 1990 and 2000 for older adults. Mortality rates during that period changed little for those with a high school education or less, while death rates declined among those with more than a high school education. The growing educational disparity in smoking rates is a likely contributor to these mortality differences (Meara, Richards, and Cutler, 2008), as are other health protective behaviors that are more common among more educated older adults. Increasing education is also associated with larger social networks, which in turn are associated with better health (Cutler and Lleras-Muney, 2008).

Additionally, the effect of education on health is partly a result of the social position that people with higher education (and usually incomes) occupy during their lives. Those are life spaces that promote and reward health behaviors like not smoking, provide supports such as access to healthy food and opportunities for physical activity, and offer a range of services that can enhance health. Residential neighborhoods are an important life space for older adults because they spend more time in their neighborhoods than employed younger adults. Neighborhoods are highly segregated by race and socioeconomic status (Massey and Denton, 1993), and neighborhood socioeconomic status is associated with mortality, disability, and self-assessed health (Riva, Gauvin, and Barnett, 2007). The conditions that are likely to affect older adults in lower-income neighborhoods include determinants of health such as the lack of availability of grocery stores and alternatives to fast food (Walker, Keane, and Burke, 2010). Low-income communities also have fewer and lower-quality sources of medical care, higher crime rates, lower-quality housing, and weaker social support networks.

SOCIAL DETERMINANTS OF HEALTH CARE

Link and Phelan (1995) provide a compelling analysis of mortality rates by social position for potentially fatal conditions where highly effective prevention or treatment is known (e.g., colon cancer) and for those with little effective prevention or treatment (e.g., brain cancer). They document a strong relationship between socioeconomic status and mortality for conditions with known treatment options, but little or no relationship in those without effective treatments (Link and Phelan, 1995), supporting the conclusion that unequal socioeconomic resources provide unequal access to medical care that can save lives. The Institute of Medicine's landmark report *Unequal Treatment* (Smedley, Stith, and Nelson, 2003) similarly documented pervasive racial differences in the quality and quantity of health services provided.

Having no insurance is not a major factor in access to care since almost all older adults in the United States have Medicare. However, there are a number of services that Medicare does not cover, and for a number of covered services there are deductibles and copayments. Vision, dental, and hearing care, for example, are not currently covered by Medicare. Yet as people get older, poor vision increases the risk of falls and driving accidents, poor oral health can affect nutrition as well as be the source of pain and social stigmata, and uncorrected hearing loss reduces social interaction (Gift and Atchison, 1995; Crews and Campbell, 2004; Campbell, Sanderson, and Robertson, 2010). Table 5.4 shows differences in the use of preventive services and delay in getting care due to its cost among older adults. Preventive services use varies by income, with those in the highest-income categories more likely to report receiving an eye exam and being able to afford dental care compared with lower-income groups. Although Medicare covers preventive services like influenza vaccinations and many health departments provide outreach to make immunizations easier to obtain, vaccination rates still vary by income.

The distribution of medical services is uneven across the population, with low-income and minority neighborhoods usually having the fewest health

TABLE 5.4

Preventive and health services use, by household income as percentage of poverty (FPL), age 65 and over

	<100% FPL	100%– 199% FPL	200%– 299% FPL	300%+ FPL
Eye exam past year, U.S.	55.9%	60.8%	63.7%	67.1%
Could not afford needed dental care past year, California	23.1	17.5	10.9	4.3
Influenza vaccination within the past year, U.S.	50.6	51.8	65.5	70.8
Delay care due to cost, U.S.	8.8	7.6	5.4	2.4

Source: United States–Agency for Healthcare Research and Quality, 2010; California–UCLA Center for Health Policy Research, 2010

Note: FPL = Federal Poverty Threshold levels.

care providers despite having the highest needs. Older adults can also face barriers due to race and income in the accessibility of that care (e.g., cost or able to get appointments in a timely manner), as well as in the acceptability of the care provided (e.g., language and cultural competence) (Wallace and Enriquez-Haass, 2001; Ponce, Hays, and Cunningham, 2006). The lack of health insurance receives the most attention in health care policy, overlooking these other barriers that are consequential to health care for older adults.

AGEISM AS A SOCIAL DETERMINANT OF HEALTH CARE

There is a continuing bias against older adults in health-related settings. In particular, there is a pervasive devaluing of older persons in the health professions (Reuben, Fullerton, Tschann, and Croughan-Minihane, 1995; Kane, 2002). Treatment decisions for older people are often influenced by the person's age, rather than a consideration of the costs and benefits of treatment for the particular individual. Older persons, for example, are less likely to receive recommendations for cancer treatments than younger people, even when there is no medical reason to avoid those treatments. The pattern of undertreatment is exacerbated by the underrepresentation of older persons in most clinical trials (Witham and McMurdo, 2007).

In social policy, older adults are often devalued in discussions of the costs of health and social programs that older persons use (Binstock, 2005). Older adults are commonly blamed for the rising costs of Medicare, even though most medical treatments are driven more by physician recommendations than patient demands. In addition, the rapidly rising costs of prescription medications appear to be driven in part by manufacturer-induced demand (particularly direct-to-consumer ads) for higher-cost drugs, rather than the use of new drugs that improve the treatment of disease (Mintzes et al., 2003; Frosch, Grande, Tarn, and Kravitz, 2010).

One example of the interaction between the devalued status of older persons and the structure of the health care system is the current treatment of older persons with incontinence. Having trouble with urination is socially embarrassing, contributes to social isolation, and is a risk factor for deconditioning, falls, and institutionalization, while often erroneously seen as a "normal" part of growing old (Mitteness and Barker, 1995). Behavioral therapy, including pelvic exercise, is the most effective treatment of urinary incontinence, but drug therapy, surgery, and the use of adult diapers continue to be common treatments (Landefeld et al., 2008). Only about half of women age 60 and over had talked with a physician about their condition, with the women usually initiating the discussion (Diokno et al., 2004). As a nonfatal condition, it is not prioritized by many physicians, despite its prevalence and impact for older adults (Wallace, 2005).

HOW SOCIAL DETERMINANTS MAY WORK TO IMPACT HEALTH AND HEALTH CARE

A critique of the traditional epidemiological risk factor approach comes from the perspective of fundamental causes (Link and Phelan, 1995). This analysis argues that the proximal risk factors of health behaviors such as smoking, physical activity, and diet are more usefully understood in the context of the social environment that encourages those behaviors. Socioeconomic status and social support are described as fundamental causes of health since they work on multiple risk factors and health outcomes through multiple mechanisms (Frieden, 2010). For example, the gap in life expectancy at age 65 is 1.6 years between the top and bottom deciles of deprivation across counties in the United States, a gap that has increased over the past 20 years (Singh and Siahpush, 2006). The growing health gap over time is attributed primarily to the improved longevity of the most-advantaged decile, suggesting an unequal distribution of health-promoting circumstances over that time.

Inequality also creates psychological stress through social comparisons, and this stress may impact the immune and other systems. The most common theory of how stress impacts health over the life course is through the bioregulatory mechanisms involved in allostatic load. Whether caused by in-equality, poverty, racism, sexism, or the lack of work autonomy, regulatory hormones such as cortisol and inflammation factors such as C-reactive pro-tein rise and, because of the chronic nature of the stress, do not return to normal levels. The cumulative impact of these factors results in increased mortality, morbidity, and disability (Seeman, Epel, Gruenewald, Karlaman-gla, and McEwen, 2010).

Attention to the impact of neighborhood contexts on health is also grow-ing (see also chap. 15) and is generally consistent with a fundamental cause analysis. The relationship between lower socioeconomic status neighbor-hoods and a wide variety of health outcomes is well documented (Diez Roux and Mair, 2010), and the few studies specifically on older adults also find a relationship between place and health (Yen, Michael, and Perdue, 2009).

The World Health Organization has embarked on a program on the social determinants of health, producing its inaugural report in 2008 (Marmot, 2007; CSDH, 2008). The report explains that the conditions under which people live and die are shaped by political, social, and economic forces. It pro-poses three principles of action: (1) improve the conditions of daily life—the circumstances in which people are born, grow, live, work, and age; (2) tackle the inequitable distribution of power, money, and resources—the structural drivers of those conditions of daily life—globally, nationally, and locally; and (3) measure the problem, evaluate action, expand the knowledge base, de-velop a workforce that is trained in the social determinants of health, and raise public awareness about the social determinants of health. This initiative has a strong focus on early childhood development; educational attainment; healthy living environments; safe adult employment with a living wage; so-cial protection for illness, disability, and loss of income; and universal access to health care. This focus on the social determinants of health can also be applied to older adults.

SOCIAL DETERMINANTS OF HEALTH AND THE LIFE COURSE

Aging and the life course are relevant to the impact of the social determinants on health through at least three different pathways. First, socioeconomic in-fluences during the prenatal period and early childhood may have an impact on health later in life, even if there is no immediately obvious effect (McEnry and Palloni, 2010). This work on critical periods of the life course finds that some socioeconomic exposures have a "latent" impact that may be either directly causal or predisposing by increasing the sensitivity of persons to risks later in life.

Second, there can be a "cumulative health impact" of social disadvantage over the life course that has been described as "weathering" in reference to the life course impact of racism (Geronimus, Hicken, Keene, and Bound, 2006); others examine the cumulative impact of economic disadvantage (Ferraro and Shi, 2009). Less common is a focus on how privilege protects health across the life course, a cumulative advantage (O'Rand, 1996). Self-assessed health, for example, falls less quickly with aging for those with more education and in higher social statuses (Mirowsky and Ross, 2008).

Third, social determinants of health may work through sorting people into different life course trajectories. Those born into disadvantaged positions are less likely to have adequate access to education, job opportunities, and other life chances as they age, leading to an entire life course trajectory that places them at a health disadvantage (Berkman, 2009).

LOOKING TO THE FUTURE: IMPROVING HEALTH EQUITY FOR OLDER ADULTS

The future holds both hopeful and discouraging potential trends for influencing the social determinants of health to reduce health inequities among older adults. On the hopeful side, the CDC has long supported consensus panels to summarize the evidence on community-level interventions, helping guide planners and policy makers toward effective population-level interventions (Centers for Disease Control and Prevention, 2010a). The CDC has also funded projects to reduce racial and ethnic health disparities, called the REACH program. The grants made in September 2010 called REACH CORE adopted a more explicit social determinants approach than previously, providing support for "evidence-based policy, system and environmental change strategies" (Centers for Disease Control and Prevention, 2010b, p. 4). With priorities that included cardiovascular disease, breast and cervical cancer, and older adult immunizations, this new program should bring new efforts to addressing health inequities that impact older adults.

The social determinants of health in old age are embedded and reproduced through social institutions, the most important one being the state. Government policies for social welfare, employment, housing, and health care are organized around the social arrangements that reinforce social inequality and privilege. For older adults, public programs in income maintenance, health care, and housing are structured in ways that reinforce inequitable social arrangements of the group's earlier life (Estes and Wallace, 2010).

Retirement policy is a clear example. Social Security is a universal program that is mildly redistributive since it pays a higher percentage of preretirement earning to low-wage than high-wage earners. Social Security accounts for 80% of the income for older persons in the bottom two-fifths of the income distribution, yet the median benefit for individuals and couples puts them right at the poverty line. Thus, low-income workers remain low-income retirees. Those with irregular work histories and the lowest wages qualify for public assistance, Supplemental Security Income (SSI), which does not bring an older adult even up to the poverty line in most states. Higher-income workers are subsidized to create personal retirement accounts (401[k]s, IRAs, etc.) through tax-advantaged savings and employer contributions (Wallace and Villa, 2009). Thus, even though the extremes of income converge somewhat among older adults, retirement policies reproduce inequality. Recent proposals to change the Social Security retirement age to reduce expenditures would further disadvantage low-income and minority older adults (who have considerably more chronic illnesses than same-aged, nonminority, higher-income older adults) while not materially affecting the wealthiest older adults or their heirs (Wallace and Villa, 2009).

To reduce income inequality and improve the resources of the poor, policy changes could increase the incomes of the poorest older adults, reduce the incomes of the wealthiest, or both (Dow, Schoeni, Adler, and Stewart, 2010). Short-term approaches could improve the incomes of older adults through increasing Social Security benefits, providing Social Security credits to those who leave the labor force for caregiving, or enhancing noncash supports like expanding affordable housing. The link to health is shown by a study that found that increased income made available through public assistance (SSI) was associated with lower levels of disability (Herd, Schoeni, and House, 2008). Long-term approaches would work to restructure the economy so the poorest could improve their educational achievement and earn higher minimum wages, and at the top end they could reduce the most extreme inherited wealth and salaries not directly related to performance through taxation.

To reduce disparities, it is important to examine the distributional impact of all new policies and innovations that address determinants of health, such as smoking, diet, and physical activity. Voluntary health behavior change innovations are more likely to be adopted by and benefit more privileged groups, whether owing to their higher education, incomes, or other resources. In cardiovascular disease prevention, for example, focusing on individual-level interventions and new medical treatments may result in *greater* health inequities when those with more education and wealth adopt the new practices first. In contrast, population-level approaches that require policy innovations and social change, such as banning smoking in public places or eliminating trans fats from commercially prepared foods, are more likely to reach those in the lowest socioeconomic positions and have the greatest impact on reducing health inequities (Capewell and Graham, 2010). Policy changes that address particular sources of poor health can also improve the health of low-income and minority communities. Those communities, for example, are disproportionately located on busy travel corridors that expose them to high levels of air pollutants (Morello-Frosch and Jesdale, 2006; Hricko, 2008). Policies to reduce diesel pollution from all trucks and trains will have the greatest impact on low-income and minority communities, improving the health of older adults (Brook et al., 2010). Finally, targeted population approaches in low-income neighborhoods can also be effective, such as increasing low-income neighborhood parks or reducing liquor store licenses (Dow et al., 2010).

Public health has a particular responsibility for addressing the social determinants of health because the necessary changes are social goods, not market goods (Beauchamp, 1976). Many companies work on developing drugs and other treatments for diseases that can be sold at a profit, and as long as those affected by the diseases can afford the treatments, the market can work effectively to produce them. But reducing urinary incontinence, changing sedentary lifestyles among poor older adults, and improving food availability in low-income communities are not efforts that are being promoted in the market, much less poverty reduction, eliminating racism, and addressing the gender disadvantages in retirement policies. Instead, efforts to address these social determinants of health need to take on the characteristics of social movements, bringing together diverse actors that include the public health sector to work to change existing policies and practices. The tobacco control movement provides one model of changing policies to promote health against the resistance of those who profited from the earlier, health-harming arrangements (see chap. 11). When a top-down approach to restricting tobacco failed, despite the scientific consensus that smoking was harmful to health, a grassroots movement developed that started by changing local ordinances and changed public perceptions of the acceptability of smoking (Wolfson, 2001).

The lessons from tobacco control can be taken to heart by those concerned with the social determinants of health in the older population. No one public health agency or a single policy will be able to address the health inequities driven by class, race, and gender inequalities in our society, but a broad-based effort to reduce health inequities could reduce the social determinants of health inequality, making real the saying that "public health is social justice."

REFERENCES

Agency for Healthcare Research and Quality. 2010. *National Healthcare Disparities Report, 2009*. Rockville, MD: Agency for Healthcare Research and Quality.

Backlund, E., G. Rowe, J. Lynch, M. C. Wolfson, G. A. Kaplan, and P. D. Sorlie. 2007. Income inequality and mortality: A multilevel prospective study of 521 248 individuals in 50 US states. *International Journal of Epidemiology* 36(3):590–96.

Bassuk, S. S., L. F. Berkman, and B. C. Amick. 2002. Socioeconomic status and mortality among the elderly: Findings from four US communities. *American Journal of Epidemiology* 155:520–33.

Beauchamp, D. E. 1976. Public health as social justice. *Inquiry* 13(1):3–14.

Beller, E., and M. Hout. 2006. Intergenerational social mobility: The United States in comparative perspective. *Opportunity in America* 16(2):19–36.

Berkman, L. F. 2009. Social epidemiology: Social determinants of health in the United States: Are we losing ground? *Annual Review of Public Health* 30:27–41.

Binstock, R. H. 2005. Old-age policies, politics, and ageism. *Generations* 29(3):73–78.

Braveman, P. 2006. Health disparities and health equity: Concepts and measurement. *Annual Review of Public Health* 27:167–94.

Brennan Ramirez, L. K., E. A. Baker, and M. Metzler. 2008. *Promoting Health Equity: A Resource to Help Communities Address Social Determinants of Health*. Atlanta: U.S. Department of Health and Human Services, Centers for Disease Control and Prevention.

Brook, R. D., S. Rajagopalan, C. A. Pope, III, J. R. Brook, A. Bhatnagar, A. V. Diez-Roux, F. Holguin, Y. Hong, R. V. Luepker, M. A. Mittleman, A. Peters, D. Siscovick, S. C. Smith, Jr., L. Whitsel, and J. D. Kaufman. 2010. Particulate matter air pollution and cardiovascular disease: An update to the scientific statement from the American Heart Association. *Circulation* 121:2331–78.

Campbell, A. J., G. Sanderson, and M. C. Robertson. 2010. Poor vision and falls. *BMJ* 340:1313–15.

Capewell, S., and H. Graham. 2010. Will cardiovascular disease prevention widen health inequalities? *PLoS Med* 7(8):e1000320.

Centers for Disease Control and Prevention. 2010a. *Guide to Community Preventive Services*. Retrieved July 28, 2010, from www.thecommunityguide.org/index.html.

Centers for Disease Control and Prevention. 2010b. *Racial and Ethnic Approaches to Community Health for Communities Organized to Respond and Evaluate (REACH CORE)*. CDC-RFA-DP10–1014. Retrieved June 12, 2010, from www.grants.gov/search/search.do?mode=VIEW&oppId=55146.

Commission on Social Determinants of Health (CSDH). 2008. *Closing the Gap in a Generation: Health Equity through Action on the Social Determinants of Health.*

Final Report of the Commission on Social Determinants of Health. Geneva: World Health Organization.

Crews, J. E., and V. A. Campbell, 2004. Vision impairment and hearing loss among community-dwelling older Americans: Implications for health and functioning. *American Journal of Public Health* 94:823–29.

Crimmins, E. M., J. K. Kim, and T. E. Seeman. 2009. Poverty and biological risk: The earlier "aging" of the poor. *Journals of Gerontology Series A: Biological Sciences and Medical Sciences* 64A:286–92.

Cutler, D. M., and A. Lleras-Muney. 2008. Education and health: Evaluating theories and evidence. In *Making Americans Healthier: Social and Economic Policy as Health Policy*, ed. R. F. Schoeni, J. S. House, G. A. Kaplan, and H. Pollack, pp. 29–60. New York: Russell Sage Foundation.

Diez Roux, A. V., and C. Mair. 2010. Neighborhoods and health. *Annals of the New York Academy of Sciences* 1186:125–45.

Diokno, A. C., K. Burgio, N. H. Fultz, K. S. Kinchen, R. Obenchain, and R. C. Bump. 2004. Medical and self-care practices reported by women with urinary incontinence. *American Journal of Managed Care* 10:69–78.

Dow, W. H., R. F. Schoeni, N. E. Adler, and J. Stewart. 2010. Evaluating the evidence base: Policies and interventions to address socioeconomic status gradients in health. *Annals of the New York Academy of Sciences* 1186:240–51.

Employee Benefit Research Institute. 2010. Health insurance coverage of the elderly. In *EBRI Databook on Employee Benefits* (Chap. 36). Washington, DC: Author.

Estes, C. L., and S. P. Wallace. 2006. Older people. In *Social Injustice and Public Health*, ed. B. S. Levy & C. W. Sidel, pp. 113–29. New York: Oxford University Press.

Estes, C. L., and S. P. Wallace. 2010. Globalization, social policy and ageing: A North American perspective. In *The SAGE Handbook of Social Gerontology*, ed. C. Phillipson and D. Dannefer, pp. 513–24. London: SAGE.

Ferraro, K. F., and T. P. Shi. 2009. Aging and cumulative inequality: How does inequality get under the skin? *Gerontologist* 49:333–43.

Forum. 2010. *Older Americans 2010: Key Indicators of Well-Being*. Washington, DC: Federal Interagency Forum on Aging-Related Statistics.

Frieden, T. R. 2010. A framework for public health action: The health impact pyramid. *American Journal of Public Health* 100:590–95.

Frosch, D. L., D. Grande, D. M. Tarn, and R. L. Kravitz. 2010. A decade of controversy: Balancing policy with evidence in the regulation of prescription drug advertising. *American Journal of Public Health* 100:24–32.

Geronimus, A. T., M. Hicken, D. Keene, and J. Bound. 2006. "Weathering" and age patterns of allostatic load scores among blacks and whites in the United States. *American Journal of Public Health* 96:826–33.

Gift, H. C., and K. A. Atchison. 1995. Oral health, health, and health-related quality of life. *Medical Care* 33(11):NS57–77.

Hajat, A., J. S. Kaufman, K. M. Rose, A. Siddiqi, and J. C. Thomas. 2010. Do the wealthy have a health advantage? Cardiovascular disease risk factors and wealth. *Social Science & Medicine* 71:1935–42.

Herd, P., R. F. Schoeni, and J. S. House. 2008. Upstream solutions: Does the supplemental security income program reduce disability in the elderly? *Milbank Quarterly* 86:5–45.

Horner, M. J., L. A. G. Ries, M. Krapcho, N. Neyman, R. Aminou, N. Howlader, S. F. Altekruse, E. J. Feuer, L. Huang, A. Mariotto, B. A. Miller, D. R. Lewis, M. P. Eisner, D. G. Stinchcomb, and B. K. Edwards, eds. 2009. *SEER Cancer Statistics Review, 1975–2006.* Bethesda, MD: National Cancer Institute.

Hricko, A. 2008. Global trade comes home: Community impacts of goods movement. *Environmental Health Perspectives* 116:A78–81.

Kane, R. L. 2002. The future history of geriatrics: Geriatrics at the crossroads. *Journals of Gerontology A: Biological Sciences and Medical Sciences* 57:M803–5.

Kondo, N., G. Sembajwe, I. Kawachi, R. M. van Dam, S. V. Subramanian, and Z. Yamagata. 2009. Income inequality, mortality, and self rated health: Meta-analysis of multilevel studies. *BMJ* 339:b4471.

Landefeld, C. S., B. J. Bowers, A. D. Feld, K. E. Hartmann, E. Hoffman, M. J. Ingber, J. T. King, W. S. McDougal, H. Nelson, E. J. Orav, M. Pignone, L. H. Richardson, R. M. Rohrbaugh, H. C. Siebens, and B. J. Trock. 2008. National Institutes of Health state-of-the-science conference statement: Prevention of fecal and urinary incontinence in adults. *Annals of Internal Medicine* 148:449–58.

Lindheim, R., and S. L. Syme. 1983. Environments, people, and health. *Annual Review of Public Health* 4:335–59.

Link, B. G., and J. Phelan. 1995. Social conditions as fundamental causes of disease. *Journal of Health and Social Behavior* 35(Extra Issue):80–94.

Markides, K. S., L. Rudkin, and S. P. Wallace. 2007. Racial and ethnic minorities. In *Encyclopedia of Gerontology*, ed. J. E. Birren, pp. 532–38. San Diego: Elsevier.

Marmot, M. 2007. Achieving health equity: From root causes to fair outcomes. *Lancet* 370:1153–63.

Massey, D. S., and N. A. Denton. 1993. *American Apartheid: Segregation and the Making of the Underclass.* Cambridge, MA: Harvard University Press.

McEnry, M., and A. Palloni. 2010. Early life exposures and the occurrence and timing of heart disease among the older adult Puerto Rican population. *Demography* 47:23–43.

Meara, E. R., S. Richards, and D. M. Cutler. 2008. The gap gets bigger: Changes in mortality and life expectancy, by education, 1981–2000. *Health Affairs* 27:350–60.

Mintzes, B., M. L. Barer, R. L. Kravitz, K. Bassett, J. Lexchin, A. Kazanjian, R. G. Evans, R. Pan, and S. A. Marion. 2003. How does direct-to-consumer advertising (DTCA) affect prescribing? A survey in primary care environments with and without legal DTCA. *Canadian Medical Association Journal* 169:405–12.

Mirowsky, J., and C. E. Ross. 2008. Education and self-rated health—cumulative advantage and its rising importance. *Research on Aging* 30:93–122.

Mitteness, L. S., and J. C. Barker. 1995. Stigmatizing a "normal" condition: Urinary incontinence in late life. *Medical Anthropology Quarterly* 9:188–210.

Morello-Frosch, R., and B. M. Jesdale. 2006. Separate and unequal: Residential segregation and estimated cancer risks associated with ambient air toxics in U.S. metropolitan areas. *Environmental Health Perspectives* 114:386–93.

National Center for Health Statistics. 2010. *Health Data Interactive*. Centers for Disease Control and Prevention, Retrieved August 1, 2010, from www.cdc.gov/nchs/hdi.htm.

Omi, M., and H. Winant. 1994. *Racial Formation in the United States: From the 1960s to the 1990s*, 2nd ed. New York: Routledge.

O'Rand, A. M. 1996. The precious and the precocious: Understanding cumulative disadvantage and cumulative advantage over the life course. *Gerontologist* 36:230–38.

Ponce, N. A., R. D. Hays, and W. E. Cunningham. 2006. Linguistic disparities in health care access and health status among older adults. *Journal of General Internal Medicine* 21:786–91.

Rehkopf, D. H., L. T. Haughton, J. T. Chen, P. D. Waterman, S. V. Subramanian, and N. Krieger. 2006. Monitoring socioeconomic disparities in death: Comparing individual-level education and area-based socioeconomic measures. *American Journal of Public Health* 96:2135–38.

Reuben, D. B., J. T. Fullerton, J. M. Tschann, and M. Croughan-Minihane. 1995. Attitudes of beginning medical students toward older persons: A five-campus study. *Journal of the American Geriatrics Society* 43:1430–36.

Riva, M., L. Gauvin, and T. A. Barnett. 2007. Toward the next generation of research into small area effects on health: A synthesis of multilevel investigations. *Journal of Epidemiology and Community Health* 61:853–61.

Rouse, C. E., and L. Barrow. 2006. U.S. Elementary and secondary schools: Equalizing opportunity or replicating the status quo? *Opportunity in America* 16:99–123.

Schoeni, R. F., L. G. Martin, P. M. Andreski, and V. A. Freedman. 2005. Persistent and growing socioeconomic disparities in disability among the elderly: 1982–2002. *American Journal of Public Health* 95:2065–70.

Seeman, T., E. Epel, T. Gruenewald, A. Karlamangla, and B. S. McEwen. 2010. Socio-economic differentials in peripheral biology: Cumulative allostatic load. *Annals of the New York Academy of Sciences* 1186:223–39.

Sen, A. 1998. Mortality as an indicator of economic success and failure. *Economic Journal* 108:1–25.

Singh, G. K., and M. Siahpush. 2006. Widening socioeconomic inequalities in US life expectancy, 1980–2000. *International Journal of Epidemiology* 35:969–79.

Smedley, B. D., A. Y. Stith, and A. R. Nelson. 2003. *Unequal Treatment: Confronting Racial and Ethnic Disparities in Health Care*. Washington, DC: National Academies Press.

UCLA Center for Health Policy Research. 2010. *AskCHIS*. Retrieved July 28, 2010, from www.chis.ucla.edu/main/default.asp.

U.S. Census Bureau. 2010. American Community Survey, 2008. Retrieved August 1, 2010, from http://usa.ipums.org/usa/.

Walker, R. E., C. R. Keane, and J. G. Burke. 2010. Disparities and access to healthy food in the United States: A review of food deserts literature. *Health & Place* 16:876–84.

Wallace, S. P. 2005. The public health perspective on aging. *Generations* 29(2):5–10.

Wallace, S. P., and V. Enriquez-Haass. 2001. Availability, accessibility, and acceptability in the evolving health care system for older adults in the United States of America. *Pan American Journal of Public Health* 10:18–28.

Wallace, S. P., D. I. Padilla-Frausto, and S. E. Smith. 2010. Older adults need twice the federal poverty level to make ends meet in California. Los Angeles: UCLA Center for Health Policy Research.

Wallace, S. P., and V. V. Villa. 2009. Healthy, wealthy and wise? Challenges of income security for elders of color. In *Social Insurance and Social Justice*, ed. L. Rogne, C. L. Estes, B. R. Grossman, B. A. Hollister, and E. Solway, pp. 165–78. New York: Springer.

Wider Opportunities for Women (WOW). 2010. The *Elder Economic Security Standard Index*. Retrieved November 10, 2010, from www.wowonline.org/ourprograms/eesi/eess.asp.

Williams, K. 2010. *NIH Announces Institute on Minority Health and Health Disparities*. Retrieved September 27, 2010, from www.nih.gov/news/health/sep2010/nimhd-27.htm.

Witham, M. D., and M. E. T. McMurdo. 2007. How to get older people included in clinical studies. *Drugs & Aging* 24:187–96.

Wolfson, M. 2001. *The Fight against Big Tobacco: The Movement, the State, and the Public's Health*. New York: Aldine de Gruyter.

Yen, I. H., Y. L. Michael, and L. Perdue. 2009. Neighborhood environment in studies of health of older adults: A systematic review. *American Journal of Preventive Medicine* 37:455–63.

Zarit, S. H., and L. I. Pearlin. 2005. Special issue on health inequalities across the life course. *Journals of Gerontology Series B: Psychological Sciences and Social Sciences* 60:S6.

CHAPTER 6

Disability and Functional Status

Laurence G. Branch, PhD
Hongdao Meng, PhD
Jack M. Guralnik, MD, PhD

Disability is an issue that affects every individual, community,
neighborhood, and family in the United States. It is more than a
medical issue; it is a costly social, public health, and moral issue.
—*Pope and Tarlov, 1991*

At the beginning of the 1990s, the Institute of Medicine (IOM) published
Disability in America: Toward a National Agenda for Prevention (Pope and
Tarlov, 1991), which called for the development of a national program for the
prevention of disability by incorporating personal, social, and environmental
factors in helping the research community and the general public understand the importance and complexity of the issue. Although the stage for
more research into the causes and consequences of disability has been set,
since its initial publication and two subsequent updates, the challenge of disability prevention at the population level has not been well met. This is due,
in part, to the enormous growth in several of the major risk factors and causes
of disability: obesity and the host of chronic conditions related to obesity (e.g.,
diabetes, cardiovascular diseases). In this chapter, we provide a brief overview

of the various definitions of disability and functional status and the issues surrounding their measurement, particularly in older populations. We then summarize present trends in disability in the U.S. population from a public health perspective, including the incidence and prevalence of types and levels of disability in different demographic older populations. We also briefly discuss how public health and aging makes use of disability data for determining resource needs of older adults such as home- and community-based services and nursing home placement. We conclude by reviewing current evidence regarding disability prevention and discussing future directions.

CONCEPTUAL MODELS OF DISABILITY

Considerable research has focused on the process of transition from health to disability in older adults, which has resulted in several useful models of disability and aging. The first and perhaps the most widely used is the impairment model, in which individuals were asked if specific activities can be performed or whether there is a departure from "normal" functions. This is sometimes referred to as the medical model. It has long been the standard measurement of disability in health, welfare, and rehabilitation literature. The second model is the functional limitation/disablement model proposed by Nagi (1976) and extended by Verbrugge and Jette (1994). This model describes a four-stage linear progression: pathology, impairment, functional limitation, and disability. The contribution of the Nagi model is that it extends the medical model beyond an individual's physical status or mental state and highlights the dynamic nature of the disablement process. Under this model, disability is the interaction between performance capacity and social, psychological, and environmental factors. In parallel to the development of the Nagi model, Lawton and Nahemow (1973) proposed a general ecological model of aging that connects epidemiology with gerontology under the concept of "person-environment fit." Therefore, ability/disability is the result of an individual's functional competency in meeting the demands of the environment, as well as the adaptation of the person to the environment. As a result, disability is considered to have the following characteristics: (1) it is an indicator of the function and ability of the older adult; (2) both individual competencies and the demand of the environment have considerable ranges; and (3) the relationship between "person" and "environment" is a dynamic process, depending on social environmental and other contextual factors. Extensions of these models have been proposed. For example, Stewart (2003) has suggested that the disablement model be expanded to incorporate physiologic aging. Finally, future research needs to explore to what extent mental functioning, cognitive capacity, and depression affect disability, as well as how to incorporate these broad indicators of mental and emotional disability in public health research and practice.

DEFINITIONS OF DISABILITY

It has been well recognized for half a century that disease diagnosis alone does not provide sufficient information necessary for public health planning and management (Katz, Ford, Moskowitz, Jackson, and Jaffe, 1963). Within the same diagnosis, people can differ greatly in disability levels or functional status. As noted above, defining disability has not been easy; disability is complex, and its definitions reflect that complexity. It also depends on its purpose or use. For example, the Social Security Administration has had a long-standing need to define disability for the purpose of making compensatory payments. It uses "inability to work due to any physical or mental impairment expected to result in death or lasting continuously for at least 12 months" as its conceptual base (Wunderlich, Rice, and Amado, 2002). Another example is the Americans with Disabilities Act (ADA), which defines disability as a substantial limitation in a major life activity such as walking, seeing, hearing, learning, breathing, caring for oneself, or working (Fleischer and Zames, 2001). Psychiatric disorders, including both alcoholism and recovered drug addiction, are also included under this definition. The Office of the Surgeon General defines disability as "characteristics of the body, mind, or senses . . . [that] affect a person's ability to engage independently in some or all aspects of day-to-day life" (U.S. Department of Health and Human Services, 2005). The National Center for Health Statistics has relied on the concept of restricted activity days for decades (U.S. Department of Health and Human Services, 1981).

Other definitions of disability are comprehensive and cover a wide range of abilty. The IOM defines disability as requiring assistance with certain tasks normally accomplished independently (Pope and Tarlov, 1991). This definition follows the Nagi Disablement Model by conceptualizing disability as having a pathologic origin that causes impairment and leads to functional limitations and disability (Nagi, 1964). The 1991 IOM report used the following definitions of stages in the process by which people acquire disabilities or improve their functioning in the context of a particular social and physical environment:

- Pathology: "interruption or interference of normal bodily processes or structures caused by disease, trauma, or other conditions"
- Impairment: "loss and/or abnormality of mental, emotional, physiological, or anatomical structure or function; includes all losses or abnormalities, not just those attributable to active pathology; also includes pain"
- Functional limitation: "restriction or lack of ability to perform an action or activity in the manner or within the range considered normal that results from impairment"
- Disability: "inability or limitation in performing socially defined activity and roles expected of individuals within a social and physical environment"; also, a "gap between a person's capacities and the demands of relevant, socially defined roles and tasks in a particular physical and social environment" (Pope and Tarlov, 1991, pp. 79–81)

One of the earliest broad measures of disability is the Index of Independence in Activities of Daily Living (or Index of ADL; Katz et al., 1963; Katz and Akpom, 1976). Its use as a research tool is likely second to none. However, the past 50 years have witnessed a plethora of disability measures. Excellent summaries of the various measures of health and disability are available. One of the most useful is *Measuring Health: A Guide to Rating Scales and Questionnaires* by McDowell (2006). This book covers a variety of domains, including physical disability, social health, psychological well-being, anxiety, depression, mental status testing, pain measurements, and general health status and quality of life.

The lack of consensus in the definition of disability has made it difficult to measure and compare its incidence and prevalence across various groups and over time. Therefore, in an effort to standardize the definition of disability, including physical and mental functioning, the World Health Organization (WHO) developed the International Classification of Functioning, Disability and Health, known more commonly as ICF (World Health Organization, 2001). The ICF provides a standard language and framework for the description of health and health-related states as a foundation for collecting, analyzing, and comparing the level of functioning and disability across populations. According to ICF, disability is broadly defined as the continuum ranging from "full health" (free of any physical, mental, and social limitations) to impairments, activity limitations, and disability. However, it has been noted that the ICF was designed as a classification framework and therefore does not explain the disability etiology, i.e., the dynamic process of enablement and disablement (Verbrugge and Jette, 1994).

MEASUREMENT ISSUES

Acknowledging that common definitions are a necessary foundation for comparing disability levels across populations and over time, it is also necessary to understand that the measurement options can also influence the reliability, validity, and even the rates of disability data. One set of measurement issues is conceptual; the other is practical. Concerning some of the conceptual measurement issues, an important limitation of the ICF model is that unlike the Nagi model, its current version lacks internal coherence and ability to differentiate among concepts and categories within the framework (Jette, 2009). Therefore, continued efforts are needed to operationalize and differentiate the ICF concepts (for example, activity vs. participation) and make it more useful in scientific investigations (Noonan, Kopec, Noreau, Singer, and Dvorak, 2009). Nevertheless, it has been shown that disability assessment tools developed based on the ICF framework have acceptable psychometric properties for clinical research (Rejeski, Ip, Marsh, Miller, and Farmer, 2008).

A second conceptual issue is that the individual's environment, as well as adaptations to that environment, can influence practical and daily functional abilities. As early as the 1972 annual meeting of the American Public Health Association, M. Powell Lawton spoke of "the basically simple-minded idea that the context in which people behave is a significant determinant of how they perform" (Lawton, 1974, p. 257). This simple idea became the basis of his "environmental competence press theory," which states that the more compromised people are in their functional abilities, the more sensitive they are to negative aspects of the physical environment—and a balance must be achieved between the psychosocial competence of the individual and the challenge of the environment. While the field of rehabilitation has focused on changing the individual's functional status, Lawton argues that adaptations to the environment are equally as efficacious for improving the quality of life. It is important that our approaches to the measurement of disability and functional status respect this important interplay between the personal functional status and the demands of the environment the person must navigate. Measurement techniques need to include this important but often neglected aspect of functional status.

The practical measurement options include performance tests or self-reports, self-reports of usual capacity or maximal performance, and self-reports or proxy reports. The response options can rely on nominal, ordinal, or interval scaling, as well as on dichotomous or continuous alternatives. Each of these measurement decisions will have an influence on the disability data obtained.

Performance tests of physical function have obvious benefits compared with self-reports. Performance tests have better face validity and are a reflection of current performance. Self-reports may inquire about behaviors (such as walking a half mile or a flight of 10 stairs) that the respondent has not attempted for some time. The self-report can also suffer from at least two other sources of inaccuracy: older individuals may have cognitive limitations that compromise their ability to respond to questions accurately, and they may be in denial about their disability and respond based on their perceptions rather than the reality of their functional abilities.

Performance tests can be superior to self-report surveys of disability in certain other ways. For example, most older adults would not be able to self-report their ability to perform certain balance tasks such as forward reach, tandem or semi-tandem stand, or their distance covered in the 6–minute walk test. While measures such as the 400–meter test (Sayers, Guralnik, Newman, Brach, and Fielding, 2006) and the Short Physical Performance Battery (Guralnik, Ferrucci, Simonsick, Salive, and Wallace, 1995) are valued lower-body mobility measures of disability for older adults, respondents would not be capable of providing an accurate estimate of their capabilities on these measures.

While performance tests have several advantages, they do require considerable time and resources and may not be practical in large-scale assessments such as national telephone surveys such as the Behavioral Risk Factor Surveillance System (BRFSS) survey. In addition, the type of disability being assessed may be more practicably determined through a survey item rather than direct observation. For example, if the investigator wanted to know if the person was able to manage their own finances, self-reports of whether the person had unintentionally neglected to pay a bill might be superior to asking the person to read a bill and prepare a check for mailing.

Reports of functional performance or of disability ideally come from the person him- or herself for the obvious reason that they know what they can and cannot do. But sometimes the older individuals themselves are unable to self-report, typically because of cognitive impairments. In these instances, the investigator is faced with missing data from those selected individuals, or relying on proxy reporters. Some investigators opt for the proxy respondent. Proxy reports should only be used to report observed behaviors, not to assess or rate things like pain, attitudes, or satisfaction that are not directly observable to a third party; only behaviors that are directly observable by a third party should be asked of the proxy respondent. A proxy could be asked to report if a third person has climbed a flight of stairs during the last week (that is an observable behavior) but should not be asked if a third person *could* climb a flight a stairs (i.e., capacity), or how much difficulty or how much pain the third person had in doing an activity. Of course, a negative proxy report does not necessarily mean that the third person cannot do the activity; it just means that the proxy has not observed it.

The use of proxy responses is cautioned, however, because proxy reports are intended to be surrogates for self-reports, and definitive research on the accuracy of the surrogate proxy reports is lacking. In addition, the use of proxy reports by definition is not random, is correlated with levels of physical and cognitive disability of the target person, and therefore can be problematic. For example, Todorov and Kirchner (2000) have found that in the National Health Interview Survey on Disability, proxy respondents tend to overreport disabilities for older adults. The major issue is that while proxy data on disability measures are better than no data at all, steps should be taken to assure that the use of proxy data in disability research does not influence the findings.

The choice of response options is also important in the measurement of physical function and disability. One of the original disability measures (noted earlier)—the Katz Activities of Daily Living (ADL) Scale (Katz et al., 1963; Katz and Akpom, 1976)—was cast as an ordinal scale: (1) was the person independent of special equipment or personal assistance, (2) was the person dependent on special equipment only, (3) was the person dependent on another person, and (4) was the person dependent on both special equipment and another person in the performance of each of the basic activities (bathing, dressing, toileting, eating, transferring from a bed to a chair, and continence). For assessments of individuals, this scale in this format allows the identification of those who are not independent. For assessments of whole populations, this scale is often summarized to indicate the percentage of the population who are not independent in every ADL domain, and this percentage is often used as an indication of the disability level in the assessed population. This ordinal scale has been useful in many situations. Researchers at the National Center for Health Statistics converted the ordinal scale into an interval scale and included it in the national Health Interview Scale (HIS) in the 1980s when the HIS was expanded to include older respondents. The interval scale was developed as a four-point-degree-of-difficulty option to the stem of "How much difficulty do you usually have [bathing, dressing eating, transferring from a bed to a chair, toileting; asked one at a time]?"

One by-product of the multiple measure options is that estimates of the rates of ADL problems among older adults in the United States can vary by as much as 60% from one national study to another (Medical Encyclopedia, n.d.). Using results from a single study in which different versions of ADL questions were asked of the same respondents, Rodgers and Miller (1997) demonstrated that prevalence rates can range from a low of 6% to a high of 28%. With the same data, Freedman, Martin, and Schoeni (2002) found that the prevalence of one or more ADL difficulties varies from 17% to nearly 30%, depending on whether the approach reflects residual difficulty (i.e., even with help or the use of an assisting device) or underlying difficulty (i.e., without help or using an assisting device).

In the midst of all this variability, Latham et al. (2008) report that the validity, sensitivity, and responsiveness of self-report measures of physical function are comparable to performance-based measures on a sample of patients followed after fracturing a hip. The measurement of disability continues to focus on the medical conceptualization of disability, i.e., a problem that is located within the individual. Other components of the disability process (participation and the interaction between the individual and the environment as previously mentioned) need to be considered in order to form a strong common basis and language to guide future research (Wunderlich, 2009).

PREVALENCE AND TRENDS IN DISABILITY AMONG OLDER ADULTS

Not only do the definitions of disability vary greatly, but so do the measurement options, and both can contribute greatly to variations in the estimates. Nevertheless, some consistencies and trends can be noted. Two of the major questions that drive research examining trends in disability in older adults are as follows: (1) Is there evidence that the level of disability among older adults is decreasing over time? (2) Are the race/ethnicity and gender gaps in health disparities in disability among older adults decreasing or increasing over time?

Prevalence and Change in Disability

A panel of prominent experts in the field reviewed disability data from five national data sets and investigated inconsistencies among the population aged 70 and older from 1980 to 2001. The panel concluded that the prevalence of disability (defined as difficulty or help with daily activities) had small declines (1%–2.5% per year) between the 1980s and 1990s (Freedman et al., 2004). However, there is conflicting evidence regarding the trend in disability during the past decade, owing to the differences in time period, definition of disability, treatment of the institutionalized population, and age standardizing used in these studies. For example, using data from the American Community Survey and the National Nursing Home Survey, Fuller-Thomson, Yu, Nuru-Jeter, Guralnik, and Minkler (2009) found that the prevalence of basic ADL disabilities and functional limitations increased by 9% between 2000 and 2005. Similarly, Seeman, Merkin, Crimmins, and Karlamangla (2010) analyzed data from the National Health and Nutrition Examination Surveys (NHANES) in the periods 1988–1994 and 1999–2004. They found significant increases in the prevalence of basic ADLs, instrumental activities of daily living (IADLs), and mobility disabilities, with the only nonsignificant results on functional limitations. Martin, Freedman, Schoeni, and Andreski (2010) found that among people aged 50–64, the proportions needing help with personal care activities increased slightly from 1997 to 2007. On the other hand, data from the Survey of Income and Program Participation (SIPP) suggest that the prevalence of disability remained stable, with ADL difficulties at 12.8% and 12.5% in 1999 and 2005 and IADL difficulties at 19.7% and 19.1% in 1999 and 2005, respectively (Centers for Disease Control and Prevention, 2001, 2009). In addition, data from the National Long-Term Care Survey (NLTCS) suggest that the prevalence of ADL and IADL disabilities may have declined from the 1980s to 2004 (Manton, Gu, and Lamb, 2006).

From a public health perspective, it is crucial to recognize that regardless of the trend in the prevalence of disability over the past few decades, the large impact of population aging on the increase in the absolute number of older adults with disabilities is likely to dominate other factors, such as differences in measurements. For example, as members of the baby boom generation (those born between 1946 and 1964) start turning 65 in 2011, the number of older adults is expected to increase dramatically in the next few decades. It is estimated that the size of the older adult population (age 65+) is projected to increase from 35 million in 2000 to 72 million by 2030. This will be followed by a rapid growth in the oldest-old (85+) population as the baby boomers move into this age group after 2030 (Federal Interagency Forum on Aging-Related Statistics, 2010). Given these impeding major shifts in demographics, the total number of persons with disabilities is expected to rise dramatically.

Evidence of Changing Disparities in Disability

The socioeconomic gradient in morbidity, mortality, and overall health status across the life span has been well documented. The disability trend study using NHANES data (Seeman et al., 2010) found that the increase in the prevalence of ADL disability from the early 1990s to the early 2000s was greater among non-Hispanic blacks and Mexican Americans and also among adults aged 60 years and older. In a study of adults aged 70 years and older using multiple cross-sectional data, Schoeni, Martin, Andreski, and Freedman (2005) reported that all socioeconomic and racial/ethnic groups experienced some decline in disability as measured by two general questions about ADL and IADL between 1982 and 2002, but the average decline was smaller among low-income or low-education subgroups compared with the more advantaged groups; no significant differences between racial and ethnic groups were detected. With a longitudinal study of Medicare beneficiaries between 1992 and 2004, Ciol et al. (2008) reported slight improvement in the proportion of respondents with ADL and IADL difficulties for all racial/ethnic groups over time, but blacks had a higher probability of reporting difficulties in ADL/IADL and slightly different trajectories in ADL/IADL compared with other minority groups. In a separate study of adults aged 65 years and older from the Health and Retirement Study (HRS), Dunlop, Song, Manheim, Daviglus, and Chang (2007) reported a higher ADL disability incidence rate over a 6-year period among African Americans and Hispanics compared with whites. They also reported that these differences were due largely to differences in socioeconomic and initial health status (for example, income, education, and chronic diseases). Therefore, future research in disability prevention should take into consideration the socioeconomic barriers and racial/ethnic differences in disability development across these subpopulations.

PUBLIC HEALTH CHALLENGES IN DISABILITY PREVENTION

Recognizing the importance of addressing public health challenges posed by disability and functional limitations, the Office of the Surgeon General, U.S. Department of Health and Human Services published a report in 2005 titled "The Surgeon General's Call to Action to Improve the Health and Wellness of Persons with Disabilities." This Call to Action delineates four specific goals:

1. People nationwide understand that persons with disabilities can lead long, healthy, productive lives.
2. Health care providers have the knowledge and tools to screen, diagnose, and treat the whole person with a disability with dignity.
3. Persons with disabilities can promote their own good health by developing and maintaining healthy lifestyles.

4. Accessible health care and support services promote independence for
persons with disabilities.

According to a recent IOM report, "the future of disability is part of the
future of public health because public health initiatives are important to
monitor disability trends, prevent primary and secondary disability, and reduce disparities in health and well being in the population" (Field and Jette,
2007, p. 27). However, the trend of increasing disability during the past 10
years suggested by some implies that disability remains one of the major public health challenges in our time.

The awareness of the importance of the disability issue in public health
was evident by 2000. Healthy People 2010 (http://healthypeople.gov/2020/)
devoted a chapter on disability and secondary conditions that are now epidemic among younger age groups as well. However, despite the progress
made in the understanding of the importance of disability issues in public
health policy, research on effective prevention strategies at the population
level is still lacking. In addition, policy initiatives aiming at reducing the impact of disability on quality of life remain elusive, in part because of disagree-
ment in the research community about the definition of disability, its linkage
with chronic medical conditions, the role of physical and social environments, and the relationship between disability prevention and altering the
environment to reduce the impact of disability on dependencies.

In December of 2010, Healthy People 2020 (http://healthypeople.gov/
2020/) was released. As with its predecessors in 1979, 1990, 2000, and 2010,
it intended to identify the most significant preventable threats to health in the
United States and to establish goals and objectives to reduce these threats. In
a departure from predecessors that focused solely on goals that had measurement systems available, the Healthy People 2020 reports contain goals for
which no measurement systems currently exist; such goals are labeled developmental. Table 6.1 provides 16 of the 20 Disability and Health (DH) objectives in Healthy People 2020 and the status of these objectives: the first three
pertain to systems and policies, the next four address barriers to health care
(two pertain to older people), the next five are concerned with the environment, and the last eight are labeled activities and participation (six pertain to
older adults).

Overall, the objectives do not seem to stretch very far, and the inclusion of
developmental objectives for which there are no baselines and therefore no
stated targets seems less than helpful. As argued in chapter 17, the establishment of reliable and valid public health information systems is a prerequisite

TABLE 6.1
Disability- and aging-related objectives in Healthy People 2020

DH-1	Include in the core of Healthy People 2020 population data systems a standardized set of questions that identify "people with disabilities." Only 2 of 26 data systems used to monitor Healthy People 2020 objectives have standardized sets of questions in 2010; the goal for 2020 is a modest improvement to four systems.
DH-2	Increase the number of tribes and states that have public health surveillance and health promotion programs for people with disabilities and caregivers. In 2010 16 states and the District of Columbia had such systems; the goal for 2020 is to add two more states.
DH-3	Increase the proportion of U.S. master of public health (MPH) programs that offer graduate-level courses in disability and health. Developmental–no estimates of the baseline level or target increase are available.
DH-4	Reduce the proportion of people with disabilities who report delays in receiving primary and periodic preventive care due to specific barriers. Developmental—no baseline estimates or target levels provided.
DH-7	Reduce the proportion of older adults with disabilities who use inappropriate medications. Developmental—no baseline estimates or target levels provided.
DH-8	Reduce the proportion of people with disabilities who report physical or program barriers to local health and wellness programs. Developmental–no baseline estimates or target levels provided.
DH-9	Reduce the proportion of people with disabilities who encounter barriers to participating in home, school, work, or community activities. Developmental—no baseline estimates or target levels provided.
DH-10	Reduce the proportion of people with disabilities who report barriers to obtaining the assistive devices, service animals, technology services, and accessible technologies that they need. Developmental–no baseline estimates or target levels provided.
DH-11	Increase the proportion of newly constructed and retrofitted U.S. homes and residential buildings that have visitable features. The baseline rate was 42.1%; the goal is a modest 10% increase to 46.3%.
DH-12	Reduce the number of people with disabilities living in congregate care residences. The baseline was reported as 57,462 adults; the goal is a reduction to 31,604 adults.
DH-13	Increase the proportion of people with disabilities who participate in social, spiritual, recreational, community, and civic activities to the degree that they wish. Developmental—no baseline estimates or target levels provided.
DH-15	Reduce unemployment among people with disabilities. Base rate was 14.5%; the goal is a 10% improvement to 13.1%.
DH-16	Increase employment among people with disabilities. The base rate was 19.2%; the goal is a 10% improvement to 21.1%.
DH-17	Increase the proportion of adults with disabilities who report sufficient social and emotional support. The base rate was 69.5%; the goal is a 10% increase to 76.5%.
DH-18	Reduce the proportion of people with disabilities who report serious psychological distress. Developmental–no baseline estimates or target levels provided.
DH-19	Reduce the proportion of people with disabilities who experience nonfatal unintentional injuries that require medical care. Developmental—no baseline estimates or target levels provided.

to improvements in the health status of populations and individuals. The United States should be chagrined that it does not have appropriate information systems to measure health objectives that a blue ribbon panel identified as among the most significant preventable threats to health in the country.

PUBLIC HEALTH INTERVENTIONS TO PREVENT DISABILITY CAUSED BY CHRONIC CONDITIONS

Because of the tremendous impact disability has on an individual's quality of life, mortality, morbidity, and long-term care medical and nonmedical costs (e.g., informal caregiving), research and public policy on disability prevention should become a public health priority until ameliorated. From a public health perspective, it is helpful to distinguish three different approaches of prevention in targeting subgroups in the population who are at high risk of developing disabilities or who already have disabilities: primary, secondary, and tertiary preventions (Gordis, 2008). Primary prevention refers to actions taken to prevent the development of disability by lowering the probability that disabilities will develop in the first place. For example, by promoting regular physical activities and healthy eating behaviors, many individual-level lifestyle risk factors (such as obesity and diabetes) can be prevented, and as a result disability might also be prevented. On the other hand, secondary prevention can be described as identifying individuals who are at early stages of the disablement process (i.e., at the functional impairment or limitation stages) through screening and monitoring and then intervening to minimize the development of subsequent disability. For example, various screening tests used to identify health conditions, such as hypertension screening, a functional reach test, or a balance test, are effective approaches in early detection and treatment, which can thereby lead to interventions to minimize the development of the disability. Finally, tertiary prevention focuses on reducing the negative consequences of disability among people who have already developed disabilities, and the literature is replete with examples of interventions leading to remission of the disabilities.

The primary prevention of disability is sometimes difficult to verify. All those who gave up smoking in their forties, all those who began rigorous aerobic exercises in their fifties, all those who altered their diets and consumed fewer fats and calories in their sixties, and all those who took up weight and balance training in their seventies and have no disability in their eighties may be the beneficiaries of primary prevention. While these changes in lifestyle decades earlier may account for their lack of disabilities in their eighties, for some it could also be a result of a good genetic constitution.

As noted above, secondary prevention of disability focuses on early detection of disability. It aims at interrupting the pathological progression of underlying diseases or conditions. Because chronic conditions are one of the primary determinants of disability burdens in the population, secondary prevention of disability coincides with the goals for proper management of chronic conditions (such as arthritis, hypertension, and diabetes) among older adults. The past decade has seen increasing interest in chronic disease management from public and private insurers, as a result of both the potential benefits on patient health and costs outcomes. For example, Medicare has been conducting demonstration projects aimed at evaluating various chronic disease management programs since 2002 (Foote, 2003). Disease management protocols often utilize a case manager, most often a nurse, who usually engages in an initial assessment, education, activation or empowerment, and periodic monitoring of the patient. However, evidence regarding the effectiveness of disease management interventions on disability prevention remains mixed (see chap. 8).

Tertiary prevention of disability focuses on providing supportive and rehabilitative services to reduce the impact of disability on the quality of life. For example, it has been shown that a six-month home-based physical therapy program is effective in reducing the progression of functional decline among physically frail older persons (Gill et al., 2002). A recent review found that 5 of 10 randomized controlled trials that evaluated disease management activities and evaluated disability outcomes of patients who were already disabled reported significantly better disability outcomes for the treatment group compared with the control group (Liebel, Friedman, Watson, and Powers, 2009). In addition, a secondary analysis of data from a randomized controlled trial found that a multicomponent disease management intervention resulted in better disability status for the intervention group than for the control group at 22 months after study entry, but only among participants with normal body weight (Meng et al., 2010). In addition, a number of intervention studies have found that weight loss and exercise may slow the progression of disability in older adults (Jensen, Roy, Buchanan, and Berg, 2004; Villareal, Banks, Sinacore, Siener, and Klein, 2006; Wong, Wong, Yusoff, Karunananthan, and Bergman, 2008), and one study has reported that obese patients had better functional outcome after a rehabilitation intervention compared with normal-weight patients (Jain, Al-Adawi, Dorvlo, and Burke, 2008). Daniels, van Rossum, de Witte, Kempen, and van den Heuvel (2008) reviewed nine randomized controlled trials aiming at disability (ADL/IADL) prevention among community-living, frail older persons. They found that three of the eight physical exercise interventions produced positive disability outcomes while nutritional interventions or lower-extremity strength training alone did not have a significant effect on disability outcomes. Specific features of the effective interventions included longer duration (9–12 months) with at least three sessions per week. Thus, there is support in the literature for interventions that maintain or improve disability status among persons who already are disabled.

FUTURE DIRECTIONS

Public health efforts to mitigate the impact of disability on population health rely on a number of key factors: the ability to monitor the trend of disability through surveillance systems, which in turn would be facilitated by consensus in definitions and measurements; the ability to identify modifiable risk factors for preventing disability; and effective intervention strategies aiming at social behavioral, medical, and environmental factors. For example, at the individual behavioral level, obesity has been identified as a strong independent predictor for disability (Al et al., 2007; Balzi et al., 2010). A population-based study of 3,717 adults aged 60 and above who participated in NHANES found that obesity was associated with significantly higher odds of having ADL and IADL disabilities among women even after controlling for major chronic conditions (Chen and Guo, 2008). Unfortunately, despite the fact that obesity is among the easiest conditions to be recognized and diagnosed, it has been extremely difficult to reverse, as evidenced by the continued increase in the rate of obesity across all age groups and among all racial-ethnic groups. Based on the strong linkage between obesity and disability, the effectiveness of disability prevention will in part be dependent on whether and to what extent the obesity epidemic can be halted. Some of the key reasons for the failure to stem the obesity epidemic are tremendous growth in energy intake and concomitant decline in physical activities, changes in social behavioral norm (i.e., the conscious and unconscious acceptance of being overweight or obese) as the entire distribution of population body weight increases, and lack of accountability among individual consumers and medical care providers.

The two most common forms of arthritis (osteoarthritis [wear and tear] and rheumatoid [inflammatory]) present another example of a disease that contributes greatly to disability among the U.S. population, but regrettably both the medical model and the public health model are limited in their interventions to ameliorate the arthritis-disability association. Arthritis currently affects 46 million adults in the United States, mostly older, and is projected to affect 67 million by 2030. From the perspective of the medical model, there is no medicinal cure for arthritis, nor does the evidence support systematic efforts at primary or secondary prevention, and tertiary prevention is limited. From the public health perspective, interventions are rarely targeted to those with arthritis.

CONCLUSION

Reducing the impact of disability among the older population in the United States will remain one of the major challenges in the next few decades. Disability is both conceptualized and measured differently by many of the participants who seek to ameliorate its rates and severity. But regardless of the orientation or measures, a plethora of studies have provided irrefutable evidence that certain interventions are successful in reducing disability in certain people. With that as a starting point, we need to expand the interventions that are effective and explore further the strengths and weaknesses of targeting the interventions to all those with a certain level of disability regardless of the etiology, or whether our interventions can be more effective if targeted to subgroups whose origins of disability are similar.

REFERENCES

Al, S. S., K. J. Ottenbacher, K. S. Markides, Y. F. Kuo, K. Eschbach, and J. S. Goodwin. 2007. The effect of obesity on disability vs. mortality in older Americans. *Archives of Internal Medicine* 167:774–80.

Balzi, D., F. Lauretani, A. Barchielli, L. Ferrucci, S. Bandinelli, E. Buiatti, Y. Milaneschi, and J. M. Guralnik. 2010. Risk factors for disability in older persons over 3–year follow-up. *Age and Ageing* 39:92–98.

Centers for Disease Control and Prevention. 2001. Prevalence of disabilities and associated health conditions among adults—United States, 1999. *Morbidity and Mortality Weekly Report* 50:120–25.

Centers for Disease Control and Prevention. 2009. Prevalence and most common causes of disability among adults—United States, 2005. *Morbidity and Mortality Weekly Report* 58:421–26.

Chen, H., and X Guo. 2008. Obesity and functional disability in elderly Americans. *Journal of the American Geriatrics Society* 56:689–94.

Ciol, M. A., A. Shumway-Cook, J. M. Hoffman, K. M. Yorkston, B. J. Dudgeon, and L. Chan. 2008. Minority disparities in disability between Medicare beneficiaries. *Journal of the American Geriatrics Society* 56:444–53.

Daniels, R., E. van Rossum, L. de Witte, G. I. Kempen, and W. van den Heuvel. 2008. Interventions to prevent disability in frail community-dwelling elderly: A systematic review. *BMC Health Services Research* 8:278.

Dunlop, D. D., J. Song, L. M. Manheim, M. L. Daviglus, and R. W. Chang. 2007. Racial/ethnic differences in the development of disability among older adults. *American Journal of Public Health* 97:2209–15.

Federal Interagency Forum on Aging-Related Statistics. 2010. *Older Americans 2010: Key Indicators of Well-Being.* Washington, DC: U.S. Government Printing Office.

Field, M. J., and A. M. Jette, eds. 2007. *The Future of Disability in the United States, Institute of Medicine Committee on Disability.* Washington, DC: National Academies Press.

Fleischer, D. Z., and F. Zames. 2001. *The Disability Rights Movement: From Charity to Confrontation.* Philadelphia: Temple University Press.

Foote, S. M. 2003. Population-based disease management under fee-for-service Medicare. *Health Affairs* W3:342–56.

Freedman, V. A., E. Crimmins, R. F. Schoeni, B. C. Spillman, H. Aykan, E. Kramarow, K. Land, J. Lubitz, K. Manton, L. G. Martin, D. Shinberg, and T. Waidmann. 2004. Resolving inconsistencies in trends in old-age disability: Report from a technical working group. *Demography* 41:417–41.

Freedman, V. A., L. G. Martin, and R. F. Schoeni. 2002. Recent trends in disability and functioning among older adults in the United States: A systematic review. *Journal of the American Medical Association* 288:3137–46.

Fuller-Thomson, E., B. A. Yu, J. M. Nuru-Jeter, J. Guralnik, and M. Minkler. 2009. Basic ADL disability and functional limitation rates among older Americans from 2000–2005: The end of the decline? *Journals of Gerontology Series A: Biological Sciences and Medical Sciences* 64A:1333–36.

Gill, T. M., D. I. Baker, M. Gottschalk, P. N. Peduzzi, H. Allore, and A. Byers. 2002. A program to prevent functional decline in physically frail, elderly persons who live at home. *New England Journal of Medicine* 347:1068–74.

Gordis, Leon, ed. 2008. *Epidemiology*, 4th ed. Philadelphia: Elsevier Saunders.

Guralnik, J. M., L. Ferrucci, E. M. Simonsick, M. E. Salive, and R. B. Wallace. 1995. Lower extremity function in persons over the age of 70 years as a predictor of subsequent disability. *New England Journal of Medicine* 332:556–61.

Jain, N. B., S. Al-Adawi, A. S. S. Dorvlo, and D. T. Burke. 2008. Association between body mass index and functional independence measure in patients with deconditioning. *American Journal of Physical Medicine & Rehabilitation* 87:21–25.

Jensen, G. L., M. A. Roy, A. E. Buchanan, and M. B. Berg. 2004. Weight loss intervention for obese older women: Improvements in performance and function. *Obesity Research* 12:1814–20.

Jette, A. M. 2009. Toward a common language of disablement. *Journals of Gerontology Series A: Biological Sciences and Medical Sciences* 64:1165–68.

Katz, S., and C. A. Akpom. 1976. Index of ADL. *Medical Care* 14:116–18.

Katz, S., A. Ford, R. Moskowitz, B. Jackson, and M. Jaffe. 1963. Studies of illness in the aged. *Journal of the American Medical Association* 185:914–19.

Latham, N. K., V. Mehta, A. M. Nguyen, A. M. Jette, S. Olarsch, D. Papanicolaou, and J. Chandler. 2008. Performance-based or self-report measures of physical function: Which should be used in clinical trials of hip fracture patients? *Archives of Physical Medicine and Rehabilitation* 89:2146–55.

Lawton, M. P. 1974. Social ecology and the health of older people. *American Journal of Public Health* 64(3):257–60.

Lawton, M. P., and L. Nahemow. 1973. The psychology of adult development and aging. In *Ecology and the Aging Process*, ed. C. Eisdorfer and M. P. Lawton, pp. 619–74. Washington, DC: American Psychological Association.

Liebel, D. V., B. Friedman, N. M. Watson, and B. A. Powers. 2009. Review of nurse home visiting interventions for community-dwelling older persons with existing disability. *Medical Care Research and Review* 66:119–46.

Manton, K. G., X. Gu, and V. L. Lamb. 2006. Change in chronic disability from 1982 to 2004/2005 as measured by long-term changes in function and health in the U.S. elderly population. *Proceedings of the National Academy of Sciences USA* 103:18374–79.

Martin, L. G., V. A. Freedman, R. F. Schoeni, and P. M. Andreski. 2010. Trends in disability and related chronic conditions among people ages fifty to sixty-four. *Health Affairs* 29:725–31.

McDowell, I. 2006. *Measuring Health: A Guide to Rating Scales and Questionnaires,* 3rd ed. New York: Oxford University Press.

Medical Encyclopedia, n.d. *Surveys—Limitations of Survey Research and Problems with Interpretations.* Retrieved October 25, 2010, from http://medicine.jrank.org/pages/1728/Surveyshtml#ixzz13NvQkOwb.

Meng, H., B. R. Wamsley, B. Friedman, D. Liebel, D. A. Dixon, S. Gao, D. Oakes, and G. M. Eggert. 2010. Impact of body mass index on the effectiveness of a disease management-health promotion intervention on disability status. *American Journal of Health Promotion* 24:214–22.

Nagi, S. Z. 1964. A study in the evaluation of disability and rehabilitation potential: Concepts, methods, and procedures. *American Journal of Public Health* 54:1568–79.

Nagi, S. Z. 1976. An epidemiology of disability among adults in the United States. *Milbank Memorial Fund Quarterly* 54:439–67.

Noonan, V. K., J. A. Kopec, L. Noreau, J. Singer, and M. F. Dvorak. 2009. A review of participation instruments based on the International Classification of Functioning, Disability and Health. *Disability and Rehabilitation* 31:1883–901.

Pope, A. M., and A. R. Tarlov, eds. 1991. *Disability in America: Toward a National Agenda for Prevention.* Washington, DC: National Academies Press.

Rejeski, W. J., E. H. Ip, A. P. Marsh, M. E. Miller, and D. F. Farmer. 2008. Measuring disability in older adults: The International Classification System of Functioning, Disability and Health (ICF) framework. *Geriatrics & Gerontology International* 8:48–54.

Rodgers, W., and B. Miller. 1997. A comparative analysis of ADL questions in surveys of older people. *Journals of Gerontology Series B: Psychological Sciences and Social Sciences* 52:21–36.

Sayers, S. P., J. M. Guralnik, A. B. Newman, J. S. Brach, and R. A. Fielding. 2006.

Concordance and discordance between two measures of lower extremity function: 400 meter self-paced walk and SPPB. *Aging Clinical and Experimental Research* 18:100–106.

Schoeni, R. F., L. G. Martin, P. M. Andreski, and V. A. Freedman. 2005. Persistent and growing socioeconomic disparities in disability among the elderly: 1982–2002. *American Journal of Public Health* 95:2065–70.

Seeman, T. E., S. S. Merkin, E. M. Crimmins, and A. S. Karlamangla, 2010. Disability trends among older Americans: National Health and Nutrition Examination Surveys, 1988–1994 and 1999–2004. *American Journal of Public Health* 100:100–107.

Stewart, A. L. 2003. Conceptual challenges in linking physical activity and disability research. *American Journal of Preventive Medicine* 25:137–40.

Todorov, A., and C. Kirchner. 2000. Bias in proxies' reports of disability: Data from the National Health Interview Survey on disability. *American Journal of Public Health* 90:1248–53.

U.S. Department of Health and Human Services. 1981. *Prevention '80*, Public Health Service, DHHS (PHS) Publication No. 81–50157.

U.S. Department of Health and Human Services. 2005. *The Surgeon General's Call to Action to Improve the Health and Wellness of Persons with Disabilities*. Rockville, MD: Office of the Surgeon General.

Verbrugge, L. M., and A. M. Jette. 1994. The disablement process. *Social Science & Medicine* 38:1–14.

Villareal, D. T., M. Banks, D. R. Sinacore, C. Siener, and S. Klein. 2006. Effect of weight loss and exercise on frailty in obese older adults. *Archives of Internal Medicine* 166:860–66.

Wong, C. H., S. F. Wong, A. M. Yusoff, S. Karunananthan, and H. Bergman. 2008. The effect of later-life health promotion on functional performance and body composition. *Aging Clinical and Experimental Research* 20:454–60.

World Health Organization. 2001. *ICF: International Classification of Functioning, Disability, and Health*. Geneva, Switzerland: World Health Organization.

Wunderlich, G. S. 2009. *Improving the Measurement of Late-Life Disability in Population Surveys: Beyond ADLs and IADLs: Summary of a Workshop*. Washington, DC: National Academies Press.

Wunderlich, G. S., D. P. Rice, and N. L. Amado, eds. 2002. *The Dynamics of Disability: Measuring and Monitoring Disability for Social Security Programs*. Washington, DC: National Academies Press.

CHAPTER 7

Behavioral Risk Factors and
Evidence-Based Interventions

Susan L. Hughes, PhD
Marcia G. Ory, PhD, MPH
Rachel B. Seymour, PhD

A better understanding of the nature, determinants, and consequences of behavioral risk factors and the identification of different evidence-based strategies for encouraging health-promoting behaviors are critical for advancing public health and aging research and practice. Most of the medical research conducted in the twentieth century focused on searches for cures to specific diseases that were associated with high morbidity and mortality rates. Only during the past few decades has systematic attention been paid to underlying behavioral risk factors that give rise to chronic conditions that cause substantial amounts of morbidity and disability (McGinnis and Foege, 1993; Institute of Medicine, 2001; Ory, Jordan, and Bazzarre, 2002). Even more recent is the appreciation that behavioral risk factors remain potent as well as modifiable late in life (Haber, 2010), debunking myths that older adults are unable or unwilling to change their behaviors (Ory, Hoffman, Hawkins, Sanner, and Mockenhaupt, 2003). Thus, it is now apparent that focused attention on behavioral risk factors and their dynamic interplay with biological, social, and environmental factors has the potential to postpone or prevent the incidence of disability among future cohorts of older adults and constrain the rate of growth in health and long-term care expenditures (Fries, Bloch, Harrington, Richardson, and Beck, 1993).

This chapter briefly reviews the prevalence and associated outcomes for current *major* modifiable behavioral risk factors. We then review several theories of behavior change. Building on this knowledge base, we describe steps used to develop and test successful evidence-based behavior change interventions. Finally, we conclude with topics needing future research and action in the field. Also, while acknowledging that behavioral risk factors are inextricably linked to social, environmental, and policy contexts, this chapter focuses on *behavioral* risks. A companion chapter in this section focuses on social determinants of health and disability and functional status (see chap. 5). Additionally, we do not focus on translational research since that is the focus of chapter 8.

RISK FACTORS: PREVALENCE AND CONSEQUENCES

U.S. national health statistics document proven links between behaviors and health outcomes, which should give direction to public health action (e.g., Healthy People 2010: U.S. Department of Health and Human Services, 2000; Behavioral Risk Factor Surveillance System [BRFSS]: Centers for Disease Control and Prevention [CDC], 1991–2009). A comprehensive review of studies published between 1980 and 2002 that linked risk behaviors and mortality found that the leading causes of death in 2000 were tobacco (18.1%) and poor diet and physical inactivity (16.6%), followed by alcohol consumption (3.5%) (Mokdad, Marks, Stroup, and Gerberding, 2004). These figures underscore the importance of these risk factors for health promotion efforts.

Physical Inactivity

The 2008 Physical Activity Guidelines for Americans issued by the U.S. Department of Health and Human Services (2008) designated older adults as a specific population target for concern. The guidelines provide tailored recommendations for persons aged 65 years and older. In order to derive substantial health benefits, older adults are encouraged to participate in 150 minutes of moderate-intensity or 75 minutes of vigorous-intensity physical activity per week or an equivalent combination of moderate and vigorous physical activity throughout the week. The guidelines suggest that additional health benefits can be gained through greater amounts of physical activity and that the recommended activity levels be viewed as the *minimum* amount required to achieve health benefits.

Currently, the number of older adults who engage in regular physical activity falls far short of meeting these guidelines. Traditionally, older adults are among the most sedentary segment of the population. In 2007–2008, 22% of persons aged 65 years and older reported engaging in leisure-time physical activity (LTPA) (Forum, 2010). The percentage of older persons engaging in LTPA declined with age, ranging from 25% among persons aged 65–74 years to 11% among persons aged 85 years and older (Forum, 2010). Older men were more likely than women in the same age group to participate in LTPA (27% vs. 18%, respectively). Older non-Hispanic white adults reported higher levels of physical activity than non-Hispanic blacks (23% vs. 13%, respectively). Finally, although strength training is strongly recommended to improve balance and reduce risk for falls, data from 2007 to 2008 show that only 14% of older adults reported participating in strength training activities.

For older adults with certain chronic conditions the rate of sedentary behavior is even higher. Recent data have shown that persons with osteoarthritis (OA) who also have diabetes or heart disease, which are common comorbidities, are significantly less likely than counterparts without OA to participate in doctor-recommended physical activity (Bolen et al., 2008, 2009). Importantly, it is now possible for public health practitioners to access prevalence data for their own state and select local areas by accessing BRFSS data on the CDC Healthy Aging Program's interactive website (www.cdc.gov/aging).

Poor Diet

Diet and nutrition have a major impact on health and well-being, including substantially reducing risk factors for chronic conditions such as hypertension, diabetes, and heart disease. The Dietary Guidelines for Americans are published and updated every 5 years by the U.S. Department of Agriculture (www .health.gov/dietaryguidelines/dga2005/report). Unfortunately, older Americans failed to meet or exceed federal recommendations on 9 of 12 components of what is considered to constitute a "healthy diet" (Forum, 2010). Specifically, older adults meet or exceed recommendations for intake of fruit, total grains, and meats and beans but do poorly with regard to intake of vegetables, whole grains, milk, and whole fruits. Older adults also consume more saturated fat, sodium, solid fats, alcoholic beverages, and added sugars than recommended. There are also differences in diet quality between the young old (65–74 years of age) and the old old (75 years and older). Diet quality among those aged

75 and older was superior to those aged 65–74 years on several indicators including total fruit, dark green and orange vegetables and legumes, whole grains, milk, and oils; however, for total vegetables, those aged 65–74 years fared better than those aged 75 and older (Forum, 2010).

Obesity and Overweight

Obesity, defined as an excessively high amount of body fat or adipose tissue in relation to lean body mass, is associated with the onset or exacerbation of most chronic illnesses and disabilities (Stunkard and Wadden, 1993; Forum, 2010). Recent levels of overweight and obesity among older adults in the United States are unprecedented. The prevalence of obesity assessed by a body mass index (BMI) of 30 or greater has increased rapidly among older adults in recent years. In 2007–2008, 32% of persons aged 65 and over were obese, compared with 22% in 1988–1994. Although obesity is slightly more prevalent among older men than older women, the increases in obesity rates have affected both genders similarly. Although the trend toward increased prevalence has leveled off during the nine years between 1999–2000 and 2007–2008, it remains alarmingly high. Importantly, older adults with less than a high school education have the highest rate of obesity, followed by older adults who completed high school. The prevalence of overweight defined by a BMI of 25–29.9 declines by age cohort such that the prevalence of overweight is significantly higher for those aged 65–74 and those aged 75–84 than for those 85 and older (Li, Fisher, and Harmer, 2005).

Overweight and obesity have been identified as causal or exacerbating factors with respect to diabetes, hypertension, heart disease, and OA among older adults. Diabetes alone is one of the leading causes of morbidity and mortality among adults over the age of 65 (Desai, Zhang, and Hennessey, 1999). OA is one of the most common chronic conditions among older adults and the number one cause of disability among them (Hootman, Brault, Helmick, Theis, and Armour, 2009). Lower-extremity joint symptomatology related to OA can be either caused or exacerbated by obesity. Nationally, in 2002, 35% of persons with arthritis were obese, compared with 21% of the total population. The interrelationship between obesity and lower-extremity knee OA at least in part explains rapid increases in the use of total hip and knee replacement surgery in the United States. In 2004, more than 650,000 of these procedures were performed at the cost of $9.1 billion for this condition alone (Kim, 2008). These figures demonstrate that chronic conditions stemming from or complicated by overweight and obesity are linked to substantial amounts of morbidity and disability, as well as major drivers of health care use and cost. Finally, and potentially tragically, morbidity associated with overweight and obesity may be reversing a decade of progress in decreasing rates of disability among older adults.

Disability rates among older adults reported by national longitudinal surveys showed consistent declines between 1982 and 2004 (Manton, Gu, and Lamb, 2006; Manton, Gu, and Lowrimore, 2008). However, recent studies question whether that trend will continue and have identified overweight and obesity as important factors that are helping to reverse it. A seminal paper by Olshansky et al. (2005) postulates a potential decline in life expectancy as a result of increased levels of obesity experienced by younger cohorts in the United States over the past 30 years. Supporting this hypothesis, recent analyses of National Long Term Care Survey data have shown that obesity increased the risk of disability (Wu, McCrone, and Lai, 2008). Similarly, data from the National Health Interview Survey revealed that the proportion of people aged 50–64 who report needing help with personal care activities increased significantly from 1997 to 2007 (Martin, Freedman, Schoeni, and Andreski, 2010). These studies raise substantial concerns about our ability to maintain previous gains in life expectancy and *active* life expectancy among older adults and underscore the important role that behavioral and lifestyle changes play in countering the obesity epidemic.

Tobacco Use

Tobacco use, including cigarette smoking, cigar smoking, and smokeless tobacco use, remains the leading preventable cause of death in the United States (www.cdc.gov/tobacco/data_statistics/mmwrs/byyear/2009mm5802a2/highlights.htm). Tobacco use harms nearly every major organ in the body and causes mortality from cancer, cardiovascular disease, and lung disease (Centers for Disease Control and Prevention, 2004). While smoking tends to be lower among older age groups, around 10% for those aged 65 years and older (BRFSS 2008), the health consequences associated with it remain detrimental. This is contrary to the false belief by some that smoking is no longer a risk factor for those who reach late life (Weinstein, 1999).

For older adults, chronic lower respiratory disease is the fourth leading cause of death among people aged 65 and over. There was a 50% increase in rates of death from respiratory diseases between 1981 and 2006, reflecting, in part, the effects of cigarette smoking (Forum, 2010). The percentage of older Americans who are current cigarette smokers declined between 1965 and 2008, largely as a result of declines in cigarette smoking among men, whereas rates for women were relatively constant (Forum, 2010). Among older men, blacks have a higher rate of smoking than whites (18% vs. 10%, respectively). The current standard for successful smoking cessation is total abstinence. In 2008, 55% of men and 31% of women 65 years of age and older were former smokers.

Alcohol Consumption

The Center for Substance Abuse Treatment and the National Institute on Alcohol Abuse and Alcoholism (1995) recommend that men aged 65 years and older consume no more than one standard drink per day with a maximum of two drinks on any one occasion, or seven drinks on average per week. A standard drink is equal to 13.6 grams of pure alcohol, which is the amount of pure alcohol found in drinks such as 12 ounces of beer (www.cdc.gov/alcohol/faqs.htm#moderatedrinking). The recommendations for older women are less than one drink per day and a maximum of four drinks per week. Recent research has found that exceeding drinking guidelines is associated with increased risk of alcohol-use disorders and that for some older drinkers risky alcohol use is part of a larger pattern of health risks, including current smoking, major depression, and alcohol abuse or dependence history (Sacco, Bucholz, and Spitznagel, 2009). The National Social Life, Health, and Aging Project examined the prevalence of alcohol consumption among older adults in 2005–2006 and found that consumption differed substantially by age and by gender. Frequency of drinking was significantly higher among men than among women. Women were more likely than men to drink one or fewer days per week and less likely to drink daily. Frequency of drinking was also significantly higher among older compared with younger men but did not differ by age among women. The majority of respondents (77.2%) did not engage in heavy drinking behavior (four or more alcoholic drinks on one occasion, known as binge drinking) within the prior three months, but men were significantly more likely than women at all ages to report doing so. However, this risk behavior decreased with age, particularly for men.

Other Prevention Behaviors

In addition to the behaviors described above, several other behaviors are important in protecting the health of older Americans. These include participation in vaccinations and screenings. Data suggest that about 40% of adults 65 years of age and older are *not* up-to-date on a core set of clinical preventive services despite coverage of the services by Medicare. A paper by Maciosek, Coffield, Flottemesch, Edwards, and Solberg (2010) found that increasing the use of these services from current levels to 90% in 2006 would have resulted in a savings of $3.7 billion. The recently enacted Patient Care and Affordable Care Act eliminates co-pays for Medicare-covered screenings, but major gaps are expected to remain in use of these life-saving services.

THE SCIENCE OF BEHAVIOR CHANGE

The past two decades have identified key behavior change concepts and tested different theoretical models to explain behavior change (Ory et al., 2002; Ory, Smith, Mier, and Wernicke, 2010). Table 7.1 identifies commonly used theoretical models and associated constructs for explanatory and change theories. While these theoretical frameworks are also used by public health researchers, there is an increasing trend to pose research problems in terms of "the theory of the problem" (Black and Laflin, 2009). Public health research is guided by evaluation models that call attention to the steps in evaluation practice (i.e., engage the stakeholders, describe the problem, focus on the evaluation design, gather credible evidence, justify conclusions, and ensure and share lessons learned) (Centers for Disease Control and Prevention, 1999) and logic models that specify linkages between inputs, outputs, and outcomes (Centers for Disease Control Evaluation Working Group, 2010).

Specific behavior change strategies have been identified, especially related to behavioral and lifestyle factors (Ory et al., 2002, 2010; Cress et al., 2004). Table 7.2 lists several frequently used behavior change strategies and provides some specific examples for implementing such strategies. Evidence-based programs often adopt one or more of these strategies, with debate in the literature on whether similar or different strategies are needed for initiating versus maintaining recommended health behaviors (Seymour et al., 2010).

PLANNING AND EVALUATING EVIDENCE-BASED INTERVENTIONS

We now turn to the important topic of designing and testing interventions to reduce these behavioral risk factors. It is important to note that interventions can be designed to affect many different levels of the social-ecological model. For example, policy interventions such as excise taxes have been very effective in promoting smoking cessation at the population level (Prohaska et

TABLE 7.1
Widely utilized theoretical frameworks for behavior change

Theoretical frameworks	Description	Constructs
Health belief model	This model seeks to understand how the individual views the health problem by describing perceived levels of susceptibility and severity. The model then seeks to understand the individual's motivation to act by examining barriers, cues to action, and self-efficacy.	1) Perceived susceptibility 2) Perceived severity 3) Perceived barriers 4) Perceived benefits
Precaution adoption process model	This model is composed of seven stages of progression from unawareness of a health problem to maintenance of behavioral change addressing a health problem.	1) Unaware of issue 2) Unengaged by issue 3) Deciding about acting 4) Decided not to act 5) Decided to act 6) Acting 7) Maintenance
Social-cognitive	This model describes the interplay between personal factors, environmental factors, and human behavior.	1) Reciprocal determinism 2) Behavioral capability 3) Expectations 4) Self-efficacy 5) Observational learning 6) Reinforcements
Stages of change (transtheoretical model)	This model describes behavior change as a process of moving through five stages.	1) Precontemplation 2) Contemplation 3) Preparation 4) Action 5) Maintenance
Theory of planned behavior	This model believes that a person's intention to change behaviors is driven by their attitude toward change and the approval or disapproval of those whose opinion the individual values.	1) Behavioral/intention 2) Attitude 3) Subjective norm 4) Perceived behavioral control

Source: National Cancer Institute, 2005

al., 2009). Similarly, the strategic placement of benches and lengthening the intervals of stoplights in heavily trafficked downtown spaces may have a substantial impact on mobility among older adults. Because other chapters deal with policy and environmental issues in greater detail, this chapter focuses on the design of interventions that affect the person and groups.

Several evidence-based interventions have been developed and tested to address many of the behavioral risk factors described in this chapter. The at-

TABLE 7.2
Behavioral change strategies and specific examples

Strategies	Example(s)
Active choices	Customized options for improvement
Goal setting	Setting concrete goals Making goals achievable and realistic
Health contracts	Health calendar Health goals collaboratively determined with a professional
Monitoring and tracking	Visualizing attainment of goal Daily or weekly tracking of goals
Perceived safety	Education about intervention(s) Self-monitoring by the individual
Positive reinforcement	Recruitment incentives Rewards for reaching goals
Problem solving	Identification of barriers and challenges Self or group brainstorming to overcome barriers
Regular performance feedback	Recognition of positive changes and successes
Relapse prevention	Planning for anticipated relapse Reviewing behavioral change interventions
Self-efficacy	Identifying opportunities to succeed Increasing sense of mastery through rehearsal
Social support	Peer support Health educator support

Source: Strategies compiled from Ory et al., 2002; Cress et al., 2004; and Guide to Community Preventive Services, 2010

tributes of successful programs are described in greater detail in sections to follow, along with steps involved in designing and testing an intervention.

Intervention Design

Designing and testing interventions can be a lengthy process. Evidence-based programs generally target an important and relevant *risk factor* and *target population*. The risk factor selected should affect sufficiently large numbers of older adults to be socially significant and, if modified, should also have the potential to substantially enhance the independent functioning of older adults over multiple years of active life. Importantly, most interventions are embedded within conceptual models or theories described in tables 7.1 and 7.2. These conceptual models describe how the intervention will mediate social and behavioral processes that will lead to improved health status and functioning.

Other attributes of evidence-based programs that contribute to their success include the comparative simplicity of the intervention and community-based participation in its design. The RE-AIM framework was developed and proposed by Glasgow, Vogt, and Boles (1999) as a method of increasing the impact of public health interventions. The framework has five dimensions: reach, effectiveness, adoption, implementation, and maintenance. Reach refers to the number, proportion, and representativeness of persons enrolled in the intervention trial. Effectiveness is concerned with the impact of the intervention, including any untoward or negative effects. Adoption refers to the uptake of the intervention among the universe of potential host sites. Implementation refers to treatment fidelity during the trial along with fidelity and adaptations made when a successful intervention is translated into multiple adopting sites (going to scale). Finally, maintenance refers to both the durability of program effects at the level of the individual and the survivability of the program across adopting sites during the translation phase.

Careful consideration of the RE-AIM components during the design of an intervention can have enormous payoffs down the road, once the intervention has demonstrated efficacy. For example, the cost of the intervention is important to consider at the design stage. Although it may be necessary to design a "Cadillac" version of the intervention for testing efficacy, as soon as efficacy is demonstrated it is essential to examine whether a "stripped-down" version of the intervention can also produce similar results. Another crucial consideration is the need for trained versus lay leaders or other nonprofessional instructors (Lorig, Ritter, Laurent, and Plant, 2006; Seymour, Hughes, Campbell, Huber, and Desai, 2009). Generally, the more simple the type of instruction required, consistent with the maintenance of program effects, the greater the likelihood that the program will be widely adopted in practice (Glasgow et al., 1999). The characteristics of the site required are also very important to consider at the design stage, as is the frequency of program contact and its duration (*dose*). All things being equal, programs that can be conducted over the phone or in an average senior center or church basement are more likely to be successful in the long run, as are programs that meet less frequently and for shorter durations of time.

Intervention Testing

In this section we examine a number of critical issues related to piloting of interventions, efficacy, and cross-cutting issues concerning recruitment, duration retention, treatment fidelity, effectiveness, and protocol fidelity.

Pilot Testing

Before testing for efficacy, it is critically important to pilot test the intervention. Pilots can provide information that is needed for the successful implementation of an intervention in a clinical trial. The pilot enables investigators to test participant enrollment and recruitment procedures and assess participant satisfaction with elements such as the program format, time of day offered, day of week, and site and instructor characteristics. A pilot also enables investigators to assess the feasibility of a variety of outcome measures and instruments. Most importantly, the pilot enables investigators to collect preliminary participant baseline and outcome data that can indicate whether the intervention has a strong probability of impacting desired outcomes. The conduct of a time-limited pilot also enables investigators to meet with participants after the first iteration of the intervention to assess their views on the comparative success of different program components and offers the important opportunity to refine components, consistent with participant input. The importance and value of this opportunity for refinement cannot be overstated. In fact, this type of program evaluation should be a continuous feature of the intervention from this point forward.

Efficacy

After the pilot test has been conducted and any necessary modifications have been made, the next step is to test the intervention for efficacy. Randomized controlled trials (RCTs), when feasible and appropriate, are considered to be the gold standard for evidence regarding efficacy for the following reasons (Shadish, Cook, and Campbell, 2002). At this stage in the development of the intervention, the investigator seeks to test as unequivocally as possible whether the intervention achieves an intended outcome or outcomes with a carefully specified target population. At this stage of intervention development, the investigator's main concern is controlling for all other possible causes of change in the outcomes tested. Thus, the paramount need at this stage is maximizing *internal validity* by minimizing exposure to common threats to internal validity. Internal validity means that one can be reasonably confident that changes in the outcome measure, if observed, are attributable to the intervention. Simple pretest-posttest designs are ambiguous with respect to attributions of causality. It is simply not possible to unequivocally attribute pretest-posttest changes experienced within a single group to the intervention. Without a baseline and posttest measures from a comparison group, it is impossible to know whether the changes observed would have happened anyway (maturation, regression to the mean) without the intervention.

Although use of a comparison group has advantages over a single-group design, it is possible that the comparison group may differ systematically on some variable that is unmeasured at baseline but still relevant to trial outcomes. For example, if a treatment is offered to persons in one geographic area and the comparison group is recruited from a neighboring town or area, it is possible that persons in the comparison group are systematically wealthier, poorer, or more or less well educated, for example. Any of these differences could be more powerful in affecting outcomes than the intervention tested. A randomized design, in contrast, ensures that all members of a selected target group have an equal probability of being in the treatment group or being in the control group. Thus, the selection process is known as opposed to unknown or partially known. Although several threats to internal validity such as maturation, regression to the mean, history, and testing are still present, they are less plausible threats because they are distributed randomly over treatment and control conditions (Shadish et al., 2002). It is important to acknowledge that the tight inclusion criteria commonly used in randomized trials can reduce the external validity or generalizability of trial findings. However, this trade-off can be addressed in subsequent effectiveness studies that test the replicability of the efficacy findings in other populations and settings.

Cross-Cutting Issues

Several other cross-cutting issues are salient both to testing intervention efficacy and also to testing intervention effectiveness.

Recruitment

Consideration of the population being targeted and enrolled in a study or program is a crucial step in program planning. Several recruitment strategies have been used successfully by different types of behavioral interventions for older adults (Ory et al., 2002; Yancey, Ory, and Davis, 2006). The importance of partners during the recruitment process cannot be overstated. Cultivating partnerships with community members and organizations that can assist with the recruitment process is vital. Partners can include announcements about the new program or trial in their newsletters, post flyers in their organizations, send targeted mailings to their mailing list, and provide forums for research staff to make announcements and/or talk to constituents about the research. Also, given the need to enroll more diverse populations in health behavior trials, it is important to engage in a community-based participatory research perspective (Israel, Eng, Schulz, and Parker, 2005) and to use culturally sensitive recruitment approaches (Yancey et al., 2004; Mier, Ory, and Medina, 2009).

Duration

A major limitation of many intervention trials with older adults until recently has been their short duration, in many cases no longer than 8 or 12 weeks. Although it is important to demonstrate short-term proximal benefits of an intervention, an equally pressing question is whether the intervention has lasting benefits. Thus, it is important, if resources allow, to extend the posttest out to 6, 12, 18, or 24 months and/or to obtain supplemental funding for longer-term follow-up if initial findings are promising. If the intervention includes an education component or frequent social contact, it also may be necessary to plan an attention control. In this case the investigator provides a similar dose of contact but the content of the sessions is unrelated to and not anticipated to impact the trial outcomes.

Retention

Another critical factor for success is retention—both program retention and measurement retention (Seymour et al., 2010). Program retention refers to maintaining participant involvement in the intervention, while measurement retention refers to retaining participants in data collection at scheduled follow-ups. Most programs recognize that there will not be 100% adherence to all program components but have designated what successful completion means. This definition varies by whether the program is time limited or ongoing to foster longer-term behavior change. The ability of a study to retain participants in the intervention and in measurement also impacts the generalizability of the findings.

Several strategies can help maximize program retention, including taking attendance, providing incentives for attendance (e.g., certificates of completion, lottery system), and calling participants who miss intervention sessions. The primary way to maximize measurement retention is to make measurement easy by conducting interviews at the program location, going to participants' homes, and offering flexible times for completion and flexible ways to complete the survey. Incentives matter and can include compensation for completion or a lottery system that provides the possibility of additional compensation to participants whose time and energy are valuable.

Treatment Fidelity

It is also very important to monitor the delivery of the intervention closely through multiple visits to the program as it is being implemented on site. Lack of close supervision at this stage can lead to an assumption that the concept driving the intervention is faulty when, in fact, a no-treatment finding reflects implementation issues.

Effectiveness

Assuming that an intervention has demonstrated substantial benefits, the next step in the development of an evidence-based intervention is testing effectiveness under different conditions with respect to more diverse participant populations, sites, geographic locations, and instructors. During this stage of continued intervention development, it may be appropriate to use a *single-group pretest-posttest design* since efficacy has already been demonstrated and the main objective at this point is to test whether the same findings demonstrated in the RCT are replicable under increasingly generalizable conditions (Wilcox et al., 2006, 2008; Hughes et al., 2010).

Protocol Fidelity

Depending on the nature of the intervention, it is very important at this point to invest resources in standardizing instructor training procedures and developing printed or online instructor and participant manuals, as well as site program implementation guidelines. These efforts help ensure that the program will be implemented faithfully across sites and instructors. This consistency of program delivery across settings is referred to as *program fidelity*, which encompasses adherence to the program protocol. However, as the program expands to address the needs of more diverse populations and settings, it is also important to *adapt* the program to make it culturally sensitive. At this point the research team needs to seriously consider which program elements are essential versus modifiable. For example, a low-impact aerobic program may need to be of a specified duration, intensity, and frequency to achieve a standardized benefit on a 6–minute distance walk test. However, the specific steps and routines involved and the music can vary substantially, depending on the preferences of participants, who usually are quite vocal in this respect. In order to assess treatment fidelity and ensure that adaptations or modifications are appropriate, investigators must design and implement mechanisms to monitor and maximize fidelity. Bellg et al. (2004) have defined five types of treatment fidelity to consider when examining whether interventions are delivered as intended: treatment design, provider training, treatment delivery, treatment receipt, and enactment of treatment. Treatment delivery is the dimension that has been most studied, with several assessment methodologies being employed, including observations, checklists, and self-assessments.

The development of a standardized instrument that monitors fidelity can provide important data that can be used to provide feedback, share successful modifications or adaptations, and improve quality. Periodic "boosters" for intervention delivery agents, such as meetings, conference calls, or webinars to provide continuing education, can be used to maintain fidelity over time. The feedback received from providers and instructors in the field provides a unique opportunity for program designers to simplify instruction requirements and test different delivery modes (Web vs. group based) while continuing to track and monitor attendance, program evaluation, and a limited but consistent set of participant outcomes. Finally, developing a program license also helps to ensure that providers who offer the program have been trained in and comply with program procedures.

SUMMARY AND RECOMMENDATIONS

This review of behavioral risk factors and evidence-based interventions designed to reduce them clearly highlights the importance of developing and disseminating more evidence-based interventions, particularly those designed to impact healthy diets and obesity. The need for new evidence-based programs that can reverse the current obesity epidemic cannot be overemphasized.

In 2010, Healthy People 2020 included a topic area devoted to older adults and identified 12 new objectives, of which three are developmental (www.healthy people.gov/2020/topicsobjectives2020/objectiveslist.aspx?topicid=31). Among the new objectives are the following:

- "Increase the proportion of older adults who use the Welcome to Medicare benefit"
- "Increase the proportion of older adults who are up to date on a core set of clinical preventive services"
- "Increase the proportion of older adults with reduced physical or cognitive function who engage in light, moderate, or vigorous leisure-time physical activities"
- "Reduce the rate of emergency department visits due to falls among older adults"
- "Increase the proportion of older adults with one or more chronic

health conditions who report confidence in managing their conditions" (developmental)
- "Reduce the proportion of unpaid caregivers of older adults who report an unmet need for caregiver support services" (developmental)

These new objectives also present important challenges that can be expected to guide the development of interventions and translation research over the coming decade.

As this chapter demonstrates, we have made substantial progress with respect to the development and testing of evidence-based programs, but several important challenges remain. While national statistics monitor and report prevalence rates for major risk factors separately, there is growing awareness of the co-occurrence of many risk factors. Growing evidence regarding the co-occurrence of risky behaviors indicates that interventions that assess multiple behaviors may have greater impact on health; however, little is known at present about the successful design, impact, adoption, and maintenance of multiple-behavior interventions. At present, we do not have a good understanding of the additive effects of multiple behavioral risk factor interventions, nor do we have a good way of appreciating the effects of interventions that address multiple levels of the social-ecological model (e.g., those affecting individuals and communities simultaneously; Kaplan, 1997). This is a very fruitful area for future research since change in one behavior may also serve as the gateway to action regarding the companion behavior and interventions that address multiple levels of the social-ecological model would be expected to be considerably more powerful than those that address a single level (Prohaska, Spring, and Nigg, 2008).

On the practice side, it is vitally important to have multiple programmatic options that appeal to different populations with different needs. This array of evidence-based program options can reinforce and translate behavioral skills learned in one setting to another—for example, enabling Chronic Disease Self-Management Program graduates to move on to a physical activity program like Fit & Strong! for older adults with arthritis (Hughes et al., 2004, 2006). It is also important for consumers, providers, and payers to be able to refer to a common set of definitions/criteria for credentialing evidence-based programs. Thus, it will be critically important for potential public and private funders to consider the endorsement of a common set of criteria and/or processes for the approval, dissemination, and adoption as well as reimbursement, maintenance, and ongoing quality of evidence-based programs. It is also important to improve the access of providers to approved evidence-based programs deemed to have met a nationally agreed-upon standard or standards. The development of a national clearinghouse for this purpose would appear to be a very logical development in the future.

Further, it is critically important to develop reliable funding streams that will enable proven programs to go to scale and benefit their target populations nationally. The Centers for Medicare and Medicaid Services are currently evaluating the possibility of reimbursing providers to offer the Stanford Diabetes Self-Management Program. Medicare reimbursement for approved evidence-based programs would be totally consistent with the intent of the Patient Protection and Affordable Care Act to substitute health promotion for more expensive services that are currently reimbursed (Government Printing Office, 2010). While many community organizations now sponsor evidence-based programs, the future sustainability of these programs depends on the development of a stable funding stream that will enable community providers to keep offering the programs once demonstration funding ceases. Finally, the question arises as to how to integrate evidence-based programs within the broader constellation of social, behavioral, and biological processes that are reinforced by environmental and policy contexts. These questions provide substantial scope for future research, demonstrations, and public health debate.

REFERENCES

Bellg, A. J., B. Borrelli, B. Resnick, J. Hecht, D. S. Minicucci, M. G. Ory, G. Ogedegbe, D. Orwig, D. Ernst, and S. Czajkowski. 2004. Enhancing treatment fidelity in health behavior change studies: Best practices and recommendations from the NIH Behavior Change Consortium. *Health Psychology* 23:443–51.
Black, D. R., and M. T. Laflin. 2009. ViewPoint: Conversation with Kenneth R. McLeroy, PhD. *American Journal of Health Behavior* 33:466–78.
Bolen, J., J. Hootman, C. G. Helmick, L. Murphy, G. Langmaid, and C. J. Caspersen. 2008. Arthritis as a potential barrier to physical activity among adults with diabetes—United States, 2005 and 2007. *Morbidity and Mortality Weekly Report* 57:486–89.
Bolen, J., L. Murphy, K. Greenlund, C. G. Helmick, J. Hootman, T. J. Brady, G. Langmaid, and N. Keenan. 2009. Arthritis as a potential barrier to physical activity among adults with heart disease—United States, 2005 and 2007. *Morbidity and Mortality Weekly Report* 58:165–69.
Centers for Disease Control and Prevention. 1991–2009. *Behavioral Risk Factor Surveillance System Survey Data*. Atlanta: U.S. Department of Health and Human Services, Centers for Disease Control and Prevention.
Centers for Disease Control and Prevention. 1999. Framework for Program Evaluation in Public Health. *Morbidity and Mortality Weekly Report* 48(No. RR-11).
Centers for Disease Control and Prevention. 2004. *The Health Consequences of*

Smoking: A Report of the Surgeon General. Atlanta: U.S. Department of Health and Human Services.

Centers for Disease Control Evaluation Working Group. 2010. *Logic Model Resources.* Retrieved November 16, 2010, from www.cdc.gov/eval/resources.htm#logic model.

Cress, M. E., D. M. Buchner, T. Prohaska, J. Rimmer, M. Brown, C. Macera, L. De-Pietro, and W. Chodzko-Zajko. 2004. Physical activity programs and behavior counseling in older adult populations. *Medicine & Science in Sports & Exercise* 36:1997–2003.

Desai, M. M., P. Zhang, and C. H. Hennessy. 1999. Surveillance for morbidity and mortality among older adults—United States 1995–1996. *Morbidity and Mortality Weekly Report* 48:7–25.

Federal Interagency Forum on Aging-Related Statistics (Forum). 2010. *Older Americans 2010: Key Indicators of Well-Being.* Washington, DC: U.S. Government Printing Office.

Fries, J. F., D. A. Bloch, H. Harrington, N. Richardson, and R. Beck. 1993. Two-year results of a randomized controlled trial of a health promotion program in a retiree population: The Bank of America study. *American Journal of Medicine* 94:455–62.

Glasgow, R. E., T. M. Vogt, and S. M. Boles. 1999. Evaluating the public health impact of health promotion interventions: The RE-AIM framework. *American Journal of Public Health* 89:1322–27.

Government Printing Office (GPO). 2010. Public Law 111–148, 2010. Patient Protection and Affordable Care Act. GPO website: www.gpo.gov.

Guide to Community Preventive Services. 2010. *Promoting Physical Activity: Behavioral and Social Approaches.* Retrieved November 16, 2010, from www.thecommunity guide.org/pa/behavioral-social/index.html.

Haber, D. 2010. *Health Promotion and Aging: Practical Applications for Health Professionals*, 5th ed. New York: Springer.

Hootman, J. M., M. W. Brault, C. G. Helmick, K. A. Theis, and B. S. Armour. 2009. Prevalence and most common causes of disability among adults—United States, 2005. *Morbidity and Mortality Weekly Report* 58:421–26.

Hughes, S. L., R. B. Seymour, R. T. Campbell, G. Huber, P. Desai, and J. H. Chang. 2010. Fit and Strong!: Bolstering maintenance to physical activity among older adults with lower-extremity osteoarthritis. *American Journal of Health Behavior* 34:750–63.

Hughes, S. L., R. B. Seymour, R. T. Campbell, N. Pollak, G. Huber, and L. Sharma. 2004. Impact of the Fit and Strong! intervention on older adults with osteoarthritis. *Gerontologist* 44:217–28.

Hughes, S. L., R. B. Seymour, R. T. Campbell, N. Pollak, G. Huber, L. Sharma, and P. Desai. 2006. Long term impact of Fit and Strong! on older adults with osteoarthritis. *Gerontologist* 46:801–14.

Institute of Medicine. 2001. *Health and Behavior: The Interplay of Biological, Behavioral, and Societal Influences.* Washington, DC: National Academies Press.

Israel, B. A., E. Eng, A. E. Schulz, and A. Parker, eds. 2005. *Methods in Community-Based Participatory Research for Health.* San Francisco: Jossey-Bass.

Kaplan, G. A. 1997, Behavioral, social, and socioenvironmental factors adding years to life and life to years. In *Public Health and Aging*, ed. T. Hickey, M. A. Speers, and T. R. Prohaska, pp. 37–52. Baltimore: Johns Hopkins University Press.

Kim, S. 2008. Changes in surgical loads and economic burden of hip and knee replacements in the US: 1997–2004. *Arthritis and Rheumatism* 59:481–88. PMID: 18383407.

Li, F., K. J. Fisher, and P. Harmer. 2005. Prevalence of overweight and obesity in older US adults: Estimates from the 2003 Behavioral Risk Factor Surveillance System Survey. *Journal of the American Geriatrics Society* 53:737–39.

Lorig, K. R., P. L. Ritter, D. D. Laurent, and K. Plant. 2006. Internet-based chronic disease management: A randomized trial. *Medical Care* 44:964–71.

Maciosek, M. V., A. B. Coffield, T. J. Flottemesch, N. M. Edwards, and L. I. Solberg. 2010. Greater use of preventive services in U.S. health care could save lives at little or no cost. *Health Affairs* 29:1656–60.

Manton, K. G., X. Gu, and V. L. Lamb. 2006. Change in chronic disability from 1982 to 2004/2005 as measured by long-term changes in function and health in the U.S. elderly population. *Proceedings of the National Academy of Science USA* 103:18374–79.

Manton, K. G., X. Gu, and G. R. Lowrimore. 2008. Cohort changes in active life expectancy in the U.S. elderly population: Experience from the 1982–2004 National Long-Term Care Survey. *Journal of Gerontology: Social Sciences* 63B:S269–81.

Martin, L. G., V. A. Freedman, R. F. Schoeni, and P. M. Andreski. 2010. Trends in disability and related chronic conditions among people ages fifty to sixty-four. *Health Affairs* 29:725–31.

McGinnis, J. M., and W. H. Foege. 1993. Actual Causes of Death in the United States. *Journal of the American Medical Association* 270:2207–12.

Mier, N., M. G. Ory, and A. Medina. 2009. Anatomy of culturally sensitive interventions promoting nutrition and exercise in Hispanics: A critical examination of existing literature. *Health Promotion and Practice*, Epub. 2009 Feb. 4. PMID: 19193933.

Mokdad, A. H., J. S. Marks, D. F. Stroup, and J. L. Gerberding. 2004. Actual causes of death in the United States, 2000. *Journal of the American Medical Association* 291:1238–45.

National Cancer Institute. 2005. *Theory at a Glance: A Guide for Health Promotion Practice*. Retrieved December 28, 2010, from http://rex.nci.nih.gov/NCI_Pub_Interface/Theory_at_glance/HOME.html.

National Institute on Alcohol Abuse and Alcoholism. 1995. *The Physicians' Guide to Helping Patients with Alcohol Problems*, NIH Publication No. 95–3769. Bethesda, MD: Author.

Olshansky, S. J., D. J. Passaro, R. C. Hershow, J. Layden, B. A. Carnes, J. Brody, L. Hayflick, R. N. Butler, D. B. Allison, and D. S. Ludwig. 2005. A potential decline in life expectancy in the United States in the 21st century. *New England Journal of Medicine* 352:1138–45.

Ory, M. G., M. K. Hoffman, M. Hawkins, B. Sanner, and R. Mockenhaupt, 2003. Challenging aging stereotypes: Strategies for creating a more active society. *American Journal of Preventive Medicine* 25:164–71.

Ory, M. G., P. Jordan, and T. Bazzarre. 2002. Behavioral Change Consortium: Setting the stage for a new century of health behavior change research. *Health Education Research* 17:500–511.

Ory, M. G., M. L. Smith, N. Mier, and M. Wernicke. 2010. The science of sustaining health behavior change: The Health Maintenance Consortium. *American Journal of Health Behavior* 34:647–59.

Prohaska, J., K. Bigsby, J. Burdine, M. G. Ory, J. Sharkey, K. McLeroy, N. Mier, and B. Colwell. 2009. The impact of a community-wide smoke-free ordinance in smoking among older adults. *Preventing Chronic Disease*. Epub. 6:A17. PMID: 19080023.

Prohaska, J., J. B. Spring, and C. R. Nigg. 2008. Multiple health behavior change research: An introduction and overview. *Preventive Medicine* 46:181–88. Epub. 2008 Feb. 6.

Sacco, P., K. K. Bucholz, and E. L. Spitznagel. 2009. Alcohol use among older adults in the National Epidemiologic Survey on Alcohol and Related Conditions: A latent class analysis. *Journal of Studies on Alcohol and Drugs* 70:829–38.

Seymour, R. B., S. L. Hughes, R. T. Campbell, G. M. Huber, and P. Desai. 2009. Comparison of two methods of conducting Fit and Strong! *Arthritis Care and Research* 61:876–84.

Seymour, R. B., S. L. Hughes, M. G. Ory, D. Elliot, K. Kirby, J. Migneault, H. Patrick, J. Roll, and G. Williams. 2010. A lexicon for measuring maintenance of behavior change. *American Journal of Health Behavior* 34:660–68.

Shadish, W. R., T. R. Cook, and D. T. Campbell. 2002. *Experimental and Quasi-Experimental Designs for Generalized Causal Inference*, 2nd ed. Boston: Houghton Mifflin.

Stunkard, A. J., and T. A. Wadden, eds. 1993. *Obesity: Theory and Therapy*, 2nd ed. New York: Raven Press.

U.S. Department of Health and Human Services. 2000. *Healthy People 2010*, 2nd ed. With Understanding and Improving Health and Objectives for Improving Health. 2 vols. Washington, DC: U.S. Government Printing Office.

U.S. Department of Health and Human Services. 2008. *Physical Activity Guidelines for Americans*. Hyattsville, MD.

Weinstein, N. D. 1999. What does it mean to understand a risk? Evaluating risk comprehension. *JNCI Monographs* 25:15–20.

Wilcox, S., M. Dowda, S. F. Griffin, C. Rheaume, M. G. Ory, L. Leviton, A. C. King, A. Dunn, D. M. Buchner, T. Bazzarre, P. A. Estabrooks, K. Campbell-Voytal, J. Bartlett-Prescott, D. Dowdy, C. M. Castro, R. A. Carpenter, D. A. Dzewaltowski, and R. Mockenhaupt. 2006. Results of the first year of Active for Life®: Translation of two evidence-based physical activity programs for older adults in community settings. *American Journal of Public Health* 96:1201–9.

Wilcox, S., M. Dowda, L. Leviton, J. Bartlett-Prescott, T. Bazzarre, K. Campbell-Voytal, R. A. Carpenter, C. M. Castro, D. Dowdy, A. L. Dunn, S. F. Griffin, M. Guerra, A. C. King, M. G. Ory, C. Rheaume, J. Tobnick, and S. Wegley. 2008. Active for Life: Results from the translation of two physical activity programs. *American Journal of Preventive Medicine* 35:340–51.

Wu, Y., S. H. McCrone, and H. J. Lai. 2008. Health behaviors and transitions of physical disability among community-dwelling older adults. *Research on Aging* 30:572–91.

Yancey, A. K., S. K. Kumanyika, N. A. Ponce, W. J. McCarthy, J. E. Fielding, J. P. Leslie, and J. Akbar. 2004. Population-based interventions engaging communities of color in healthy eating and active living: A review. *Preventing Chronic Disease* 1:A09.

Yancey, A. K., M. G. Ory, and S. M. Davis. 2006. Dissemination of physical activity promotion interventions in underserved populations. *American Journal of Preventive Medicine* 31:S82–91.

PART III

Societal Applications

CHAPTER 8

Translation

Dissemination and Implementation Issues

Thomas R. Prohaska, PhD
Renae Smith-Ray
Russell E. Glasgow, PhD

There has been considerable advancement in our understanding of the impact of lifestyle and behavioral risk factors on the health and well-being of older adults. Early longitudinal evidence from the Alameda County Population Study demonstrated the association between behavioral risk factors such as smoking and physical activity and mortality and change in physical functioning in older adults (Kaplan, Seeman, Cohen, Knudsen, and Guralnik, 1987; Kaplan, Strawbridge, Camacho, and Cohen, 1993). More recent reviews of epidemiological, clinical, and longitudinal studies continue to confirm the impact of behavioral risk factors, especially the use of tobacco, poor diet, physical inactivity, and alcohol consumption, not only on the major causes of death and disability, but also on health and well-being (Mokdad, Marks, Stroup, and Gerberding, 2004). We also have considerable surveillance data on the prevalence of these risk factors and the demographic distribution of these risk factors among subgroups of older adults (see chap. 7). Given the known impact of behavioral risk factors on health, the translation of efficacious interventions on these and other behavioral risk factors into programs that can be disseminated at the community level is a primary public health concern. At present, there are relatively few feasible, generalizable, effective, and sustainable health promotion interventions for use in applied health and community settings (Glasgow, Klesges, Dzewaltowski, Bull, and Estabrooks, 2004). In this chapter, we examine interventions to promote health and manage chronic conditions and refer to this class of programs as health promotion interventions. Consistent with social-ecological models, we recognize the importance of policy and systems-level interventions but do not include such examples of approaches given that other chapters have a policy focus.

Many of these efficacious interventions are being considered for translation and implementation as community-based programs. However, while randomized controlled trials of successful health promotion interventions are a common first step, they are often neither sufficient nor feasible for translating into practice. The majority of these interventions have not been translated into effective programs, and fewer yet become widely disseminated to older populations in community and clinic settings (Glasgow, Lichtenstein, and Marcus, 2003). Traditionally, it has taken many years to move interventions to widespread practice because they required taking a highly controlled trial and making it applicable for wide distribution in real-world settings (Prohaska, Peters, and Warren, 2000a).

In this chapter we address several critical questions and offer insights into how to move the field forward. Why is there a disconnection between health promotion and disease prevention research and the transition of this research to practice? Why do some successful health promotion interventions become adopted by public health and aging services practitioners while other equally successful interventions never reach the community? And for health promotion interventions that are adopted, what factors are associated with widespread application in community settings? We examine the process of going beyond the establishment of efficacy and effectiveness of health promotion interventions to translation, implementation, and dissemination in the context of community-based health promotion interventions for older adults. We identify factors used to determine whether a program is "evidence-based" and propose factors to enhance the likelihood of translating research to practice. Examples of successful and widely disseminated programs are presented and include characteristics contributing to their success. Finally, we offer recommendations to facilitate dissemination and improve the public health impact of these programs.

Translation involves multiple phases for integrating research practices into established organizations, settings, or practice (Rogers, 2003; Smith-Ray et al., 2009). Translational research examines the process of enhancing adoption and implementation of effective practice and the program characteristics and community practice system processes that facilitate translation and sustainability of health promotion interventions (Khoury et al., 2007). This is consistent with the Centers for Disease Control and Prevention (CDC) perspective of translational research as a process and sequence of events in which the intervention is successfully institutionalized and integrated into established practice (Briss et al., 2000). To date, translational research in health promotion interventions for older adults has focused primarily on characteristics and processes contributing to successful implementation and dissemination, with relatively little research on the speed of translation, long-term sustainability, or public health impact.

THE PROCESS FROM RESEARCH TO PRACTICE

Community-based health promotion interventions are typically multilevel, multifaceted interventions that include a therapeutic element (treatment) and a well-developed strategy for implementing the treatment (program delivery) (Prohaska and Etkin, 2010). The intervention may target a specific behavior (physical activity), multiple interrelated behaviors (chronic disease management, falls prevention), or different targeted groups based on chronic health problems (depression, diabetes) and demographic and cultural background. The intervention has been justified based on sound empirical support that has (1) established links between behaviors and health outcomes, (2) developed methods for measuring the behaviors (and behavior change), and (3) identified the demographic, psychosocial, and environmental correlates that influence the behavior (Sallis, Owen, and Fotheringham, 2000).

No matter how well designed, no single randomized controlled trial is sufficient for determining its potential for translation and wider community application. Interventions that have been replicated (Glasgow, 2010) and continue to demonstrate efficacy, and preferably effectiveness, are prime candidates for an evidence-based review. Once the intervention has been replicated in randomized and nonrandomized trials, the research enters a phase in which there are a sufficient number of studies to review the strength and consistency of the evidence (Sallis et al., 2000). While there are several review tools and procedures, more common strategies include meta-analyses, expert panels, and consensus conferences. The Institute of Medicine, the Guide to Community Preventive Services, and the Cochrane Collaboration are well-known sources of evidence-based reviews, whose basic objective is to determine whether the evidence of the treatment effect on outcomes is sufficient to recommend adoption. These reviews may also comment on the strength of the evidence for demographic subgroups such as gender and age categories. Although evidence-based reviews may vary in quality and rigor, an intervention receiving a favorable review is more likely to be considered for implementation in community settings and, in turn, more widely disseminated. For example, an expert panel reviewed interventions on community-based treatment of late-life depression and rated the evidence. Depression care management was determined to be an effective intervention. The Program to Encourage Active Rewarding Lives for Seniors (PEARLS) was one of the interventions determined to be effective (Frederick et al., 2007). Subsequently, findings on a subset of interventions from this review were presented to the Task Force on Community Preventive Services. The Task Force decided to recommend depression care management at home for older adults with depression on the basis of strong evidence of effectiveness in improving short-term depression outcomes. Additionally, following an extensive independent review of the evidence supporting PEARLS, the National Registry of Evidence-based Programs and Practices (NREPP), sponsored by the U.S. Substance Abuse and Mental Health Services Administration, added PEARLS to its searchable online registry of mental health and substance abuse interventions. Finally, PEARLS has been placed on the recommended list of programs by the National Council on Aging (2008), which in turn was listed as one of the qualifying programs offered under initiatives by the Administration on Aging to implement and disseminate across the United States.

Evidence-based reviews have been criticized for focusing almost exclusively on randomized controlled trials with highly restrictive inclusion criteria, resulting in limited external validity and generalizability to real-world application (Rothwell, 2005). The fundamental concern is that, while internal validity and treatment fidelity must be established, external validity is also critical (Green and Glasgow, 2006). With randomized controlled trials focused on health promotion, both the therapeutic element (behavior change) and the implementation strategy (program delivery) may result in compromised efficacy when applied to diverse settings and populations under less controlled conditions by less highly trained individuals, and with more complex or less highly motivated participants. In short, there is insufficient information on the robustness and flexibility of the therapeutic element and program delivery to determine its potential in real-world settings (Green, Ottoson, Garcia, and Hiatt, 2009; Glasgow, 2010). This reality requires evidence of the representativeness of the participants, environments, and settings where the program will be implemented and the conditions, resources, and intervention staff involved (Glasgow et al., 2004). *Fidelity* is the term used to describe whether the essential elements of the program are maintained through subsequent iterations of implementation. In his seminal work on the Diffusion of Innovations, Rogers (2003) wrote that transformation of the program is necessary for taking efficacious interventions into real-world settings. This process as described by Rogers is *reinvention* of the intervention. He asserts that a program with rigid, inadaptable features is simply not practical when the goal is to use that program in a variety of settings with highly diverse populations. Such programs do not provide an opportunity for potential participants to benefit from the tacit knowledge practice professionals develop through experiences with the given target population. Hence, interventions should allow for reinvention by balancing the provision of essential elements of the intervention while retaining strong detailing of the intervention's underlying mechanisms of effectiveness—fidelity—with the expectation that local adaptation will occur to improve the fit of the intervention for new settings and audiences. The challenge to public health and aging researchers, then, is to find the balance between *reinvention* and *fidelity*.

WHAT MAKES FOR SUCCESSFUL TRANSLATION, IMPLEMENTATION, AND DISSEMINATION?

Although there are no agreed-upon standards or criteria, researchers have identified several program characteristics that generally contribute to successful translation, implementation, and dissemination (Glasgow and Emmons, 2007). The intervention must have demonstrated efficacy and some level of effectiveness across diverse populations. Also, the essential elements required for program success should be clearly identified. These are the empirically supported components found to be critical for maintaining the integrity and efficacy of the intervention. Most of these programs share key principles and strategies for behavior change such as increasing self-efficacy, the use of problem solving, social support, self-regulation, self-monitoring, and development of action plans. These theoretical constructs form the essential elements. Incorporation of the priorities and realities of community practitioners and agency directors can also be considered as criteria for adoption of the intervention. It is believed that programs with detailed implementation manuals are likely to lead to more rapid dissemination, and those that include information on the principles that the procedures are based on are more likely to ensure fidelity to those principles. Although not always provided or required, it is believed that interventions that provide estimates of cost, cost-effectiveness, or data on "return on investment" may help support institutional adoption and implementation. At the organizational level, programs that use existing community resources are sensitive to the resources of the sponsoring agency and are aligned with agency priorities that are likely to be adopted and implemented (Estabrooks and Glasgow, 2006). For example, the Strong for Life exercise program for frail older adults has been successfully implemented into community Faith in Action sites using volunteer resources available to these charitable organizations serving the community (Etkin, Prohaska, Harris, Latham, and Jette, 2006). Lastly, community-based interventions that have demonstrated flexibility in terms of the settings where the programs can be delivered, the level of expertise required of practitioners delivering the program, and the mode of program delivery are more likely to be implemented and widely disseminated. For example, the Stanford Chronic Disease Self-Management Program has been successfully implemented in health care systems using health professionals (Lorig, Hurwicz, Sobel, Hobbs, and Ritter, 2005) and community settings led by peer leaders (Druss et al., 2010) and using the Internet and e-mail (Lorig, Ritter, Laurent, and Plant, 2006). While this list of emerging standards and criteria is not exhaustive, it does suggest a growing understanding of the program characteristics that facilitate implementation of interventions into community settings.

Rogers (2003) and others have reviewed setting characteristics of "potential adopting agents" that make uptake of a given program more likely. Most importantly, there needs to be a good fit among the potential participants, program characteristics, the potential adopting setting, and staff to implement the program (Rogers, 2003; Estabrooks and Glasgow, 2006).

EXAMPLES OF EVIDENCE-BASED PROGRAMS

We reviewed the characteristics of six health promotion interventions aimed at addressing the needs of older adults that have received considerable attention. These are the Chronic Disease Self-Management Program (CDSMP; http://patienteducation.stanford.edu/programs/cdsmp.html), EnhanceFitness (Senior Services, 2007; www.projectenhance.org), Matter of Balance (www .mainehealth.org/pfha), Healthy IDEAS (http://careforelders.org/default.aspx/ MenuItemID/501/MenuGroup/Healthy+IDEAS.htm), Fit & Strong! (www .fitandstrong.org), and Active Choices and Active Living Every Day (AC and ALED; www.activeliving.info). All have been part of one or more evidence-based reviews and have been recommended as interventions by CDC programs or endorsed for wider dissemination in community settings by various organizations including the National Council on Aging. These programs share demonstrated effectiveness, clearly defined essential elements of the program, use of lay leaders, and use of program manuals and have been implemented in community settings and embedded within a service network (medical facility, community recreation facilities, etc.). Moreover, all have an underlying framework based on established theoretical constructs. With the exception of CDSMP, none of these programs have been widely implemented without external funding support. CDSMP, EnhanceFitness, Matter of Balance, and AC and ALED have provided cost data; very few (e.g., CDSMP) have provided information on cost-effectiveness. With the exception of EnhanceFitness requiring a certified fitness instructor, these programs have developed and tested options for nonprofessional staff to implement the program. CDSMP and AC and ALED offer multiple forms of program delivery, including in-person, telephone, or Internet-based sessions. Finally, each of these evidence-based programs has been conducted in diverse older populations and has extensive documentation and materials for implementation.

EVALUATION OF PUBLIC HEALTH IMPACT

The impact of evidence-based health promotion programs for older adults has been examined using the RE-AIM framework (Glasgow, Vogt, and Boles, 1999; www.re-aim.org), which identifies five dimensions, Reach, Effectiveness, Adoption, Implementation, and Maintenance (RE-AIM), used to evaluate translatability and public health impact (Glasgow, Klesges, Dzewaltowski, Estabrooks, and Vogt, 2006). Reach examines the number and percent of persons recruited and the degree to which the participants recruited represent those most in need and who would consequently benefit most from the program. Effectiveness is evaluated on how well the intervention obtains outcomes comparable to the original trials. While not typically addressed, Glasgow et al. (2006) suggest that quality of life, unanticipated outcomes, and generalizability of effects should also be considered as indices of effectiveness. Quality-of-life outcomes are valued by participants and provide a method for comparing impact across diverse programs. Adoption reflects the number and range of settings where the program is implemented and the representativeness of those settings. Implementation is the consistency and the fidelity of adherence to program essential elements, as well as the costs and resources required to deliver the program or policy. Finally, maintenance is the extent to which the participants continue the health behaviors and skills learned and to which settings/agencies continue to offer the program over time. When the impact of any one of these domains is minimal, the overall public health impact is also minimal.

RECOMMENDATIONS FOR ENHANCING OVERALL IMPACT

The RE-AIM framework provides a useful strategy to determine the impact of community programs, practitioners, and agencies but has yet to provide much guidance on how to determine whether an acceptable overall level of program impact has been obtained or how impact can be enhanced across the domains. We offer the following recommendations, which are summarized here and listed in table 8.1.

1. *Greater focus on reach.* Practitioners in aging services routinely define reach by the number of participants they serve given financial resources and availability of sites for recruitment and implementation. If the number of participants is emphasized over representativeness, external validity can be compromised. In addition, if metrics such as number of brochures distributed are used, it is unclear if participants are actually reached. Recruitment attrition is not random, and knowing the true number and level of need in a community and how to best target recruitment is difficult to determine. Not knowing the "denominator" or extent of need in the community and number of persons who would benefit from the program makes it difficult to determine acceptable reach. Determining reach and recruitment strategies involves both cost and ethical considerations. It is often more costly to recruit in disadvantaged communities where existing resources for implementing programs will be fewer than in other, more resource-rich settings. However, the need for such programs is often greater (Warren-Findlow, Prohaska, and Freedman, 2003).

   We offer four recommendations for research and practice to improve reach. The first is to examine recruitment as stages of readiness to participate. Passive, less costly recruitment messages may be sufficient for older adults who are considering or are taking steps to address their health concerns. Active (typically more costly) recruitment practices can be applied to encourage those less prepared to participate. For example, a recruitment strategy may be based on identifying factors associated with those not exposed to the recruitment message, those exposed and who decided not to participate, and those who decided to

TABLE 8.1
Recommendations for enhancing impact

1. Provide greater focus on reach
    Examine recruitment as stages of readiness to participate
    Recruit in settings where diverse and underrepresented older persons are likely
        to be found
    Use interactive technologies to expand reach
    Be aware of how program attrition impacts reach
2. Focus on essential elements
3. Consider contextual factors within the environment
4. Improve prospect for long-term sustainability
5. Engage key stakeholders
6. Develop interventions with dissemination in mind
7. Include continued development and refinement of the program
8. Investigate new modalities for program delivery

participate (Prohaska, 1998). Analyses of motivational and resource differences between these groups may reduce recruitment attrition at each stage of recruitment. Second, consider reach in the context of the environmental settings where diverse and underrepresented populations are likely to be found. For example, the Strong for Life exercise program was designed to be administered in the home of frail older adults who typically do not participate in group-based programs (Jette et al., 1999). Third, the use of alternative delivery mechanisms, such as the use of interactive technologies to attain traditionally underrepresented individuals, can improve reach often with less cost and effort. The CDSMP and AC and ALED are two examples of programs making use of the telephone, e-mail, and the Internet for program delivery and maintenance.

The fourth overlooked threat to program reach is loss of participants during program participation. Participant attrition is common across all programs, and participants will drop out no matter how well designed the program. Attrition is not random and affects reach. Prohaska et al. (2000a) found that program attrition was associated with increases in caregiving responsibilities and deteriorating health status among older African American participants in group-based exercise programs. As a result, those most in need of such programs (caregivers, frail older adults) are more likely not to complete the program or receive its full benefits. Evaluations of program and participant characteristics associated with attrition are recommended.

2. *Focus on essential elements.* As noted earlier, program essential ele-

ments are the empirically supported intervention components identified as critical for maintaining the integrity and effectiveness of the intervention. Developers should identify the program essential elements and stress the importance of staying true to these elements, previously referred to as fidelity. Researchers and practitioners should also identify and communicate program elements that may be reinvented for successful application within a variety of settings. Program flexibility is a desirable characteristic of community-based health promotion programs, and identifying the essential elements will allow for this flexibility while staying true to the intervention.

3. *Consider contextual factors within the environment.* Health promotion programs have been primarily at the individual level and focus on motivational behavior change theories. While the evidence-based programs reviewed here have an ecological perspective as part of the intervention strategy, they are limited in their ecological approach. Programs such as falls prevention interventions incorporate proximal environmental enhancement (home improvement) but rarely address more distal, upstream strategies such as changes in the built environment, neighborhoods, and policy for addressing prevention of falls (see chap. 15). Environmental factors directly and indirectly affect the individual, suggesting that these contextual factors may be a fundamental cause of the health risk (Link and Phelan, 1995). For this reason, Frieden (2010) suggests that the greatest public health impact may be achieved when interventions are directed at these fundamental causes, including socioeconomic and environmental factors. A practical example of influence at the contextual level concerns the adaptation and dissemination of CDSMP into the Expert Patients Program (EPP) in the United Kingdom (UK). EPP adapted CDSMP to fit the British culture and the health care system structure and then disseminated at the national level. The results showed that EPP did not fit well with the UK National Health System and encountered problems in terms of reach and effectiveness (Kennedy, Rogers, and Gately, 2005). Specifically, the program did not result in significant reductions in health service use, and recruitment drew primarily middle-class, highly educated adults who were already committed to chronic disease management. The authors concluded that the lack of participation of disadvantaged individuals with lower economic resources potentially contributed to increased inequalities (Kennedy et al., 2004). Additional research should be directed at how

community-based programs can be reinvented to maximize the impact of these broader environmental and socioeconomic factors.

4. *Long-term sustainability.* Sustainability (setting-level maintenance) is the least investigated of the RE-AIM framework elements (Glasgow et al., 2004). A recurring theme influencing program sustainability is the availability of continued funding. Programs are often implemented initially through external funding from foundation and federal grants but are rarely sustained when these initial external funding sources expire (Prohaska and Etkin, 2004). The Robert Wood Johnson Foundation asked health care and community agencies applying for initial funding how they intended to sustain AC and ALED once their initial funding ended. Four funding strategies were noted: (1) apply for additional external funding, (2) charge participants for program services, (3) provide assurance that their agency/organization would incorporate the program into existing services, and (4) broaden community support and involve other stakeholders for support. The latter two strategies were deemed most likely to result in long-term sustainability (Prohaska and Etkin, 2004).

Evashwick and Ory (2003) tracked the factors that impacted the sustainability of 20 Archstone award-winning programs that promote the health of older adults and were maintained from 2 to 10 or more years after receiving the award. Financial factors were the most frequently noted challenge to sustainability. Organizational factors that improved the prospect for sustainability included finding program champions who were strong leaders, involving community leaders and key stakeholders in program development, effective use of the organization's infrastructure, completing marketing and outreach efforts, and continuing to gather outcome data to justify the program's effectiveness. Additional work related to this important issue is clearly needed.

5. *Key stakeholder engagement.* Another method to enhance impact is to incorporate multiple stakeholders who have insight into the program characteristics that facilitate adoption and dissemination. Stakeholders with a vested interest in the translation of research to practice include researchers whose ultimate goal is to have the program become widely used, agencies that implement the program, practitioners responsible for program delivery, and participants benefiting from the program. Traditionally these stakeholders have different goals and perspectives concerning the program, and communication between researchers and

these stakeholders has often been unidirectional (Prohaska, Peters, and Warren, 2000b). These stakeholders can also provide insight into elements of the intervention that may require reinvention to facilitate adoption and dissemination. Regular discussions between researchers and consumers should be implemented across the full transition process from research development to practice to improve reach and facilitate implementation (Glasgow et al., 2004; Prohaska and Etkin, 2010; Solberg et al., 2010). This process will also contribute to the continuous reinvention of the program as lessons learned from the community are integrated into program revisions, a process that Solberg et al. (2010) term "engaged scholarship and knowledge integration."

An example of the value of stakeholder engagement was the reinvention of a diabetes prevention program that was translated into a tangible program for dissemination reported by Smith-Ray et al. (2009). The Diabetes Prevention Program (DPP) is an intensive lifestyle intervention for individuals diagnosed with prediabetes (Diabetes Prevention Program Research Group, 2002). Individuals randomized to the DPP exhibited better management of diabetic symptoms than their counterparts randomized to the gold-standard prescription drug (Metformin). Interested in applying this intervention at an organizational level, researchers at a large health maintenance organization developed a more efficient variant of the DPP with involvement of front-line staff, including dieticians and health educators, who were able to inform the researchers of common concerns, barriers, and perceptions of recently diagnosed prediabetic patients. This resulted in a reinvention of the DPP that did not compromise the essential elements of the DPP but was effective with regard to both outcomes and cost (Smith-Ray et al., 2009).

As mentioned previously, the emerging theme seems to be retention of essential elements while simultaneously making appropriate adaptations to fit the local setting and culture (Solberg et al., 2010). Recognizing this, the RE-AIM definition of implementation has been modified to include not only fidelity or consistency of intervention delivery across sites, staff, program component, and time but also adaptations that are made throughout the program and the rationale for such changes using mixed quantitative and qualitative methods (Glasgow and Linnan, 2008). Finally, more transparent investigation and reporting of variation in program implementation across sites and the relationship of these variations to outcomes should help clarify key principles and strategies (Glasgow, 2010).

6. *Interventions should be developed with dissemination in mind*. Program developers should be mindful of potential barriers to dissemination during the earliest stages of program development, especially when broad-scale dissemination is the ultimate goal. This can be done by engaging organizations that may later deliver the intervention and avoiding features that may pose barriers to dissemination within those organizational contexts. For instance, program costs are often the greatest barrier to maintenance. For this reason the use of expensive equipment should be avoided if possible. This may not always be possible, but it could be addressed in community-based trials that test the effect of the intervention using the resources (staff, equipment). This also requires that training and supervision materials be developed so that staff from a variety of backgrounds can successfully implement the intervention and identify essential program elements. We recommend including lay persons, community health workers, front-line delivery staff, or senior volunteers to assist with these guidelines at the earliest stages of development.

   Programs designed to be aligned with health policies, especially new policies such as changes in reimbursement for services or requirements such as Healthcare Effectiveness Data and Information Set (HEDIS) performance criteria, are more likely to be disseminated and therefore have greater potential for public health impact. Similarly, programs that have practical appeal to clinicians are better candidates for dissemination. These include programs that address important clinical need but do so more efficiently than the standard approach (Smith-Ray et al., 2009).

7. *Continued development and refinement of programs*. The number, types, and quality of evidence-based programs to improve the health of older adults will continue to grow. One promising direction for program development and targeting is to design programs based on life transitions among older adults. Possible self-care and health promotion programs oriented toward life transitions may address changes in health practices and risk factors in the transition into retirement, becoming a caregiver, loss of spouse, and becoming frail and dependent (Prohaska and Clark, 1997). For example, the Care of Persons with Dementia in their Environments (COPE) program is a biobehavioral, educational, and skill-building program for family caregivers to reduce the negative consequences of caregiving (Gitlin, Winter, Dennis, Hodgson, and Hauck, 2010). Similarly, as our understanding of the variety of behavioral and psychosocial risk factors associated with cognitive impairment

becomes more acute, comprehensive evidence-based programs based on these mutable factors may emerge.

8. *Investigate new modalities for program delivery.* As mentioned above with the CDSMP and AC and ALED programs, expanding and evaluating the impact of different modalities of program delivery such as Internet-based or telephone modalities can improve the reach, scalability, and potentially the cost-effectiveness of interventions (Lorig, Ritter, Laurent, and Plant, 2006). Innovations have included automated telephone disease management (Piette, Weinberger, Kraemer, and McPhee, 2001), and several researchers are developing text messaging alternatives for program delivery. Similarly, Internet developers are exploring Web 2.0 and social media applications (Bennett and Glasgow, 2009) that have the potential to enhance peer engagement, improve cost-effectiveness, and reach many users in settings such as rural areas as more older adults become Internet and cell phone users.

   Such alternative delivery modalities should not be uncritically accepted simply because they are "the latest fad" but evaluated as to their strengths and weaknesses compared with face-to-face program delivery on their impact on the various RE-AIM dimensions (Glasgow, McKay, Piette, and Reynolds, 2001). We see numerous opportunities for research comparing delivery modalities as part of the new national emphasis on comparative effectiveness research.

Figure 8.1 provides a conceptual framework for describing the process of translation of research to practice and the dynamics in the research-practice partnership. This framework highlights the interaction that occurs at multiple levels to facilitate dissemination and reflects our recommendations for enhancing impact. The context of this framework and our recommendations primarily involves implementation within community-based organizations and health care systems, both of which may have multiple delivery sites. Our recommendations to improve reach are embedded in the partnership between researchers and practitioners noted in figure 8.1. For example, interventions that involve interactive technology to improve reach are designed and tested by the research design team with input from individuals at the partner organization, resulting in an adaptive design. While the focus on essential elements begins in the evidence-tested program (critical elements), identification of these elements is done with consideration of the fit with the organization. Contextual factors that may influence dissemination and long-term sustainability are considered for each of the community sites by the program delivery staff in partnership with the research design team. This

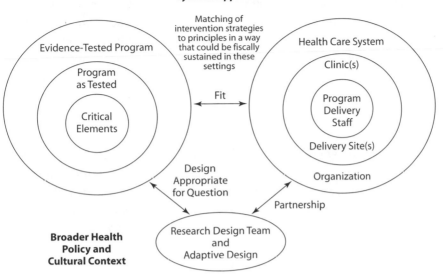

Fig. 8.1. Framework for describing the process of translation of research to practice and the dynamics in the research-practice partnership.

partnership increases key stakeholder engagement at the organization level. The research design team and key stakeholders within the organization work together to consider dissemination early in the research development phase and the continued development and refinement of the program, including, if necessary, new modalities for program delivery.

FUTURE DIRECTIONS

A critical area in need of further work is determining the relative merits and implications of "top-down" versus "bottom-up" strategies for dissemination. Top-down dissemination is driven by federal and corporate agencies. Often as a public health approach, government agencies or corporations may decide that a program has the potential to offer sufficient impact at the community level and, with this decision, award grants to smaller clinics or organizations that propose to offer the program. A bottom-up strategy of dissemination is where practitioners or researchers advocate for disseminating their program to a broad community-level audience. The bottom-up, researcher or activist-driven strategy is more commonplace in public health and has been the primary method of dissemination for many successful health promotion programs including CDSMP, Fit & Strong!, and AC and ALED. With the top-down approach, the funder typically chooses which programs will be offered and has a vested interest in a long-term commitment to the program as designed.

Although a top-down process is reasonable for wider dissemination, it can result in a fixed "gold standard" program with limited opportunities for reinvention. This potential stagnation of the program can be avoided by conducting comparative effectiveness studies. A final approach that combines elements of both the top-down and bottom-up approaches involves social networking and opinion leader approaches to identify opinion leaders in target organizations and working with them to introduce the innovation and hopefully become program champions. The rationale is that being both trusted and credible sources to others in the organization and local, their opinion is likely to carry more weight than information from outside experts. The potential implications of these strategies are significant, and research on the merits and limitations of these approaches should be conducted and the findings used to inform policy.

Another critical area is to determine the relative merits and limitations of the randomized controlled trial (RCT) relative to the practical clinical trial. The practical or pragmatic clinical trial model (Thorpe et al., 2009) has gained recent support as a method for improving dissemination. Practical clinical trials involve blending the strength of controlled research with the practicality of a dissemination study. Typically, a practical clinical trial tests the effectiveness of an intervention by randomly assigning the program to individuals or organizations in real-world settings, with the control condition consisting of the standard care or current organizational offering (Estabrooks et al., 2011). While its research design involves more rigor than a traditional effectiveness or dissemination trial, the practical clinical trial differs from an RCT in that it utilizes an existing program delivery system to disseminate the intervention. The appeal of the practical clinical trial is that if effectiveness is demonstrated using this design, then the progression to dissemination is much more rapid and natural than the less certain traditional "pipeline" from efficacy (RCT) to effectiveness to dissemination. Future research should consider the benefits of using the practical clinical trial model given its potential to bring research from bench to bedside to community much more swiftly.

CONCLUSION

Researchers in the behavioral sciences and the evolving field of implementation and dissemination research have unique roles in the translation and application of programs to promote the health of older adults. However, these roles can no longer be mutually exclusive. There is also an extensive public health and aging service network capable of implementing these evidence-based programs. This is best noted by Balsam and Bottom (1997, p. 17), who propose "a coordinated continuum of (health promotion) services formed by the integration of these two networks . . . to meet the needs of older adults." As noted by Green (2008), "If we want more evidence-based practice, we need more practice-based evidence." We have reinforced the need for a collaborative partnership model bridging the public health research and public health practice community that so many others have stressed (Prohaska et al., 2000a; Glasgow and Emmons, 2007; Solberg et al., 2010). The unfortunate state of the field in which there are relatively few feasible, generalizable, effective, and sustainable evidence-based programs promoting the health of older adults will soon change. However, with the proliferation of new evidence-based programs, there needs to be a corresponding effort to improve the quality, promote the flexibility, and enhance the public health impact of these programs. Recommendations for criteria and guidelines to promote collaboration and enhance the public health impact were suggested, and frameworks such as RE-AIM and the Integrated Dynamic Research-Practice Partnership presented in figure 8.1 are provided as useful guides to make the transition from research to dissemination and implementation of programs for older adults a smooth and expeditious one.

REFERENCES

Balsam, A. L., and C. L. Bottom. 1997. Understanding the aging and public health networks. In *Public Health and Aging*, ed. T. Hickey, M. Speers, and R. Prohaska. Baltimore: Johns Hopkins University Press.

Bennett, G., and R. Glasgow. 2009. The delivery of public health interventions via the Internet: Actualizing their potential. *Annual Review of Public Health* 30:273–92.

Briss, P. A., S. Zaza, M. Pappaloanou, J. Fielding, L. Wright-DeAguero, B. I. Truman, D. P. Hopkins, P. D. Mullen, R. S. Thompson, S. H. Woolf, V. G. Carande-Kulls, L. Anderson, A. R. Hinman, D. V. McQueen, S. M. Teutsch, and J. R. Harris, The Task Force on Community Preventive Services. 2000. Developing an evidence-based *Guide to Community Preventive Services*—methods. *American Journal of Preventive Medicine* 18(Suppl. 1):35–43.

Diabetes Prevention Program Research Group. 2002. Reduction in the incidence of type 2 diabetes with lifestyle intervention or Metformin. *New England Journal of Medicine* 346:393–403.

Druss, B.G., L. S. A. Zaho, J. R. von Esenwein, L. Bona, S. Fricks, E. Jenkins-Tucker, R. Sterling, R. DiClemente, and K. Lorig. 2010. The Health and Recovery Peer (HARP) program: A peer-led intervention to improve medical self-management for persons with serious mental illness. *Schizophrenia Research* 118:264–70.

Estabrooks, P. A., and R. E. Glasgow. 2006. Translating effective clinic-based physical activity interventions into practice. *American Journal of Preventive Medicine* 31:45–56.

Estabrooks, P. A., R. L. Smith-Ray, F. A. Almeida, M. Gonzalez, P. Schreiner, and R. Van Den Berg. 2011. Move more: Translating efficacious physical activity intervention into effective clinical practice. *International Journal of Sport and Exercise Psychology*, 9, 4–18.

Etkin, C., T. Prohaska, B. Harris, N. Latham, and A. Jette. 2006. Feasibility of implementing the Strong for Life program in community settings. *Gerontologist* 46: 284–92.

Evashwick, C., and M. Ory. 2003. Organizational characteristics of successful innovative health care programs sustained over time. *Family & Community Health* 26(3):177–93.

Frederick, J., L. Steinman, T. Prohaska, W. Satariano, M. Bruce, P. Ciechanowski, B. DeVellis, K. Leith, K. Leyden, J. Sharkey, G. Simon, N. Wilson, J. Unutzer, and M. Snowden. 2007. Community-based treatment of late life depression: An expert panel–informed literature review. *American Journal of Preventive Medicine* 33:222–47.

Frieden, T. R. (2010). A framework for public health action: The health impact pyramid. *American Journal of Public Health* 100:590–95.

Gitlin, L. N., L. Winter, M. P. Dennis, N. Hodgson, and W. W. Hauck. 2010. A biobehavioral home-based intervention and the well-being of patients with dementia and their caregivers. *Journal of the American Medical Association* 304:983–91.

Glasgow, R. 2010. HMC research translation: Speculations about making it real and going to scale. *American Journal of Health Behavior* 34:833–40.

Glasgow, R., and K. Emmons. 2007. How can we increase translation of research into practice? Types of evidence needed. *Annual Review of Public Health* 28:413–33.

Glasgow, R., L. Klesges, D. Dzewaltowski, S. Bull, and P. Estabrooks. 2004. The future of health behavior change research: What is needed to improve translation of research into health promotion practice. *Annals of Behavioral Medicine* 27(1):3–12.

Glasgow, R., L. Klesges, D. Dzewaltowski, P. Estabrooks, and T. Vogt. 2006. Evaluating the overall impact of health promotion programs: Using the RE-AIM framework to form summary measures for decision making involving complex issues. *Health Education & Research* 21:688–94.

Glasgow, R., E. Lichtenstein, and A. Marcus. 2003. Why don't we see more translation of health promotion research to practice? Rethinking efficacy-to-effectiveness transition. *American Journal of Public Health* 93:1261–67.

Glasgow, R., and L. Linnan, 2008. Evaluation of theory-based interventions. In *Health Behavior and Health Education: Theory, Practice and Research*, 4th ed., ed. K. B. Glanz, B. Rimer, and V. Vishwanath, pp. 487–92. San Francisco: Jossey-Bass.

Glasgow, R., H. McKay, J. Piette, and K. Reynolds. 2001. The RE-AIM framework for evaluating interventions: What can it tell us about approaches to chronic illness management? *Patient Education Counseling* 44:119–27.

Glasgow, R., T. Vogt, and S. Boles. 1999. Evaluating the public health impact of health promotion interventions: The RE-AIM framework. *American Journal of Public Health* 89:1322–27.

Green, L. 2008. Making research relevant: If it is an evidence-based practice, where's the practice-based evidence? *Family Practice* 25(Suppl. 1):i20–24.

Green, L., and R. Glasgow. 2006. Evaluating the relevance, generalization, and applicability of research: Issues in translation methodology. *Evaluation Health Professions* 29(1):126–53.

Green, L., J. Ottoson, C. Garcia, and R. Hiatt. 2009. Diffusion theory and knowledge dissemination, utilization, and integration in public health. *Annual Review of Public Health* 30:151–74.

Jette, A., M. Lachman, M. Giorgetti, S. Assmann, B. Harris, C. Levenson, M. Wernick, and D. Krebs. 1999. Exercise—it's never too late: The Strong for Life program. *American Journal of Public Health* 89:66–72.

Kaplan, G., T. E. Seeman, R. D. Cohen, L. P. Knudsen, and J. Guralnik. 1987. Mortality among the elderly in the Alameda County Study: Behavioral and demographic risk factors. *American Journal of Public Health* 77:307–12.

Kaplan, G., W. Strawbridge, T. Camacho, and R. Cohen. 1993. Factors associated with change in physical functioning in the elderly: A six-year prospective study. *Journal of Aging and Health* 5:140–53.

Kennedy, A., A. Rogers, and C. Gately. 2005. Assessing the introduction of the expert patients programme into the NHS: A realistic evaluation of recruitment to a national lay-led self-care initiative. *Primary Health Care Research and Development* 6:137–48.

Khoury, M., M. Gwinn, P. Yoon, N. Dowling, C. Moore, and L. Bradley. 2007. The continuum of translation research in genomic medicine: How can we accelerate the appropriate integration of human genome discoveries into health care and disease prevention? *Genetics in Medicine* 9:665–74.

Link, B. G., and J. Phelan. 1995. Social conditions as fundamental causes of disease. *Journal of Health and Social Behavior* 35(Extra Issue):80–84.

Lorig, K., M. L. Hurwicz, D. Sobel, M. Hobbs, and P. Ritter. 2005. A national dissemination of an evidence-based self-management program: A process evaluation study. *Patient Education and Counseling* 59:69–79.

Lorig, K., P. Ritter, D. Laurent, and K. Plant. 2006. Internet-based chronic disease management: A randomized trial. *Medical Care* 44(11):964–71.

Mokdad, A., J. Marks, D. Stroup, and J. Gerberding. 2004. Actual causes of death in the United States, 2000. *Journal of the American Medical Association* 291:1238–45.

National Council on Aging. 2008. *Review of Findings on Chronic Disease Self-Management Program (CDSMP) Outcomes: Physical, Emotional, and Health-Related Quality of Life, Healthcare Utilization and Costs.* Washington, DC: National Council on Aging.

Piette, J., M. Weinberger, F. Kraemer, and S. McPhee. 2001. The impact of automated calls with nurse follow-up on diabetes treatment outcomes in a Department of Veterans Affairs health care system. *Diabetes Care* 24:202–8.

Prohaska, T. 1998. The research basis for the design and implementation of self-care programs. In *Self-Care in Later Life: Research, Program, and Policy Issues*, ed. M. G. Ory and G. H. DeFriese, pp. 62–84. New York: Springer.

Prohaska, T., and M. Clark. 1997. Health behavior and the human life cycle. In *Handbook of Health Behavior Research III: Demography, Development, and Diversity*, ed. D. Gotchman, pp. 29–48. New York: Plenum.

Prohaska, T., and C. Etkin. 2004. What gets left when the funds dry up? How to sustain community advances in public health. *Aging Today* 25(2):11.

Prohaska, T., and C. Etkin. 2010. External validity and translation from research to implementation. *Generations* 34(1):59–65.

Prohaska, T., K. Peters, and J. Warren. 2000a. Health behavior: From research to community practice. In *Handbook of Social Studies in Health and Medicine*, ed. G. L. Albrecht, R. Fitzpatrick, and S. Scrimshaw, pp. 359–73. London: Sage.

Prohaska, T., K. Peters, and J. Warren. 2000b. Sources of attrition in a church-based exercise program for older African-Americans. *American Journal of Health Promotion* 14:380–85.

Rogers, E. M. 2003. *Diffusion of Innovations*, 5th ed. New York: Free Press.

Rothwell, P. 2005. External validity of randomized controlled trials: "To whom do the results of this trial apply?" *Lancet* 365:82–93.

Sallis, J., N. Owen, and M. Fotheringham. 2000. Behavioral epidemiology: A systematic framework to classify phases of research on health promotion and disease prevention. *Annals of Behavioral Medicine* 22:294–98.

Senior Services. 2007. *About EnhanceFitness Classes at Project Enhance*. Retrieved January 1, 2010, from www.projectenhance.org/ind_ef_aboutclass.html.

Smith-Ray, R., F. A. Almeida, J. Bajaj, S. Foland, M. Gilson, S. Heikkinen, H. Seagle, and P. A. Estabrooks. 2009. Translating efficacious behavioral principles for diabetes prevention into practice. *Health Promotion Practice* 10:58–66.

Solberg, L., R. Glasgow, J. Unutzer, N. Jaeckets, G. Oftedahl, A. Beck, V. Maciosek, and A. Crain. 2010. Partnership research: A practical trial design for evaluation of a national experiment to improve depression care. *Medical Care* 48:576–82.

Thorpe, K., M. Zwarenstein, A. Oxman, S. Treweek, C. Furberg, D. Altman, M. Tunis, E. Bergel, I. Harvey, D. Magid, and K. Chalkidou. 2009. A pragmatic-explanatory continuum indicator summary (RRECIS): A tool to help trial designers. *Canadian Medical Association Journal* 180(10):E47–57.

Warren-Findlow, J., T. Prohaska, and D. Freedman. 2003. Challenges and opportunities in recruiting and retaining underrepresented population into health promotion research. *Gerontologist* 43:37–46.

CHAPTER 9

Family Caregiving
of Older Adults

Laura N. Gitlin, PhD
Richard Schulz, PhD

There are only four kinds of people in the world—those who
have been caregivers, those who currently are caregivers, those
who will be caregivers and those who need caregivers.

—Former First Lady Rosalynn Carter

Providing care to an older family member is an activity that spans time, place, and cultures. Family members have been, are now, and will continue to be the primary providers of care to older adults. They are the backbone of health care systems worldwide (Spillman and Black, 2005; Institute of Medicine, 2008). Broadly speaking, family caregivers are family members, friends, fictive kin, or neighbors who provide some form of care to an older adult with whom they have a relationship. Care may involve monitoring on-site or long-distance and providing coordination, hands-on assistance, health-related services such as wound care, or financial support to someone in need or with a cognitive and/or physical impairment (Schulz and Tompkins, 2010). Family caregivers are involved in episodic, transitional, and long-term care and may need to assume responsibilities for care tasks for which they have little knowledge, training, or support (Stone, Cafferata, and Sangl, 1987; Wolff and Roter, 2008; Levine, Halper, Peist, and Gould, 2010).

Family members may be the primary care provider, the secondary or tertiary care provider, or part of a network of informal and/or formal paid caregivers (Dilworth-Anderson, Williams, and Cooper, 1999), and they may offer care full- or part-time, or live with or apart from the individual receiving care. Family caregivers are typically unpaid, in contrast to formal caregivers who are associated with a service delivery system and either volunteer or are paid.

Despite the extensive care families provide—in the United States an estimated 85% of help to older adults is provided by families—they are a neglected population. With few exceptions, family caregiving has not been systematically examined from a public health perspective (Schulz and Martire, 2004; Talley and Crews, 2007). Given that providing care has emotional, physical, and financial consequences as well as societal costs and significant implications for health policy and the organization of health delivery systems, this chapter makes the case for family caregiving as a major public health concern. Using a public health lens, we examine demographic transitions shaping caregiving, prevalence of caregiving, health risks, and preventive and supportive strategies to minimize adverse outcomes among caregivers. As caregiving is an emerging global phenomenon, we also highlight its worldwide implications and consider the key components necessary for a societal infrastructure to effectively support family caregivers and from which to advance a public health response. In this chapter we focus primarily on middle-aged or older family caregivers providing care to aging spouses, parents, or friends.

DEMOGRAPHIC TRANSITIONS

A confluence of demographic and societal factors portend that the roles and responsibilities of family caregivers will continue and expand in the future. The most important trend is the dramatic upward shift in the age structure of developing and developed countries such that people are living longer with comorbidities and complex medical conditions that require episodic and long-term help (Wolff and Kasper, 2006; United Nations, 2007). In the United States alone, in 2008, there were an estimated 39 million people aged 65 and over, over 13% of the total population. By 2030, the older population is projected to be almost twice as large (72 million), representing nearly 20% of the total population (Federal Interagency Forum on Age-Related Statistics, 2010). Other significant trends effecting caregiving include the worldwide increase in chronic diseases requiring ongoing care management (World Health Organization, 2008), technological advances supporting health care provision at home, decline in and delay of nursing home placement (particularly in the United States and developed countries; Federal Interagency Forum on Age-Related Statistics, 2010), early hospital discharge to home, emergence of medical home care models emphasizing family involvement, shortages in trained health care providers (Robert Graham Center, 2007; Institute of Medicine, 2008), and the strong desire among older adults and families to age at home (AARP, 2003).

Moreover, while greater demands for providing care are being imposed on families, there is simultaneously a shrinking pool of informal providers. This shrinking pool is due to changes in family size and composition, greater mobility of families, and increased labor force participation of women. These trends have significant implications for policies, particularly in the United States, that seek to prevent or delay nursing home placement or return nursing home residents to the community and that rely on family participation to accomplish these goals (Spillman and Long, 2009).

Although caregiving is not a new phenomenon, what has changed is the number of individuals providing care, the length of time spent caregiving, and the breadth of caregiving tasks performed and hence skills needed to be a caregiver (Schulz and Martire, 2004). The convergence of three key factors in the decades ahead—increased need for care of an aging population worldwide, decreased availability or shortages of formal care providers, and decreased number of adult children to provide care—has the makings of a perfect storm that will challenge policy makers and a public health response to family caregiving for decades to come.

PREVALENCE OF CAREGIVING

Currently, there are no precise estimates of the number of family caregivers. Existing estimates vary widely based on how caregiving is defined, the sampling strategy used, and age and conditions considered of the person receiving care. At one extreme are prevalence estimates that 28.5% of the U.S. adult population (65.7 million) provided unpaid care to an adult relative in 2009, with the majority (83%) of this care delivered to people aged 50 years or older (National Alliance for Caregiving and AARP, 2009). At the other extreme, data from the National Long-Term Care Survey suggest that as few as 3.5 million informal caregivers provided instrumental activities of daily living (IADL) or activities of daily living (ADL) assistance to people aged 65 and over (National Institute on Aging and Duke University, 2004). Intermediate estimates of 28.8 million caregivers ("persons aged 15 or over providing personal assistance for everyday needs of someone age 15 and older") have also been reported (National Family Caregivers Association and Family Caregiver Alliance, 2006). A recent national survey of individuals aged 45 and older using a large national epidemiological sample yielded a caregiving rate of 12%, or 14.9 million adults (Roth, Perkins, Wadley, Temple, and Haley, 2009).

High-end estimates tend to be generated when broad and inclusive definitions of caregiving are used (e.g., "Unpaid care may include help with personal needs or household chores. It might be managing a person's finances, arranging for outside services, or visiting regularly to see how they are doing.") (National Alliance for Caregiving and AARP, 2004). Low-end estimates tend to be generated when definitions require the provision of specific ADL or IADL assistance (e.g., Wolff and Kasper, 2006; Schulz and Tompkins, 2010; for comparison of estimates of prevalence rates see Gibson and Houser, 2007).

These estimates, however, do not account for episodic or intermittent caregiving that may be provided by family members, such as accompanying older relatives to doctor appointments or briefly caring for persons following medical events such as a hip fracture, stroke, cancer treatment, injury, or trauma (Wolff, Boyd, Gitlin, Bruce, and Roter, in press). Also, we do not have adequate estimates of the number of families providing long-distance care. It has been suggested that approximately 15% of caregivers live at least 1 hour away from their older relatives and provide care at a distance (National Alliance for Caregiving, 2004; Schulz and Tompkins, 2010).

Although family caregiving is gaining global attention, few country-specific probability surveys to determine prevalence exist (AARP, National Alliance for Caregiving, and United Nations Programme on Aging, 2008). In Europe, available data suggest a similar caregiving profile as in the United States, with 80% of long-term care being provided by informal caregivers (e.g., EuroFamCare Project). Another source of information about caregiving in European countries is national census data that include caregiving questions; an exemplar is Ireland (Care Alliance Ireland, 2010). Based on their 2006 population census, an estimated 160,917 were family caregivers, representing 4.8% of the total population. Because the question asked of respondents emphasized long-term caregiving, this figure may underestimate prevalence.

The amount of time providing some form of care to an older adult is also difficult to quantify; estimates vary by condition of the person receiving care, population surveyed, and specific care tasks considered (for comparison of estimates of hours across studies see Gibson and Houser, 2007). Gibson and Houser (2007) projected that 30–38 million family caregivers provided an average of 21 hours of care per week (that is, 1,080 hours per year). Caregivers of individuals with dementia provide slightly more hours of care on average than caregivers of other older adults. Of the close to 11 million estimated family caregivers of people with dementia, an average of 21.9 hours of care is provided per week (that is, 1,139 care hours per caregiver per year; Alzheimer's Association, 2010).

Long-distance caregivers spend on average 3.4 hours per week arranging services and another 4 hours per week checking in or monitoring care of the care recipient. One-third of long-distance caregivers visit at least once a week and provide on average 34 hours of I/ADL assistance per month (National Alliance for Caregiving, 2004; Schulz and Tompkins, 2010).

CHARACTERISTICS OF CAREGIVERS

Although prevalence estimates vary, a consistent profile of caregivers emerges across surveys. Most family caregivers worldwide are female, although the percentage of male caregivers, at least in the United States, is increasing, with estimates ranging from 34% to 40% (EuroFamCare Project, n.d.; National Alliance for Caregiving and AARP, 2009; Alzheimer's Association, 2010). Most (86%) provide care to a relative who is also primarily female, the majority are 61 years or older, and most are providing care in their own home (National Alliance for Caregiving and AARP, 2009).

In the United States, the typical caregiver is a 48–year-old woman, has some college education, works, and spends more than 20 hours per week providing unpaid care to her mother. Sixty-six percent of caregivers are women, and most work either full- or part-time (59%). Education level of caregivers is slightly higher than the U.S. adult population, with more than 90% having completed high school and 43% being college graduates (compared to 85% and 27%, respectively) (Stoops, 2004; Schulz and Tompkins, 2010).

A recent survey (National Alliance for Caregiving and AARP, 2009) suggests that the demographic characteristics of caregivers vary substantially by race and ethnic groups in the United States. For example, Hispanic caregivers tend to be younger (43 years of age) and less likely to be married, although they report having children or grandchildren in their households compared with white and African American caregivers. One survey found that long-distance caregivers were more educated and affluent and more likely to play a secondary helper role compared with in-home caregivers, but these characteristics need to be examined more closely (National Alliance for Caregiving, 2004). Moreover, data are limited concerning diverse race/ethnic groups, and we cannot characterize differences well within groups.

Although caregivers are predominantly middle-aged or older, some children also assume caregiving responsibilities for an older adult. As many as 1.4 million children in the United States between the ages of 8 and 18 provide care to an older adult. These children are more likely to come from households with lower incomes and are less likely to live in a two-parent home (Levine et al., 2005; Schulz and Tompkins, 2010).

WHO RECEIVES CARE?

It is projected that the number of older adults with functional limitations will increase from 22 million in 2005 to 38 million by 2030 (Institute of Medicine Committee on Disability in America, 2007). This demographic shift is occurring at the same time that there are critical shortages of nurses and other health care workers and increasing costs of hospitalization and long-term care (Talley and Crews, 2007) (see chap. 13).

Approximately 9.4 million adults aged 18 years and older need assistance with ADLs, with about 3.2 million needing assistance with more than one self-care activity (Agency for Healthcare Research and Quality, 2000; Kaye, Harrington, and LaPlante, 2010). Care recipients are typically women (66%) and older (80% are aged 50 years or older), and their main presenting problems or illnesses are "old age" (12%), followed by Alzheimer's disease or other dementias (10%), cancer (7%), mental/emotional illness (7%), heart disease (5%), and stroke (5%). The average length of time caregivers report providing care is 4.6 years (National Alliance for Caregiving and AARP, 2009), but the length of time may be considerably more depending on the condition of the individual receiving care. In the case of dementia, caregiving may range from 4 to 20 years.

WHAT CARE DO FAMILY CAREGIVERS PROVIDE?

Families assume a wide range of roles and responsibilities necessitated by the care recipient's health condition, which can include communicating and negotiating with others about care decisions, providing companionship and emotional support, interacting with physicians and other health care providers, coordinating care needs, driving, doing housework and home repairs, shopping, completing paperwork and managing finances, hiring nurses and aides, helping with personal care and hygiene, lifting, transferring and maneuvering the care recipient, and assisting with complex medical and nursing-related tasks (e.g., infusion therapies, tube feedings, medication monitoring). Additionally, caregivers are called upon to coordinate services from health and human service agencies, to make difficult decisions about service needs, and to determine how best to access all of the services that may be needed, including the hiring and oversight of paid care providers. Long-distance caregivers have the added challenges of identifying relevant resources in the care recipient's local environment from afar, hiring individuals to provide needed care, and monitoring from afar the care providers' performance as well as the status of the care recipient.

Figure 9.1 illustrates a common care trajectory for an older individual with cognitive or physical limitations who is living at home. Caregiving may begin sporadically by being present at routine encounters with physicians or other health care providers (Wolff and Roter, 2008; Wolff et al., in press), serving as proxy decision makers to severally ill older adults (Shalowitz, Garrett-Mayer, and Wendler, 2006), or providing transient assistance to post-acute patients discharged from hospital to home (Weinberg, Lusenhop, Gittell, and Kautz, 2007). We know little about the intensity, duration, or type of care provided or about the characteristics of informal caregivers in these instances.

Because episodic health events are often characterized by acute onset without warning, they entail different challenges than chronic or ongoing caregiving. Episodic caregivers have to quickly acquire skills related to performing specific in-home medical procedures, operating medical equipment, monitoring patient status, or coordinating care (Schulz and Tompkins, 2010). Episodic care also has implications for caregivers still in the workforce as it may require leaving work early, missing work, or using vacation days to be able to carry out periodic care tasks.

Caregiving demands and the amount of time required in care increase when the person receiving care is no longer able to perform IADLs (fig. 9.1, col. 2). Surveys suggest that caregivers provide assistance with a wide range of IADL tasks, including helping with transportation (83%), housework tasks (75%), grocery shopping (75%), and preparing meals (65%) (National Alliance for Caregiving and AARP, 2009).

As the health condition of the care recipient worsens and disabilities increase, caregiver tasks expand to include more hands-on physical assistance with ADL tasks such as dressing, bathing, ambulating, and toileting (fig. 9.1, col. 3). Fifty-six percent of all caregivers provide ADL assistance such as helping the care recipient get in and out of bed (40%), dress (32%), or bathe (26%). Caregivers may also be required to closely monitor the activity of the person receiving care to ensure their safety at home (National Alliance for Caregiving and AARP, 2009).

If we examine the effects on caregivers, care responsibilities may begin incrementally and slowly expand without full recognition by the family care-giver of the scope of support provided to the care recipient. An older adult may begin to experience seemingly small functional difficulties owing to age-related changes or chronic disease such as not being able to carry groceries, take the garbage outside, or do light housekeeping. Families typically do not self-identify as caregivers at this early stage in which some form of assistance may be necessary. Using the term "caregiver" signals a conscious recognition that one has passed a threshold from normative to extraordinary care.

The roles and responsibilities of caregivers tend to expand incrementally, with care tasks being cumulative over time (fig. 9.1, row 2). Increasing care demands often result in caregivers needing to leave the workforce, relocate to the care recipient's home, or having the individual receiving care move into caregivers' homes. Additionally, caregivers may need to participate in medi-cally related tasks such as wound care, pain management, sterilizing equip-ment, tube feeding, or monitoring infusion therapies and medical equip-ment. Few caregivers either receive adequate instruction in these forms of care or are assessed for their ability or willingness to participate in such tasks (Donelan et al., 2002).

Also, caregiving does not terminate with nursing home placement (fig. 9.1). Families continue to provide on-site monitoring and hands-on assis-tance with daily activities, be responsible for coordinating care and ongoing decision making, communicate care decisions with other family members, and monitor adequacy and quality of care. Thus, caregiving can be time in-tensive, emotional, and physically demanding even with residential place-ment (Schulz et al., 2004).

HEALTH EFFECTS OF CAREGIVING

Understanding the health effects of caregiving is important for identifying supportive strategies, developing health policies, and planning for the organi-zation and delivery of services. Figure 9.1 (row 2) highlights known health effects as they unfold along the care trajectory. As shown, the negative health effects of caregiving increase with the amount of time and type of caregiving tasks required. Psychiatric symptoms (anxiety and depression) initially emerge in the early stages of caregiving, with more intensive hands-on assistance leading to significant physical health effects. Negative health effects can con-tinue with nursing home placement but appear to resolve following the death of the person receiving care and hence termination of care responsibilities (Schulz, Boerner, Shear, Zhang, and Gitlin, 2006).

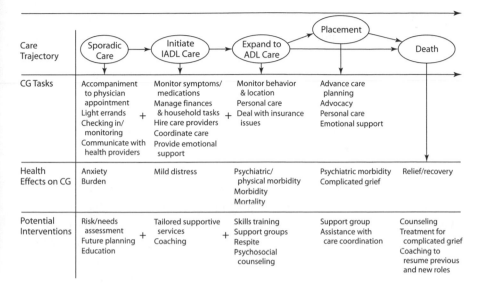

Fig. 9.1. Care task demands, health effects, and interventions along care trajectory. *Note*: CG = caregiver; IADL = instrumental activities of daily living (e.g., cooking, cleaning, shopping); ADL = activities of daily living (e.g., bathing, dressing, toileting). Entries based on research evidence.

The psychiatric and morbidity effects of caregiving are well documented (Pinquart and Sörensen, 2003a). Compared to non-caregivers, caregivers report more distress and lower quality of life. The largest differences between caregivers and non-caregivers are found for depression, stress, and self-efficacy. Differences persist with regard to physical health status again favoring non-caregivers, with the largest difference in health status occurring for dementia caregivers (Schulz, O'Brien, Bookwala, and Fleissner, 1995; Pinquart and Sörensen, 2003b). As a chronic stressor, caregiving has been shown to result in immune deregulation, poor sleep, and greater acute care utilization (for an overview see Vitaliano, Zhang, and Scanlan, 2003; Schubert et al., 2008).

High-Risk Groups

Although caregivers, compared with non-caregivers, are at risk for health and psychosocial difficulties, within the caregiving population itself, there are subgroups at elevated risk. Those at highest risk of health decline include low-income, younger caregivers and those with high levels of emotional distress. These groups experience more depression and anxiety compared with their non-caregiving counterparts and other caregivers. Stressed caregivers, especially spouses, are particularly at high risk for earlier placement of their family member in a nursing home (Spillman and Long, 2009), stroke and coronary heart disease (Haley, Roth, Howard, and Safford, 2010), and mortality (Schulz and Beach, 1999) in comparison with nonstressed caregivers.

Although the number of male caregivers is increasing, caregiving is still primarily a woman's health issue. Female caregivers are at higher health risk than their male counterparts (Yee and Schulz, 1999). They tend to report higher levels of depression, burden, distress, and poor health.

Caring for an individual with dementia places the family member at an even higher health risk level as this neurologically progressively deteriorating disease poses complex challenges requiring extraordinary care, high levels of skill, and long amounts of time spent in caregiving. Not surprisingly, dementia caregivers experience greater anxiety, depression, and poorer quality of life compared with caregivers of nondemented individuals (Ory, Hoffman, Yee, Tennstedt, and Schulz, 1999; Pinquart and Sörensen, 2003b, 2007). The relationship between dementia caregiving and depression is particularly well documented. Levels of depression range from 28% to 55% for this group, compared with 15% in the non-caregiving older adult population (Elliott, Burgio, and Decoster, 2010). Caregivers of individuals with dementia may also be at an increased risk for attaining that disease. In a sample of 2,442, spouse caregivers were six times more likely to develop dementia themselves if their spouse had dementia compared with older married adults whose spouse never developed the disease (Norton et al., 2010).

Health effects also differ by race and ethnic groups, with Hispanic populations reporting the greatest psychiatric symptoms compared with white or African American caregivers (Belle et al., 2006). There is strong evidence as well that Hispanic and African American spousal caregivers have poorer health than their white counterparts (Pinquart and Sörensen, 2005).

Inasmuch as caregiving tasks are physically, cognitively, and emotionally demanding, older, low-income, and chronically ill or disabled individuals who assume the caregiving role will also be at higher risk for adverse outcomes. Similarly, caregivers with limited experience and training may find these challenges overwhelming and be at higher risk than caregivers with greater resources, including knowledge and skills needed for caregiving (Pinquart and Sörensen, 2005).

Despite the overwhelming evidence of the negative health effects of caregiving, caution must be applied in generalizing to all caregiving populations. Most caregiver studies are restricted to volunteer samples as opposed to representative samples, are geographically limited, do not include racially/

ethnically diverse caregivers, or focus only on dementia caregivers (Pruchno et al., 2008). As studies are usually not representative of the population at large, it is not clear what the detrimental health effects of caregiving are at the population level. Existing data also provide limited understanding of the mechanisms by which caregiving increases morbidity and mortality. Most studies assume that providing care itself is responsible for poor health. However, recent population-based studies suggest that this may not be the case. For example, a population-based study found that spending 14 hours or more per week providing care to a spouse was associated with decreased mortality for caregivers, suggesting that caregiving is not uniformly an unhealthy role (Brown et al., 2009; Poulin et al., 2010).

Schulz and colleagues suggest that the health effects of caregiving may be partially determined by the amount of suffering expressed by the care recipient and the caregiver's ability to effectively decrease care recipient suffering. In the early stages of a caregiving career, when care recipient suffering may be limited and the caregiver can effectively address care recipient needs, caregiving may have salutary effects on health, whereas in later stages, when suffering is high and attempts to help the care recipient are futile, caregiving may be more likely to contribute to negative health effects (Schulz et al., 2007; Monin and Schulz, 2009).

Caregiving as a Health Disparity

Family caregivers are hidden patients (Reinhard, Brooks-Danso, and Kelly 2008) yet are rarely assessed for their own health and caregiving needs. Moreover, by virtue of time spent in caregiving, they may find that they do not have time or energy to engage in health-promoting behaviors, preventive doctor visits, or their own disease management. Spouses in particular are at risk for not engaging in health-promoting strategies (Talley and Crews, 2007). Thus, compared with non-caregivers, caregivers experience significant gaps in the quality of their health and health care. Recognizing caregiving as a health disparity provides a basis for organizing a public health response (see chap. 5).

ECONOMIC COSTS

Although the economic implications of caregiving are difficult to discern worldwide, data from the United States provide important clues. The national economic value of family caregiving is extraordinary (Arno, Levine, and Memmott, 1999). Estimated at $350 billion, it is as much as 2005 Medicare program expenditures ($342 billion) and more than 2005 Medicaid expenditures ($300 billion), nursing home and home health care ($206.6 billion), and formal home care ($76.8 billion; Gibson and Houser, 2007). As family caregiving reduces nursing home placement (Spillman and Long, 2009), this represents a cost savings from a societal perspective.

Costs associated with caregiving vary by condition of the individual receiving care. Caregivers of individuals with dementia spend much more time providing care than caregivers of individuals with other conditions. Thus, the estimated economic value of caring for the dementia population living at home is $144 billion (12.5 billion hours of care valued at $11.50 per hour) (Alzheimer's Association, 2010). The cost of caregiving is also high for adult siblings of persons with mental illness who assume primary care. An average of $1,277 and 73 hours more each year is spent by this group compared with nonprimary caregivers (Lohrer, Lukens, and Thorning, 2007).

The personal costs of caregiving are also high. The yearly expenditure for caregiving has been estimated at $10,400 (using an hourly rate of $9.63) for caregivers overall and four times that amount ($43,000) for caregivers of individuals with dementia (Gibson and Houser, 2007). The Caregiving in the U.S. 2009 survey found that while most caregivers (70%) report little to no financial hardship from caregiving, Hispanics, those with low income, and those reporting high burden are more likely to report significant financial challenges. A U.S. survey of 1,000 caregivers providing 5 or more hours of ADL or IADL care showed that they had an estimated annual out-of-pocket expense of $5,531. This represented more than 10% of the median income ($43,026) of the group. Long-distance caregivers have estimated annual expenses of $8,728, which are higher than for caregivers living with the care recipient ($5,885) or close by ($4,570). Greater financial hardship has also been linked to higher caregiver stress (National Alliance for Caregiving and Evercare, 2007).

The economic downturn in the United States has had widespread impact on caregivers. A survey of 1,005 caregivers found that 60% reported increased care expenditures and difficulty paying for basic needs and 63% reported saving less for retirement, with those providing the most intense personal care at greatest financial risk. For working caregivers (64% of sample), 50% reported increased reluctance to take time off from work to provide care in fear of losing their job, 33% reported having to work more hours or get an additional job, 43% had cuts of work hours or pay, and 15% indicated that the economic recession resulted in job loss (Evercare and National Alliance for Caregiving,

2009). Accommodations for working caregivers cost U.S. employers between $11.4 billion and $29 billion per year in lost productivity (National Alliance for Caregiving and Lifeplans, Inc., 2001).

SUPPORTING FAMILY CAREGIVERS

Figure 9.1 also outlines the needs and range of supportive services for caregivers throughout the care trajectory. A robust research literature documents that caregiver interventions at each stage along this trajectory can effectively improve caregiver well-being. Taken as a whole, these studies show that services including education, skills training, problem solving, environmental redesign, and social support can reduce stress, burden, and depression; enhance efficacy and skills; reduce health care utilization; and delay nursing home placement (see Rosalynn Carter Institute for evidence-based caregiver interventions: www.rosalynncarter.org/caregiver_intervention_database/).

Interventions can be broadly categorized as those targeting the individual being cared for or objective aspects of burden such as time spent caregiving or environmental stressors (e.g., respite, removing unsafe conditions), those that target the caregiver and address subjective burden and competency (e.g., counseling, skills training, support groups), those that target both care receiver and caregiver, and those at the societal level. Greater positive outcomes have been found for caregivers of individuals with physical versus cognitive impairments (Sörensen, Pinquart, and Duberstein, 2002; Pinquart and Sörensen, 2006).

Most intervention research has focused on caregivers of individuals with dementia (for National Institutes of Health [NIH] Resources for Enhancing Alzheimer's Caregiver Health [REACH I] studies see *Gerontologist*, 2003, vol. 43(4); for NIH REACH II study see Belle et al., 2006), as this group experiences poorer health, greater psychiatric and physical morbidity, and are at greater risk of institutionalizing their family member than caregivers of individuals with physical impairments. Randomized controlled trials suggest that multicomponent, supportive, and risk reduction approaches effectively enhance emotional and physical health, skills, self-efficacy, and sleep quality.

Although caregiver interventions vary in dose, intensity, and mode of delivery (telephone, mail, face-to-face, technology), several treatment principles can be derived across effective interventions (Zarit and Femia, 2008; Gitlin, 2009). These include active involvement of family caregivers in the treatment process versus didactic, prescriptive approaches or providing education only (Belle et al., 2003; Chee, Gitlin, Denis, and Hauck, 2007); tailoring interventions to specific needs (Richards et al., 2007); addressing multiple areas of need (Belle et al., 2006; Zarit and Femia, 2008); longer interventions or episodic support over the duration of caregiving; and adjusting dose and intensity of intervention based on risk profiles (Belle et al., 2006; Montgomery and Kwak, 2008; Czaja et al., 2009). Interventions that are client centered and tailored to specific needs are efficient and incorporate elements of emerging novel treatment models (e.g., medical home, collaborative primary care).

Despite a promising literature, most intervention studies in the United States and in low- and middle-income countries have been conducted with small sample sizes (less than 600), use nonprobability sampling, are geographically bounded, are not representative of diverse populations, and include a limited set of outcome measures. Unknown, for example, is the effect of supportive services on hospitalization rates of caregivers and care receivers, mortality, or cost savings to families or society. Also, with few exceptions (Burgio et al., 2009; Gitlin, Jacobs, and Vause-Earland, 2010; Nichols, Martindale-Adams, Burns, Graney, and Zuber, 2011), interventions have not been translated for delivery in different care settings, nor are funding streams available to sustain program delivery aside from federal or foundation grant mechanisms. Thus, proven interventions are currently not part of standard care in most clinical and social service settings, and when available, they are offered as an out-of-pocket expense or part of time-limited grant mechanisms. Therefore, despite proliferation of proven interventions, the vast majority of families continue to be underserved, have unmet needs, or receive services that are not evidence-based (Sörensen et al., 2002; Brodaty, Green, and Koschera, 2003; Centers for Disease Control and Prevention, 2008).

Another consideration is that caregiver interventions are not always aligned with the evidence generated from population-based surveys. For example, data from the 1999 National Long Term Care survey suggest that the physical demands and financial burdens of caregiving contribute to caregiver stress, a strong predictor of nursing home placement for the care recipient (Spillman and Long, 2009). Thus, developing and testing interventions that address the physical demands of caregiving or that offer economic incentives may have a stronger impact on delaying or preventing nursing home placement than other approaches tested thus far.

Interventions at the societal level are limited. In the United States all states have programs to support family caregivers such as respite or adult day services. Adult day services provide families brief time away from care responsibilities and can reduce burden. Augmenting adult day services with systematic care management can boost benefits, including delaying nursing home placement and improving caregiver well-being (Gitlin, Reever, Dennis, Mathieu, and Hauck, 2006).

Support for families through the National Family Caregiver Support Program (NFCSP) has been modest. In 2005, NFCSP provided about $155 million in grants to states, representing about $200 per caregiver served (Administration on Aging, 2004). The Lifespan Respite Care Act of 2006 provides state grants to enhance respite and other services for caregivers but only recently received funding (Spillman and Long, 2009). Some states are seeking legislation to provide federal tax credits for families.

Similar limitations and challenges are present worldwide, especially for resource-poor countries. Research on interventions to support caregivers of individuals with dementia in India, Russia, and Latin America is promising. Using lay or community-based interventionists, caregivers are provided basic education and supportive services. However, caution is advised when implementing interventions developed in one country in another as cultural variations must be accounted for within and across countries (Mittelman, Brodaty, Wallen, and Burns, 2008).

PUBLIC HEALTH RESPONSE

In the United States, Healthy People 2020 includes a new indicator specific to supporting family caregivers ("Reduce the proportion of unpaid caregivers of older adults who report an unmet need for caregiver support services"), signaling a movement toward viewing caregiving from a population-based perspective and through a public health lens (www.healthypeople.gov/2020/topicsobjectives2020/objectiveslist.aspx?topicid=31). Table 9.1 identifies eight elements of an infrastructure necessary to inform a public health response to family caregiving. It also highlights progress to date to put such an infrastructure in place. Here we highlight key elements of such an infrastructure.

A key element of a public health infrastructure concerns surveillance or data monitoring. As we discussed, the information available on the prevalence, characteristics, and health effects of family caregiving in all regions of the world, including the United States, remains fragmentary. Although in the United States some surveillance data exist, they are inconsistent and not comprehensive. Thus, to assess the comparative importance of health risks in different caregiving populations and derive comprehensive and consistent estimates of mortality, morbidity, care challenges, and unmet needs, a comprehensive surveillance approach is necessary. The approach adopted by the World Health Organization to examine the global burden of disease may serve

TABLE 9.1
Components of a public health infrastructure to support caregiving

Component	Description	Progress to date
Consistent definition not dependent on self-disclosure or self-identification	Broad uniform definition to ensure consistency in measurement and outreach	- No consensus - Inconsistency in definitions used - Most research still dependent on self-identification
National and state prevalence data	Ongoing nationwide surveillance data to trace number of careers, tasks performed, and health effects	One caregiver question included in 2009 BRFSS core questionnaire; caregivers' module (10 questions) implemented in only a few states
National public health goal to support families	Articulated national goal to ease caregiver burden	Healthy People 2020 includes goal to provide evidence-based programs
Assessment of caregiver risks and needs	Consistent, standardized statewide comprehensive needs assessments that can be linked to services and delivery of evidence-based programs	- A few states have adopted TCARE® (Montgomery comprehensive assessment) - REACH II brief risk assessment validated and can be used in variety of settings
Public health education	National campaign to raise awareness and education about caregiving and supportive services	No government sponsored programs to date
Policy initiatives and legislation that support caregivers	Federal and state policy initiatives and legislation to provide tax credits, access to evidence-based services, and reimbursement for caregiver training and education	National Family Caregiver Program
Technical support to states and community organizations	Support for aging network services and community-based agencies to assess and deliver evidence-based programs	Some technical support available through researchers of evidence-based programs, Rosalynn Carter Institute, Administration on Aging, CDC's Healthy Aging Research Network, Substance Abuse and Mental Health Services Administration
Training health and human service professionals to involve families as partners in care	Develop and implement competencies and accreditation criteria for working effectively with family caregivers	State of the Science 2008 national conference yielded published competencies for nursing and social work

as a model (World Health Organization, 2008). In the United States, epidemiologic data at both the state and local levels (Talley and Crews, 2007) will be important to better inform local policies and program implementation. State-level data in particular are necessary to enable local documentation, planning, benchmarking, and prioritizing of caregiver needs.

Another important infrastructure element is detailing more carefully the disparities in health between those who do and those who do not provide care. While a strong relationship between caregiving and health has been established, many areas require further systematic inquiry, particularly as they concern identifying mechanisms linking caregiving to health decline and mortality. Also, examining special populations of caregivers, such as those with comorbidities and geographically, racially, and ethnically diverse caregivers, is an important area for continued investigation.

Another consideration is the professional training of health care providers (doctors, nurses, social workers, occupational therapists, physical therapists, direct care workers) to adopt family-centered care models that include the assessment of caregiver needs and the skills they may have and need. The advancement of integrated health care models such as the medical home and collaborative and patient-centered care that involve partnerships with family members will require research to determine the most effective approaches to involving families and training health professionals in these best practices. Health professional groups are currently examining the competencies necessary for and professional challenges of this paradigm shift (see new competencies for nursing and social work; Given, Sherwood, and Given, 2008; Reinhard et al., 2008; Mitnick, Leffler, and Hood, 2010). The Institute of Medicine has recommended that informal caregivers receive training to reduce the burden of care and also to improve care to older adults (2008). Thus, developing an infrastructure for continuous systematic assessment of caregiver needs over the care trajectory and systematically enabling families to access evidence-based supportive services are paramount to a positive public health response to caregiving.

CONCLUSION

We stand at the crossroads of dramatic societal and demographic transitions that place increasing demands on families to provide ongoing, more intensive and complex care to older adults. Family caregiving is now longer in duration and more expansive in terms of roles and responsibilities than at any other historical juncture. Family caregivers form the backbone of health care systems in developed, low-income, and middle-income countries. Families are typically unpaid, yet their contributions to long-term care services are critical to the economies of most countries. Nevertheless, while the demands on caregivers are increasing, there has not been a coordinated, systematic public health response. Also, little formal support is made available to this group, and they have not been fully integrated in new patient-centered models of care.

A public health perspective is critical to developing an understanding of and response to this important public health issue. Critical ethical questions also emerge, including the following: (1) Under what circumstances can family care substitute for nursing home placement? (2) Are we placing undo expectations and demands on families to provide care that is too complex and medically demanding, and at what expense to the caregiver's own health and well-being? (3) How can we create a health care delivery system that balances the roles of families, recognizes what they can and cannot do, and supports families in the care tasks they provide? (4) Is the economic savings of having families provide care a societal savings when those at high risk have higher health care utilization rates? These are some of the pressing issues that must be addressed if we are to publically and equitably respond to the rising caregiver crisis.

ACKNOWLEDGMENTS

The authors were supported in part by grants from the National Institute on Aging and the National Institute of Nursing Research (R01 AG22254, R01 AG026010, R01 AG032370, R01 NR009573), the National Institute of Mental Health (P30 MH071944), the National Science Foundation (NSF0540865), the Health Research and Services Administration (UB4HP19199), the PA Department of Health, Tobacco Settlement (SAP#100027298), and the Alzheimer's Association (IIRG-07–28686). Work on this paper was conducted by Dr. Gitlin while she was the director of the Jefferson Center for Applied Research on Aging and Health, Thomas Jefferson University, Philadelphia, PA.

REFERENCES

AARP, National Alliance for Caregiving, and United Nations Programme on Ageing. 2008. *AARP International IDOP 2008: Global Perspectives on Family Caregiving Conference.*

Administration on Aging. 2004. *The Older Americans Act National Family Caregiver Support Program: Compassion in Action.* Retrieved July 10, 2010, from www.aoa .gov/AoAroot/Program_Results/docs/Program_Eval/FINAL%20NFCSP%20 Report%20July22,%202004.pdf.

Agency for Healthcare Research and Quality. 2000. *Long-Term Care Users Range in Age and Most Do Not Live in Nursing Homes.* Retrieved December 28, 2010, from http://archive.ahrq.gov/news/press/pr2000/ltcpr.htm.

Alzheimer's Association. 2010. *2010 Alzheimer's Disease Facts and Figures.* Retrieved December 28, 2010, from www.alz.org/documents_custom/report_alzfactsfigures 2010.pdf.

American Association of Retired Persons (AARP). 2003. *These Four Walls: Americans 45+ Talk about Home and Community.* Washington, DC: Author.

Arno, P. S., C. Levine, and M. M. Memmott. 1999. The economic value of informal caregiving. *Health Affairs* 18:182–88.

Belle, S. H., L. Burgio, R. Burns, D. Coon, S. J. Czaja, D. Gallagher-Thompson, L. N. Gitlin, J. Klinger, K. M. Koepke, C. C. Lee, J. Martindale-Adams, L. Nichols, R. Schulz, S. Stahl, A. Stevens, L. Winter, and S. Zhang. 2006. Enhancing the quality of life of dementia caregivers from different ethnic or racial groups: A randomized, controlled trial. *Annals of Internal Medicine* 145:727–38.

Belle, S. H., S. J. Czaja, R. Schulz, S. Zhang, L. D. Burgio, L. N. Gitlin, R. Jones, A. B. Mendelsohn, and M. Ory. 2003. Using a new taxonomy to combine the uncombinable: Integrating results across diverse interventions. *Psychology and Aging* 18:396–405.

Brodaty, H., A. Green, and A. Koschera. 2003. Meta-analysis of psychosocial interventions for caregivers of people with dementia. *Journal of the American Geriatrics Society* 51:657–64.

Brown, S. L., D. M. Smith, R. Schulz, M. U. Kabeto, P. A. Ubel, M. Poulin, J. Yi, C. Kim, and K. M. Langa. 2009. Caregiving behavior is associated with decreased mortality risk: Research article. *Psychological Science* 20:488–94.

Burgio, L. D., I. B. Collins, B. Schmid, T. Wharton, D. McCallum, and J. Decoster. 2009. Translating the REACH caregiver intervention for use by area agency on aging personnel: The REACH OUT program. *Gerontologist* 49:103–16.

Care Alliance Ireland. 2010. Family caring in Ireland. Retrieved December 28, 2010, from www.carersireland.com/userfiles/file/Family%20Caring%20in%20Ireland%20 An%20Overview%20May%202010.pdf.

Centers for Disease Control and Prevention. 2008. *Assuring Healthy Caregivers, A Public Health Approach to Translating Research into Practice: The RE-AIM Framework.* Washington, DC: Author.

Chee, Y. K., L. N. Gitlin, M. P. Dennis, and W. W. Hauck. 2007. Predictors of adherence to a skill-building intervention in dementia caregivers. *Journals of Gerontology Series A: Biological Sciences and Medical Sciences* 62:673–78.

Czaja, S. J., L. N. Gitlin, R. Schulz, S. Zhang, L. D. Burgio, A. B. Stevens, L. O. Nichols, and D. Gallagher-Thompson. 2009. Development of the risk appraisal measure: A brief screen to identify risk areas and guide interventions for dementia caregivers. *Journal of the American Geriatrics Society* 57:1064–72.

Dilworth-Anderson, P., S. W. Williams, and T. Cooper. 1999. Family caregiving to elderly African Americans: Caregiver types and structures. *Journals of Gerontology Series B: Psychological Sciences and Social Sciences* 54:S237–41.

Donelan, K., C. A. Hill, C. Hoffman, K. Scoles, P. H. Feldman, C. Levine, and D. Gould.

2002. Challenged to care: Informal caregivers in a changing health system. *Health Affairs* 21(4):222–31.

Elliot, A. F., L. D. Burgio, and J. Decoster. 2010. Enhancing caregiver health: Findings from the Resources for Enhancing Alzheimer's Caregiver Health II Intervention. *Journal of the American Geriatrics Society* 58:30–37.

EuroFamCare Project. n.d.. *Welcome to EUROFAMCARE*. Retrieved December 28, 2010, from www.uke.de/extern/eurofamcare/.

Evercare and National Alliance for Caregiving. 2009. The Evercare® Survey of the economic downturn and its impact on family caregiving. Retrieved July 15, 2010, from www.caregiving.org/data/EVC_Caregivers_Economy_Report%20 FINAL_4–28–09.pdf.

Federal Interagency Forum on Age-Related Statistics. 2010. *Older Americans 2010: Key Indicators of Well-Being*. Retrieved December 28, 2010, from www.agingstats .gov/agingstatsdotnet/Main_Site/Data/2010_Documents/Docs/OA_2010.pdf.

Gerontologist. 2003. *Special Section: Resources for Enhancing Alzheimer's Caregiver Health*. 43:514–91.

Gibson, J. J., and A. Houser. 2007. *Valuing the Invaluable: A New Look at the Economic Value of Family Caregiving*. AARP Public Policy Institute Issue Brief. Retrieved December 28, 2010, from http://assets.aarp.org/rgcenter/il/ib82_caregiving.pdf.

Gitlin, L. N. 2009. Environmental adaptations for older adults and their family members in the home and community. In *International Handbook of Occupational Therapy Interventions*, ed. I. Soderbck, pp. 53–62. New York: Springer.

Gitlin, L. N., M. Jacobs, and T. Vause-Earland. 2010. Translation of a dementia caregiver intervention for delivery in homecare as a reimbursable Medicare Service: Outcomes and lessons learned. *Gerontologist* doi:10.1093/geront/gnq057.

Gitlin, L. N., K. Reever, M. P. Dennis, E. Mathieu, and W. W. Hauck. 2006. Enhancing quality of life of families who use adult day services: Short and long-term effects of the "Adult Day Services Plus" program. *Gerontologist* 46:630–39.

Given, B., P. R. Sherwood, and C. W. Given. 2008. What knowledge and skills do caregivers need? *American Journal of Nursing* 108(Suppl. 9):28–34.

Haley, W. E., D. L. Roth, G. Howard, and M. M. Safford. 2010. Caregiving strain and estimated risk for stroke and coronary heart disease among spouse caregivers: Differential effects of race and sex. *Stroke* 41:331–36.

Institute of Medicine. 2008. *Retooling for an Aging America: Building the Health Care Workforce*. Washington, DC: National Academies Press.

Institute of Medicine Committee on Disability in America. 2007. *The Future of Disability in America*, ed. M. J. Field and A. M. Jette. Washington, DC: National Academies Press.

Kaye, H. S., C. Harrington, and M. P. LaPlante. 2010. Long-term care: Who gets it, who provides it, who pays, and how much? *Health Affairs* 9(1):11–21.

Levine, C., G. Gibson Hunt, D. Halper, A. Y. Hart, J. Lautz, and D. A. Gould. 2005. Young adult caregivers: A first look at an unstudied population. *American Journal of Public Health* 95:2071–75.

Levine, C., D. Halper, A. Peist, and D. A. Gould. 2010. Bridging troubled waters: Family caregivers, transitions, and long-term care. *Health Affairs* 29(1):116–24.

Lohrer, S. P., E. P. Lukens, and H. Thorning. 2007. Economic expenditures associated with instrumental caregiving roles of adult siblings of persons with severe mental illness. *Community Mental Health Journal* 43(2):129–51.

Mitnick, S., C. Leffler, and V. L. Hood, for the American College of Physicians Ethics and Human Rights Committee. 2010. Family caregivers, patients and physicians: Ethical guidance to optimize relationships. *Journal of General Internal Medicine* doi:10.1007/s11606–009–1206–3.

Mittelman, M. S., H. Brodaty, A. S. Wallen, and A. Burns. 2008. A three-country randomized controlled trial of a psychosocial intervention for caregivers combined with pharmacological treatment for patients with Alzheimer disease: Effects on caregiver depression. *American Journal of Geriatric Psychiatry* 16:893–904.

Monin, J. K., and R. Schulz. 2009. Interpersonal effects of suffering in older adult caregiving relationships. *Psychology and Aging* 24:681–95.

Montgomery, R., and J. Kwak. 2008. TCARE: Tailored caregiver assessment and referral. *American Journal of Nursing* 108(Suppl. 9):54–57.

National Alliance for Caregiving. 2004. *Miles Away: The MetLife Study of Long-Distance Caregiving.* Washington, DC. Retrieved December 28, 2010, from www.caregiving.org/data/milesaway.pdf.

National Alliance for Caregiving and AARP. 2004. *Caregiving in the U.S.* Washington, DC: Authors.

National Alliance for Caregiving and AARP. 2009. *Caregiving in the U.S.* Washington, DC: National Alliance for Caregiving, American Association of Retired Persons.

National Alliance for Caregiving and Evercare. 2007. *Family Caregivers—What They Spend, What They Sacrifice.* Retrieved December 28, 2010, from www.caregiving.org/data/Evercare_NAC_CaregiverCostStudyFINAL20111907.pdf.

National Alliance for Caregiving and Lifeplans, Inc. 2001. *The MetLife Study of Employed Caregivers: Does Long Term Care Insurance Make a Difference?* Retrieved December 28, 2010, from www.metlife.com/assets/cao/mmi/publications/studies/mmi-studies-does-ltci-make-a-diff.pdf.

National Family Caregivers Association and Family Caregiver Alliance. 2006. *Prevalence, Hours and Economic Value of Family Caregiving: Updated State-by-State Analysis of 2004 National Estimates* (by Peter S. Arno, PhD). Kensington, MD: NFCA; and San Francisco: FCA.

National Institute on Aging and Duke University. 2004. *National Long-Term Care Survey.* Retrieved December 28, 2010, from www.nltcs.aas.duke.edu.

Nichols, L. O., J. Martindale-Adams, R. Burns, M. J. Graney, and J. Zuber. 2011. Translation of a dementia caregiver support program in a health care system: REACH VA. *Archives of Internal Medicine,* 171(4):353–59. doi:10.1001/archinternalmed.2010.543.

Norton, M. C., K. R. Smith, T. Østbye, J. T. Tschanz, C. Corcoran, S. Schwartz, K. W. Piercy, P. V. Rabins, D. C. Steffens, I. Skoog, J. C. Breitner, and K. A. Welsh-Bohmer; Cache County Investigators. 2010. Greater risk of dementia when spouse has dementia? The Cache County study. *Journal of the American Geriatrics Society* 58:895–900.

Ory, M. G., R. R. Hoffman, J. L. Yee, S. Tennstedt, and R. Schulz, R. 1999. Prevalence and impact of caregiving: A detailed comparison between dementia and nondementia caregivers. *Gerontologist* 39:177–86.

Pinquart, M., and S. Sörensen. 2003a. Associations of stressors and uplifts of caregiving with caregiver burden and depressive mood: A meta-analysis. *Journals of Gerontology Series B: Psychological Sciences and Social Sciences* 58:112–28.

Pinquart, M., and S. Sörensen. 2003b. Differences between caregivers and noncaregivers in psychological health and physical health: A meta-analysis. *Psychology and Aging* 18:250–67.

Pinquart, M., and S. Sörensen. 2005. Ethnic differences in stressors, resources, and psychological outcomes of family caregiving: A meta-analysis. *Gerontologist* 45:90–106.

Pinquart, M., and S. Sörensen. 2006. Helping caregivers of persons with dementia: Which interventions work and how large are their effects? *International Psychogeriatrics* 18:577–95.

Pinquart, M., and S. Sörensen. 2007. Correlates of physical health of informal caregivers: A meta-analysis. *Journals of Gerontology Series B: Psychological Sciences and Social Sciences* 62:126–37.

Poulin, M. J., S. L. Brown, P. A. Ubel, D. M. Smith, A. Jankovic, and K. M. Langa. 2010. Does a helping hand mean a heavy heart? Helping behavior and well-being among spouse caregivers. *Psychology and Aging* 25(1):108–17.

Pruchno, R. A., J. E. Brill, Y. Shands, J. R. Gordon, M. W. Genderson, M. Rose, and F. Cartwright. 2008. Convenience samples and caregiving research: How generalizable are the findings? *Gerontologist* 48:820–27.

Reinhard, S. C., A. Brooks-Danso, and K. Kelly, eds. 2008. State of the science: Professional partners supporting family caregiving. *American Journal of Nursing* 108(Suppl. 9).

Richards, K. C., C. A. Enderlin, C. Beck, J. C. McSweeney, T. C. Jones, and P. K. Roberson. 2007. Tailored biobehavioral interventions: A literature review and synthesis. *Research and Theory for Nursing Practice: An International Journal* 21(4):271–85.

Robert Graham Center. 2007. *The Patient Centered Medical Home: History, Seven Core Features, Evidence and Transformational Change.* Retrieved December 28, 2010, from www.aafp.org/online/etc/medialib/aafp_org/documents/about/pcmh .Par.0001.File.dat/PCMH.pdf.

Roth, D. L., M. Perkins, V. G. Wadley, E. M. Temple, and W. E. Haley. 2009. Family caregiving and emotional strain: Associations with quality of life in a large national sample of middle-aged and older adults. *Quality of Life Research: An International Journal of Quality of Life Aspects of Treatment, Care and Rehabilitation* 18:679–88.

Schubert, C. C., M. Boustani, C. M. Callahan, A. J. Perkins, S. Hui, and H. C. Hendrie. 2008. Acute care utilization by dementia caregivers within urban primary care practices. *Journal of General Internal Medicine* 23:1736–40.

Schulz, R., and S. R. Beach. 1999. Caregiving as a risk factor for mortality: The caregiver health effects study. *Journal of the American Medical Association* 282:2215–19.

Schulz, R., H. Belle, S. Czaja, K. McGinnis, A. Stevens, and S. Zhang. 2004. Long-term care placement of dementia patients and caregiver health and well-being. *Journal of the American Medical Association* 292:961–67.

Schulz, R., K. Boerner, K. Shear, S. Zhang, and L. N. Gitlin. 2006. Predictors of complicated grief among dementia caregivers: A prospective study of bereavement. *Archives of General Psychiatry* 14:650–58.

Schulz, R., R. S. Hebert, M. A. Dew, S. L. Brown, M. F. Schheier, S. R. Beach, S. J. Czaja, L. M. Martire, D. Coon, K. M. Langa, L. N. Gitlin, A. B. Stevens, and L. Nichols. 2007. Patient suffering and caregiver compassion: New opportunities for research, practice and policy. *Gerontologist* 47:4–13.

Schulz, R., and L. M. Martire. 2004. Family caregiving of persons with dementia: Prevalence, health effects, and support strategies. *American Journal of Geriatric Psychiatry* 12(3):240–49.

Schulz, R., A. T. O'Brien, J. Bookwala, and K. Fleissner. 1995. Psychiatric and physical morbidity effects of dementia caregiving: Prevalence, correlates, and causes. *Gerontologist* 35:771–91.

Schulz, R., and C. A. Tompkins. 2010. *Informal Caregivers in the United States: Prevalence, Characteristics, and Ability to Provide Care. Human Factors in Home Health Care.* Washington, DC: National Academies Press.

Shalowitz, D., E. Garrett-Mayer, and D. Wendler. 2006. The accuracy of surrogate decision makers: A systematic review. *Archives of Internal Medicine* 166:493–97.

Sörensen, S., M. Pinquart, and P. Duberstein. 2002. How effective are interventions with caregivers? An updated meta-analysis. *Gerontologist* 42:356–72.

Spillman, B. C., and K. J. Black. 2005. *Staying the Course: Trends in Family Caregiving.* Retrieved December 28, 2010, from http://assets.aarp.org/rgcenter/il/2005_17_caregiving.pdf.

Spillman, B. C., and S. K. Long. 2009. Does high caregiver stress predict nursing home entry? *Inquiry* 46(2):140–61.

Stone, R., G. L. Cafferata, and J. Sangl, J. 1987. Caregivers of the frail elderly: A national profile. *Gerontologist* 27:616–26.

Stoops, N. 2004. *Current Population Reports. Educational Attainment in the United States: 2003 Population Characteristics.* Washington, DC: U.S. Department of Commerce, Economics and Statistics Administration, U.S. Census Bureau.

Talley, R. C., and J. E. Crews. 2007. Framing the public health of caregiving. *American Journal of Public Health* 97:224–28.

United Nations. 2007. *World Population Ageing.* Retrieved December 28, 2010, from www.un.org/esa/population/publications/WPA2007/wpp2007.htm.

Vitaliano, P. P., J. Zhang, and J. M. Scanlan. 2003. Is caregiving hazardous to one's physical health? A meta-analysis. *Psychological Bulletin* 129:946–72.

Weinberg, D., W. Lusenhop, J. H. Gittell, and C. Kautz. 2007. Coordination between formal providers and informal caregivers. *Health Care Management Review* 32(2):140–49.

Wolff, J. L., C. M. Boyd, L. N. Gitlin, M. L. Bruce, and D. L. Roter. In press. Going it together: Persistence of older adults' accompaniment to physician visits by a family companion. *Journal of the American Geriatrics Society.*

Wolff, J. L., and J. D. Kasper. (2006). Caregivers of frail elders: Updating a national profile. *Gerontologist* 46:344–56.

Wolff, J. L., and D. L. Roter. 2008. Hidden in plain sight: Medical visit companions as a resource for vulnerable older adults. *Archives of Internal Medicine* 168:1409–15.

World Health Organization. 2008. *The Global Burden of Disease: 2004 Update.* Retrieved June 15, 2010, from www.who.int/healthinfo/global_burden_disease/ GBD_report_2004update_full.pdf.

Yee, J. L., and R. Schulz. 1999. Gender differences in psychiatric morbidity among family caregivers: A review and analysis. *Gerontologist* 35:771–91.

Zarit, S., and E. Femia. 2008. Behavioral and psychosocial interventions for family caregivers. *American Journal of Nursing* 108(Suppl. 9):47–53.

CHAPTER 10

Social Engagement and a Healthy Aging Society

Nancy Morrow-Howell, PhD
Sarah Gehlert, PhD

Social engagement has always taken center stage in discussions of aging well. Successful aging and productive aging frameworks spotlight engagement in social roles that are meaningful to the individual and to society (Butler and Gleason, 1985; Rowe and Kahn, 1998). Increasing social activity among older adults is a goal of Healthy People 2020, the Older Americans Act reauthorization of 2006, and the World Health Organization (WHO) Active Ageing initiative. The World Health Organization's Active Ageing framework (WHO, 2002) posits "active ageing" as the desired outcome, which includes the optimization of opportunities for participation in social, economic, cultural, spiritual, and civic affairs, not just the ability to be physically active or to participate in the labor force.

Social engagement may play a unique role in later life. Social engagement becomes especially salient in the maintenance of physical and mental health for older adults who experience functional limitations, loss of social roles in the workplace and family, and death of friends and partners. For example, volunteering is protective of health in the face of roles loss, especially the loss of a spouse (Li, 2007; Hao, 2008). Social engagement is a critical component of reconstituting social networks after later-life residential relocation (Dupuis-Blanchard, Neufeld, and Strang, 2009) and after retirement (Harlow and Cantor, 1996). Lee, Jang, Lee, Cho, and Park (2008) demonstrated that while social participation decreases with age, the influence of participation on health is stronger among older than younger adults.

For all of these reasons, a great deal of theoretical and empirical attention has been directed toward social engagement as it occurs in later life. In general, this scholarly work has solidified the central importance of social engagement in the health of an aging society. Yet many questions deserve the ongoing attention of transdisciplinary researchers. In this chapter, we start with definitional issues. We then review current research about antecedents and outcomes of engagement, as well as mechanisms through which engagement affects health. Finally, we review current program and policy initiatives undertaken to increase social engagement and make recommendations for future directions.

WHAT IS SOCIAL ENGAGEMENT?

Social engagement is a term used quite loosely in the literature. Scholarly work has been limited by the lack of a consistent operationalization and measurement of the term. Many concepts overlap, like civic engagement and social capital. First, we present several definitions that are most representative of the concept of social engagement. We will distinguish the concepts of social network, social support, civic engagement, productive engagement, and social capital. However, we use the terms *social engagement* and *social participation* interchangeably, as these terms are not distinguished in the current literature.

Many scholars use the term *social engagement* to refer to participation in formal and informal social groups (Lindström, Hanson, and Östergren, 2001; Ellaway and Macintyre, 2007; Lee et al., 2008). Researchers assess activities within the two broad dimensions of formal (attendance at meeting/group/club, religious participation, and volunteering) and informal (social interactions with friends, neighbors, and relatives) (Utz, Carr, Nesse, and Wortman, 2002). Some researchers break it down further. For example, Brand and Burgard (2008) identified six potential arenas of participation: church-connected groups; charitable organizations; youth groups or community centers; civic, business, political, or neighborhood organizations; professional groups; and involvement in social or leisure activities, including clubs, sports teams, or weekly social gatherings with friends. As can be seen in these definitions, the assessment of social engagement lends itself to a list of specific activities and a query as to the extent of involvement.

Unfortunately, the lists of activities used to assess social engagement vary greatly and often include activities that challenge the core concept of participation in formal and informal groups. For example, reading, watching TV, and gardening have been included, although there is no indication if indeed they are done with other people. Marital status has been used as an indicator of social engagement, although no specific activity contexts are specified. Several scholars have differentiated social engagement from associated concepts of social network and social support. Berkman, Glass, Brissette, and Seeman (2000) clarify that engagement is distinct from social network and social support. In their view, participation/engagement involves the enactment of potential ties in real-life activity. Social networks (which can be described in terms of their size, density, homogeneity, frequency of contact, reciprocity, etc.) are groups of persons rather than activities or behaviors. Social networks can provide social support (instrumental, financial, emotional, etc.), as well as the opportunity for social engagement. Further, social engagement can lead to or build social networks. Bennett (2002) suggests that social aspects of aging can be considered in three broad headings, networks, support, and participation, and this argues further for distinguishing among them.

Several other terms warrant comment. *Civic engagement* often is used to mean membership in voluntary associations, volunteering, and political participation. Thus, civic engagement can be viewed as a subcomponent of social engagement, a smaller set of activities than are included in definitions of social engagement. Differentiating productive engagement is more problematic. Some activities generally categorized as productive, like volunteering and participation in education and training, are included in most assessments of social engagement. However, family caregiving and working, clear-cut productive activities, have been excluded because they are not as discretionary as other forms of participation. Caregiving and working are two critical activities for older adults that have implications for health of the individual and society, and many scholars have chosen to distinguish them from social engagement.

The burgeoning literature on social capital has also confounded the specification of social engagement. *Social capital* can be defined as the resources available to individuals and groups through their social connections to communities (Kawachi and Berkman, 2000). Most often, it is viewed as a collective good, distinguishing it from social network or social support (Cannuscio, Block, and Kawachi, 2003). Social engagement is clearly an integral part of social capital, but it has been viewed from various perspectives. For example, it has been used as an indicator of social capital (Greiner, Li, Kawachi, Hunt, and Ahluwalia, 2004) in that higher levels of engagement indicate higher levels of social capital in a community. It has been viewed as a necessary precursor to social capital. Rohe (2004) states that social capital begins with civic engagement and that those who are civically engaged will be involved in local social relationships that lead to trust and effective collective action. In sum, to achieve social capital, community residents must be socially engaged, and participation in formal and informal activities is an essential part of the social capital concept (Sundquist, Lindstrom, Malmstrom, Johansson, and Sundquist, 2004). However, social capital is a larger concept than social participation, and social capital also includes concepts of trust and reciprocity.

It may be useful to identify a set of distinct characteristics of social engagement. Engagement in *activity* is an essential element—individuals need to be doing something active, even if it is quite passive, such as conversing with another person. *Social context* is another essential element—solitary activities are not included in the definition, and at least one other person must be involved. Mars et al. (2009) suggest that in addition to social contact, there must be some sort of social exchange— contribution to society (e.g., paying a visit) or receiving from society (e.g., receiving a visit). These social activities can be formal (e.g., an association or club) or informal (e.g., a group of friends), but willful choice to participate is specified as a criterion (Bennett, 2002; Ellaway and Macintyre, 2007). This volitional aspect of social engagement has led some scholars to eliminate paid work from the construct, because in many cases it is nonvolitional (Berry, Rodgers, and Dear, 2007) (although social activities with work acquaintances outside of the job have been included). Finally, social engagement is largely viewed as outside of the immediate household and likewise outside of the workplace.

Several measurement approaches help to further define and distinguish among social engagement activities because each of them recognizes the need to identify the constituent elements of any participation concept. First, the Maasticht Social Participation Profile consists of four indices: consumptive participation (e.g., organized sports or physical activity, cultural or educational event, eating out, public event); formal social participation (e.g., committee work, volunteer work); informal social participation—acquaintances (e.g., visiting, communicating); and informal participation—family (e.g., vacationing, visiting) (Mars et al., 2009). Second, Berry et al. (2007) developed a measure of community participation with 14 categories: contact with immediate household, contact with extended families, contact with friends, contact with neighbors, social contact with workmates, adult learning, religious observation, organized community activities, voluntary sector activity, giving money to charity, active interest in current affairs, expressing opinions publically, community activism, and political protest. Finally, Baum et al. (2000) specified six types of participation in the domain of civic life (outside immediate home and work lives): informal social participation (visiting with family and friends), social activities in public spaces (social club, restaurant, theater, party), participation in social group (hobby, support, or sporting), individual civic participation (attending community meeting, contacting local officials), collective civic participation (e.g., attending political rallies or town hall meetings), and participation in other community groups (service clubs, volunteering, church-related). These examples illustrate the value of specifying type of social relationship (immediate household, extended family, friends, neighbors, and workmates), place of activity (outside of household, in public spaces), and type of activity (attending community meeting, volunteering).

The advancement of the scientific study of social engagement requires more development and use of standardized measures that capture information about social context and activity with increased specificity about the essential elements noted above. The literature to date, reviewed below, is indeed hampered by the inconsistent use and measurement of the social engagement concept.

EPIDEMIOLOGY OF SOCIAL ENGAGEMENT

A number of empirical studies help to define the epidemiology of social engagement. In a nationally representative sample of community-dwelling adults over the age of 65 years, Glass, Mendes de Leon, Bass, and Berkman (2006) documented the prevalence of various types of activities. Participation is highest in instrumental activities, such as preparing meals, shopping, and working in the yard/garden. Thirteen percent of participants in the study were involved in full- or part-time employment. Over 70% reported taking walks, and 36% reported engaging in physical exercise. In terms of social engagement, 17% said that they participated in community work, 46% attended religious services, and 41% participated in social and community groups. Over half of the participants in the study reported going out to movies, restaurants, and events (34% sometimes and 25% often). Playing cards and games was common, with 15% reporting sometimes and 21% often. About 30% reported traveling. These data support an observation made by Bukov, Maas, and Lampert (2002) that social participation is cumulative, meaning that less resource-demanding forms of engagement (social and leisure activities) are more likely to be pursued before more resource-demanding forms, like volunteering or community work. Older adults participating in more demanding social activities are at the same time likely to be participating in less demanding activities.

Another approach to understanding the extent of social participation is to identify patterns of engagement. Croezen, Haveman-Nies, Alvarado, van't Veer, and De Groot (2009) studied 17 social activities of people over the age of 65 years and identified five subgroups. About half of the sample was classified as *less socially engaged*, 20% as *leisure engaged*, and 23% as *productively engaged*. The other two groups focused on caregivers: less socially engaged caregivers (5%) and socially engaged caregivers (2%). This approach facilitates targeting in that those older adults classified as less socially engaged or those caregivers classified as less socially engaged could be approached through program interventions to increase engagement.

Researchers have demonstrated that social engagement is patterned according to individual demographic, health, personality, socioeconomic, and environmental factors (Harwood, Pound, and Ebrahim, 2000). The WHO's Active Ageing framework identifies seven determinants, including personal, behavioral, physical environment, social environment, economic, health and social service systems, and the cross-cutting context of gender and culture. Most of these determinants have been addressed in the existing literature on older adults and social engagement.

In general, females and married persons have higher levels of participation, and individuals with higher socioeconomic status tend to participate more (Harwood et al., 2000). Poorer physical health and lower functional ability are associated with lower participation (Sorensen, Axelsen, and Avlund, 2002; Jang, Mortimer, Haley, and Borenstein Graves, 2004), and sensory impairments in vision, hearing, and communication reduce participation (Resnick, Fries, and Verbrugge, 1997). The effects of falls and fractures on social activities have been studied (Miller et al., 2009), and reduced social engagement after falling, even when lower extremity function is controlled for, may be explained by depressive symptoms. Some have suggested that mental health may have a greater effect on participation than physical health (Baum et al., 2000). Personality factors also have been associated with higher levels of participation, including lower levels of neuroticism and higher levels of extroversion (Krueger et al., 2009). The above findings have been confirmed by Croezen et al.'s (2009) cluster analysis, in which the cluster of less socially active older adults proved to be older, living alone, less well educated, and in poorer physical and mental health. The leisure engaged group was more likely to include women and persons with higher levels of education and good health.

Individual factors that influence participation must be considered in light of specific types of activities. For example, older men have higher levels of participation in political activities (Berry et al., 2007). Older women have higher levels of visiting with friends and neighbors and formal volunteering. Income and education are related to social activities in public spaces (e.g., going out to events, restaurants), as well as civic participation. Compared with younger adults, older people are more likely to participate in service clubs, volunteer groups, and churches and less likely to participate in educational organizations (Baum et al., 2000).

Physical environments affect the social participation of older adults more than they do younger adults (Glass and Balfour, 2003; Wen, Hawkley, and Cacioppo, 2006). Both objective and subjective assessments of neighborhoods are related to social participation (Bowling and Stafford, 2007), and disadvantaged neighborhoods influence participation through infrastructure, crime, and poor local facilities. Krause (2006) found that older adults who live in dilapidated neighborhoods encounter more negative interactions and receive less social support than do those who live in better-maintained neighborhoods, but these relationships were moderated by social skills. That is, if older adults have strong social skills, dilapidated neighborhoods are not associated with social support and interactions.

Various aspects of social context matter as well. In general, ethnic minorities have lower levels of social engagement, especially in formal organizations and volunteering. Older African Americans are highly involved in family caregiving, neighboring, and other forms of informal social assistance (Carlton-LaNey, 2007). Further, when informal volunteering is included in addition to formal volunteering, social engagement rates of African Americans and whites are relatively similar (Musick, Wilson, and Bynum, 2000). Yet older African Americans are underrepresented in formal organizations, and barriers identified include disparities in health and economic resources, competing demands of caregiving and working, and historic segregation (McBride, 2007).

Research demonstrates that social participation decreases with age (Lee et al., 2008), but the effects are most noticeable in the 79+ age range (Lefrançois, Leclerc, and Poulin, 1998). Older old age, by itself, does not explain withdrawal from social activities, but clearly age operates through many of the factors reviewed above. Older adults are less likely to be married and more likely to have functional and sensory limitations. They are less connected to educational and work institutions and thus have less opportunity for participation in social activities. For example, in regard to volunteering, people over the age of 55 were less likely to be asked to volunteer compared with younger age groups (Independent Sector, 2000). Further, driving cessation and lack of transportation among the 65+ population are associated with reduced participation (Marottoli et al., 2000).

Clearly, engagement opportunities are not evenly distributed across the population, and there is clearly the risk of social exclusion in the older population and for certain subgroups of older adults. A vicious cycle exists in that individuals with more frequent contacts and integration have more opportunity for engagement (Berkman et al., 2000). Individuals that are socially disengaged tend to be those who are economically and socially disadvantaged. The body of literature outlined in the following section demonstrates the negative health effects of such disengagement.

OUTCOMES OF SOCIAL ENGAGEMENT

Over 20 years ago, House, Landis, and Umberson (1988) concluded that social relationships have a predictive, arguably causal, association with health in their own right. The authors noted a positive association between social integration and life expectancy across populations as diverse as African Americans in Georgia and residents of Eastern Finland, with relative risks of mortality ranging from 1.08 to 4.00. The groundbreaking work of Berkman and Syme (1979) showed that social contact, including social participation, predicts mortality, after controlling for health, health behaviors, use of health services, and other covariates. Many subsequent studies have used various measures of social engagement, various measures of health outcomes, and different control variables to establish the positive effects of engagement on older adults.

Social engagement has been associated with increased longevity (Lennartsson and Silverstein, 2001; Bennett, 2002; Ramsay et al., 2008). In regard to self-reported health and function, Everard, Lach, Fisher, and Baum (2000) documented that social activities are associated with positive self-assessments of physical health and that activity may be more important for functioning than social support. In studying social capital, Nummela, Sulander, Rahkonen, Karisto, and Uutela (2008) considered social participation and trust together, and higher levels of participation and trust were associated with higher levels of self-rated health. There was a positive relationship between social participation and self-rated health in the 11 European countries in the Survey of Health, Ageing and Retirement in Europe (SHARE), although the strength of the relationship varied between countries (Sirven and Debrand, 2008). Sundquist et al. (2004) showed that individuals with low social participation were at increased risk of coronary heart disease, and this association was strong even after controlling for education, housing tenure, and smoking habits.

Social engagement has been related to mental health and life satisfaction outcomes as well. Michael, Berkman, Colditz, and Kawachi (2001) demonstrated that higher levels of social participation were associated with fewer mental health problems, and for individuals who were not depressed at baseline, social engagement affected trajectory of depressive symptoms over time. In studying risk factors of cardiovascular disease, Ellaway and Macintyre (2007) documented that social participation was related to less psychological distress. Several studies have found that higher levels of social engagement are related to higher levels of life satisfaction (Jang et al., 2004) and lower levels of loneliness (Newall et al., 2009).

A substantial body of work relates social engagement to cognitive function (Bassuk, Glass, and Berkman, 1999; Glei et al., 2005). Formal participation in church, senior centers, and volunteer organizations has been shown to be protective of cognitive abilities (Zunzunegui, Alvarado, Del Ser, and Otero, 2003; Carlson et al., 2009). Krueger et al. (2009) demonstrated that higher levels of engagement are associated with more optimal cognitive function, but that the association varied across domains of engagement, as would be expected, because social activities vary in degree of physical and cognitive involvement.

Social isolation can be seen as the absence of social engagement. Research has linked isolation to a number of health outcomes, including first occurrence of myocardial infarction, recurrence of stroke, and death among stroke patients (Boden-Albala, Litwak, Elkind, Rundek, and Sacco, 2005); mortality among patients with coronary artery disease (Brummett et al., 2001); and a number of adverse disease outcomes in older adults (Tomaka, 2006).

This body of work provides a convincing argument that social engagement influences health outcomes. But there are many complicating issues. First of all, despite longitudinal analyses, the work is pervasively challenged by the reciprocal relationship between engagement and health (Sørensen et al., 2002). Clearly, selection is an issue in this work, as older adults with higher levels of health and function are more socially engaged. There is evidence that both forces operate — that is, older adults with higher levels of well-being are active in social activities and also experience positive effects because of this participation (Thoits and Hewitt, 2001; Hao, 2008). Yet the evidence is mixed. To illuminate the reciprocal nature of engagement and cognitive function, Saczynski et al. (2006) assessed engagement in midlife (in 1968) and in late life (in 1991) for a group of 2,513 Japanese American men and assessed for dementia in 1994 and 1997. Those individuals with consistently low levels of engagement were at a slightly increased risk of dementia. Those individuals who dropped from high to low levels of engagement over this period were at highest risk of dementia. This could mean that high engagement in late life is protective *or* that levels of engagement were modified by the dementing process and drops in engagement were associated with the early stages of dementia. On the other side of the argument, Lövdén, Ghisletta, and Lindenberger (2005) focused on perceptual speed and demonstrated that social engagement influenced subsequent changes in speed more so than speed influenced engagement.

Research on social networks and social support demonstrates that certain social relationships can be stressful and produce negative health outcomes for individuals, and this may be the case with regard to social engagement. Berry et al. (2007) found that expressing opinions publically, political participation, and community activism are related to higher distress. Yet in general, individuals choose to participate in formal and informal organizations, and the discretionary nature of social engagement may explain why social activities outside the family have more positive effects on cognitive function than social contacts within the family (Glei et al., 2005).

Social engagement may have more positive effects for certain segments of the older population. There is evidence that older adults with fewer personal and social resources benefit more from volunteering (Musick, Herzog, and House, 1999; Piliavin and Siegl, 2007; Morrow-Howell, Hong, and Tang, 2009). Greenfield and Marks (2004) found that individuals with more social role losses (those without social roles as spouses, employees, parents) gained more from volunteering. In considering social engagement more generally, Jang et al. (2004) found that the positive relationship of social engagement with life satisfaction was stronger for those with a disability. Gender and age may moderate the relationship of social engagement and health outcomes, with the relationship being stronger for older people and for women. Research has documented that the effects of social engagement were at a maximum for older women (Lee et al., 2008) and that engagement with friends was more protective for older women than older men (Zunzunegui et al., 2003).

HOW DOES SOCIAL ENGAGEMENT LEAD TO HEALTH OUTCOMES?

The evidence supports a causal relationship between social engagement and health outcomes for older adults, and several potential pathways between social engagement and health have been identified. Putnam (2004) observed that research on the effects of social capital and health has relied on prior work about the importance of social networks and social support to health, and the same is true in the study of outcomes associated with social engagement. First, social engagement builds and reinforces social networks from which social support may come. Social support may affect health through at least three pathways: by positively influencing health behavior (e.g., encouraging exercise or help-seeking behavior), by improving psychological conditions (e.g., increasing self-esteem or self-efficacy), and by altering physiologic states (e.g., decreasing allostatic load and boosting immune function) (Berkman et al., 2000).

Optimal hypothalamic-pituitary-adrenal (HPA) functioning and associated levels of cortisol have been linked favorably to cardiovascular and brain health. Psychosocial stressors alter HPA functioning, and this stress response is modified by social support, especially in the face of chronic stress. Lutgendorf et al. (2005) found that social support was associated with "natural killer" cell activity among women awaiting surgery for ovarian cancer. Laboratory experiments with animals in which social grouping is varied and physiological outcomes measured provide evidence of the links between social isolation and disease outcomes. For example, socially isolated rats developed obesity, type 2 diabetes (Nonogaki, Nozue, and Oka, 2007), and delayed immune response (Hermes, Rosenthal, Montag, and McClintock, 2005) compared with group-housed peers.

Beyond social support, social engagement may be related to health because it involves physical and cognitive activity and bodily systems may be stimulated (Glass et al., 2006). According to the cognitive reserve hypothesis, social and physical activity increases the person's ability to tolerate brain pathology through enhanced synaptic activity and more efficient brain recovery and repair (Saczynski et al., 2006). In a small pilot study, functional magnetic resonance imaging showed that compared with controls, volunteers showed changes in brain activity that corresponded to improvements in executive functioning (Carlson et al., 2009). Social engagement also affects physical activity. Volunteers became more physically active and sustained increased activity levels after three years (Tan, Xue, Li, Carlson, and Fried, 2006; Tan et al., 2009). Lindström et al. (2001) demonstrated that socioeconomic status affected social participation, which in turn affected engagement in physical activities.

Social engagement may affect health by being an effective coping strategy, especially in the face of loss or declining health. Volunteering has been viewed as a specific coping technique in response to adversity, and individuals report that their volunteer work is therapeutic (Musick and Wilson, 2008). Li (2007) found that widows who added a volunteer role after spousal loss were better protected against depressive symptoms than those who did not, and those who increased volunteer hours after widowhood experienced gains in self-efficacy. Utz et al. (2002) found that maintaining continuity in social participation is a strategy used to cope with spousal loss. Specifically, social participation decreased before death of spouse (perhaps because of poor spousal health) but increased following loss (owing to increased support from family and friends).

Social engagement can reinforce role identities and provide opportunities for meaningful interactions. Some activities, like formal and informal volunteering, may be altruistic in nature, and helping others has been associated with positive health outcomes (Brown, Brown, House, and Smith, 2008). Greenfield (2009) assessed one aspect of altruism, the felt obligation to help others, and documented its protective role against psychological losses in the face of functional decline. Some activities, like participating in social clubs or community groups, provide purpose in life or contribute to a sense of meaning, which in turn are positively related to favorable health outcomes (Piliavin and Siegl, 2007; Krause, 2009). Mendes de Leon, Glass, and Berkman (2003), however, suggest that the process of functional decline is driven by age-related chronic conditions and social engagement might not be directly involved in disease process. More likely, engagement modifies the functional consequences of disease and attenuates the impact of declining physical health on everyday function and disability. They posit that it modifies the effects of disease by providing a greater sense of purpose, control, and self-efficacy.

A possible argument for why social engagement might have a greater effect on the health of women than men comes from the literature on stress. As mentioned above, previous work has demonstrated the relationship between social isolation and stress. A number of recent studies have found that women and men respond differently to psychosocial stress (see, e.g., Chaplin, Hong, Bergquist, and Sinha, 2008), and ability to respond to psychosocial stressors has emerged as an important risk factor for diseases such as fibromyalgia and chronic pain (Rohleder, Schommer, Hellhammer, Engel, and Kirschbaum,

2001; Kajantie and Phillips, 2006). There is evidence to support a stronger immune response after a stressor among women than among men (Rohleder et al., 2001). It may well be the case that higher levels of social engagement among women that stem from their life roles as family nurturers and caregivers may produce an evolutionary advantage by allaying the effects of stress among women.

Clearly, there are multiple pathways from social engagement to health: influence on health behavior, increased physical and cognitive activity, improved physiologic functions, and increased positive psychological states. However, it is unclear what aspects of social engagement are associated with these mechanisms. Social engagement encompasses a wide range of activities — from playing cards with friends, to formal volunteering, to attending religious services. By definition, social engagement has two components: activity and social context. It is unclear what constitutes the health-producing parts. Which activities, at what levels of involvement, and under what conditions have health effects on older adults?

It will be challenging to identify the elements of social engagement that promote health. Yet this knowledge is important in developing interventions to increase public health. Maier and Klumb (2005) attempted to distinguish the relative importance of social activities from merely being in a social context and found that social context had a stronger relationship than social activity, with the effect coming from "being in the presence of friends." Similarly, Lennartsson and Silverstein (2001) discussed the challenge of distinguishing whether the positive health effects derived from the social aspect or from the content of the activity. They found that among adults over the age of 77 years, solitary activities (engaging in hobbies) were protective, suggesting that "meaningful activity" varies by the individual. Clearly, research is needed to identify and test the salient domains of social engagement for health.

INCREASING SOCIAL ENGAGEMENT THROUGH PROGRAM AND POLICY INTERVENTIONS

Increasing social engagement of the older population is an avenue to improving public health. Social activity is clearly a modifiable risk factor. However, more scholarly attention has been given to interventions to increase physical and cognitive activity. When an older adult experiences a serious health condition or personal loss, social activities may be the first to go. Yet these changes are observable, a decrease can be detected, and a wide range of strategies for reengagement are available (Everard et al., 2000).

NANCY MORROW-HOWELL AND SARAH GEHLERT

Although too numerous to review here, there are many programs at the national, state, and local level, funded by public and private money, that promote the social engagement of older adults. The Older Americans Act established a network of senior centers and congregate meal sites, where adults come together for a meal, classes, events, games, information, and discussion. In an effort to modernize the senior center notion, there are nonprofit agencies, like Mather's More than a Café in Chicago, where older adults come for food, entertainment, lectures, and discussions (see www .matherlifeways.com), or Senior Center Without Walls, a teleconferencing activities program for isolated older adults (http://seniorcenterwithoutwalls .org). The YMCA reports that people over the age of 65 represent the fastest-growing membership, and new outreach and programming for this demographic are underway (www.SeniorJournal.com/NEWS/Fitness/5–09–26Seniors JoinY.htm). National nonprofits focus on lifelong learning and volunteer opportunities for older adults, like the OASIS Institute and the Shepherd's Centers of America.

Educational activities are often at the heart of social programming for older adults. Elderhostel (now called Exploritas) is one of the oldest and largest nonprofit education and travel organizations for individuals 50 years or older. This program has expanded beyond its origins on college campuses, but many colleges and universities now commonly have lifelong learning programs. To address issues of access and inclusion, community colleges and libraries now outreach and program for older adults (Wilson and Simon, 2006). As working longer has become a desire and necessity for many older adults, educational programming has evolved from entertainment/leisure to professional development and job training.

Volunteer opportunities for older adults have grown consistently, along with the growing rate of volunteering among this subgroup of Americans. Programs vary widely. There are episodic opportunities, such as serving a Thanksgiving meal at a homeless shelter. There are time-intensive but time-limited opportunities, like preparing income tax returns or traveling to another community for disaster relief. There are programs supported by the federal government, such as Foster Grandparents, Senior Companions, and Service Corps of Retired Executives (SCORE). There are nonprofit volunteer programs, including national networks of retired professionals working in free clinics, nonprofits, schools, and faith-based organizations (e.g., Volunteers in Medicine, the Taproot Foundation, Faith in Action). There are national campaigns to advance federal and state policies to promote older adult civic engagement (e.g., Experience Wave), and there are opportunities for international service (e.g., Encore! Service Corps International and International Senior Lawyers Project).

In the arena of formal volunteering, public policies can clearly expand opportunities and facilitate the involvement of older adults. New legislation has attempted to increase the engagement of older adults in volunteer roles, with 10% of AmeriCorps funds targeted at recruiting older volunteers and with public funding of transferrable scholarships in exchange for service in nonprofit organizations (Public Law 111–13 [H.R. 1388], 2009). States are instituting various incentives to increase volunteering by older adults. For example, Illinois has granted free public transportation to senior citizens meeting financial eligibility, with the expectation that it would facilitate greater access to community volunteer opportunities. In several other states, local districts offer residents over age 60 the opportunity to volunteer in schools and earn a modest tax credit against their property taxes (Morrow-Howell, O'Neill, and Greenfield, 2010).

The challenges to increasing social engagement are numerous. Despite the long list of programs listed above, most older adults do not participate in formal groups. Programs largely exist in metropolitan areas, and for the individual, there are always logistical challenges of time and place. There are eligibility criteria in some programs. Connecting and matching older adults to existing opportunities is often challenging. Concerns exist that current programming may be less accessible to disadvantaged older adults and fail to capture the diversity of the older population in terms of ethnicity, socioeconomic status, and disability (Martinson and Minkler, 2006). Further, it is possible that the widening gaps in health and wealth among boomers may further marginalize certain subgroups of older adults who find it difficult to participate as more formal programs for social engagement come into existence (McBride, 2007). Finally, program and policy initiatives can influence formal participation, but more social engagement occurs informally—with friends and neighbors gathering for leisure, going out together, or helping each other. How can these informal social activities be promoted and facilitated?

Several new directions may help confront these challenges. Architecture and urban design can positively affect social engagement, both informal and formal (Cannuscio et al., 2003), and aging-friendly community initiatives around the country seek changes at the community level so that older adults can "achieve easy contact" (Baum and Palmer, 2002, p. 359). WHO (2007) defines an "aging-friendly city," and it is instructive to note the key role of social activity in these characteristics: outdoor spaces and buildings, transportation, housing, social participation, respect and social inclusion, civic participation and employment, communication and information, and community support and health services. Social participation and civic participation are named specifically, and essential facilitators of engagement, like transportation and communication, are also central. In a review of aging-friendly initiatives, strategies to increase informal social engagement (developing places for walking, sitting, meeting, and entertainment) and formal engagement (increasing opportunities for volunteering and civic roles) are evident (Scharlach, 2009). Demonstration projects are growing; as an example, Florida and Minnesota have established "Communities for a Lifetime" initiatives that provide funding and assistance to local communities to develop aging-friendly programs and infrastructure (National Governors Association, 2008).

The role of the Internet in increasing social engagement is growing. The Internet has clearly affected volunteering in this country, with a steady growth in online databases of volunteer opportunities (see, for example, www.volunteer match.com and www.allforgood.org). Further, virtual or remote volunteering, like editing, translating, and writing for volunteer organizations, has become a reality and has increased opportunities for older adults with inflexible work schedules, geographic constraints, or disabilities that limit travel (Vail, 2008). Beyond volunteering, the Internet is creating new ways for individuals to socialize, and the effect of the Internet on social engagement is a topic of current interest. Through e-mails, affinity lists, chat rooms, and blogs, the Internet may foster connections that increase social interactions (Uslaner, 2004; Best and Krueger, 2006). Gilleard, Hyde, and Higgs (2007) found that the use of cell phones, e-mail, and the Internet decreased attachment to local neighborhood people over the age of 50 years, but that perceived sense of trust in or perceived friendliness of people in the neighborhood did not change. They concluded that technology may be more liberating of neighborhood boundedness than destructive of social capital.

Finally, existing health and social service organizations are being challenged to increase social engagement programming. Residential facilities are striving to increase social connection within the facilities as well as to the community (Cannuscio et al., 2003). The aging network services of the federal and state governments are charged with organizational innovation, and despite slow movement, there are ideas to extend social and civic engagement opportunities to more diverse older adults through Older Americans Act structures. Area Agencies on Aging can foster engagement by creating databases for opportunities in the community, disseminating home-based volunteer opportunities, offering computer training, and providing transportation to social activities (Kahana and Force, 2008).

CONCLUDING THOUGHTS

Putnam (2004) has called into question the goodness of the evidence that supports claims of the powerful effects of social capital on many aspects of human life, including health. He suggested that intellectual sloppiness has abounded and that durability of these premises depends on conventional scientific criteria. These statements can and should be extended to the scholarly work on the antecedents and outcomes of social engagement in later life. Better knowledge is needed about the essential elements of social engagement, the types and amounts of engagement that produce positive outcomes, the conditions that maximize these effects, and the mechanisms through which outcomes occur. We need stronger research in terms of theoretical specification, measurement, causal designs, and statistical approaches.

That being said, a compelling case currently exists for increasing social engagement to maintain and improve the health of this aging society. Applied research and demonstrations on effective strategies to increase social activity are as warranted as efforts to increase physical or cognitive activity. It is widely known that recruiting and retaining older adults into traditional health promotion programs is difficult, and the most at-risk populations are less likely to participate. Yet recruiting older adults into programs that promote social engagement may be easier. People come forward to volunteer or serve in a civic role or take a class or join a book club for a variety of reasons— to find meaning and purpose, to have fun, and to meet new people, not to participate in a health promotion program per se (Carlson et al., 2008). As Tan et al. (2010) summarize, public health interventions embedded in civic engagement have the potential to engage older adults who might not respond to a direct appeal to improve their health. This rationale can be extended beyond civic engagement to other forms of social engagement.

Gene Cohen (2003) reminded us that developing a social portfolio for retirement is just as important as building a financial portfolio. He describes a social portfolio as an individual's investment in engaging activities, mental challenges, and interpersonal relationships that can carry into old age. Public policies and programs aimed at increasing social engagement can help build the social portfolios of older Americans and contribute to individual and population health. In this writing, Cohen also quoted Samuel Johnson, an eighteenth-century author and poet, who wrote, "if you are idle, be not solitary; if you are solitary, be not idle." For a long time, we have known that both social context and activity matter, and combining them in the form of social engagement may be the best prescription for a healthy aging society.

ACKNOWLEDGMENTS

The authors acknowledge the assistance of Christina Bourne and Amanda Kazmier-ski, graduate students at Washington University in St. Louis.

REFERENCES

Bassuk, S. S., T. A. Glass, and L. F. Berkman. 1999. Social disengagement and incident cognitive decline in community-dwelling elderly persons. *Annals of Internal Medicine*1313:165–73.

Baum, F. E., R. A. Bush, C. C. Modra, C. J. Murray, E. M. Cox, K. M. Alexander, and R. C. Potter. 2000. Epidemiology of participation: An Australian community study. *Journal of Epidemiology and Community Health* 54:414–23.

Baum, F. E., and C. Palmer. 2002. Opportunity structures, urban landscape, social capita, and health promotion. *Health Promotion International* 17(4):351–61.

Bennett, K. M. 2002. Low level social engagement as a precursor of mortality among people in later life. *Age and Ageing* 31:165–68.

Berkman, L. F., T. Glass, I. Brissette, and T. Seeman. 2000. From social integration to health: Durkheim in the new millennium. *Social Science & Medicine* 51(6):843–57.

Berkman, L. F., and S. L. Syme. 1979. Social networks, host resistance, and mortality: A nine-year follow-up study of Alameda County residents. *American Journal of Epidemiology* 109(2):186–204.

Berry, H., B. Rodgers, and K. Dear. 2007. Preliminary development and validation of an Australian community participation questionnaire. *Social Science & Medicine* 64:1710–37.

Best, S. J., and B. S. Krueger. 2006. Online interactions and social capital: Distinguishing between new and existing ties. *Social Science Computer Review* 24(4): 395–410.

Boden-Albala, B., E. Litwak, M. S. V. Elkind, T. Rundek, and R. L. Sacco. 2005. Social isolation and outcomes post stroke. *Neurology* 64:1888–92.

Bowling, A., and M. Stafford. 2007. How do objective and subjective assessments of neighbourhood influence social and physical functioning in older age? Findings from a British survey of ageing. *Social Science & Medicine* 64(12):2533–49.

Brand, J. E., and S. A. Burgard. 2008. Job displacement and social participation over the lifecourse: Findings for a cohort of joiners. *Social Forces* 87(1):211–42.

Brown, S. L., R. M. Brown, J. S. House, and D. M. Smith. 2008. Coping with spousal loss: Potential buffering effects of self-reported helping behavior. *Personality and Social Psychology Bulletin* 34(6):849–61.

Brummett, B. H., J. C. Barefoot, I. C. Siegler, N. E. Clapp-Channing, B. L. Lytle, H. B. Bosworth, R. B. Williams, Jr., and D. B. Mark. 2001. Characteristics of socially isolated patients with coronary artery disease who are at elevated risk for mortality. *Psychosomatic Medicine* 63(2):267–72.

Bukov, A., I. Mass, and T. Lampert. 2002. Social participation in very old age: Cross-sectional and longitudinal findings from base. *Journal of Gerontology* 57(6):P510–17.

Butler, R., and H. Gleason. 1985. *Productive Aging: Enhancing Vitality in Later Life.* New York: Springer.

Cannuscio, C., J. Block, and I. Kawachi. 2003. Social capital and successful aging: The role of senior housing. *Annals of Internal Medicine* 139:395–400.

Carlson, M. C., K. Erickson, A. Kramer, M. Voss, N. Bolea, M. Mielke, S. McGill, G. W. Rebok, T. Seeman, and L. Fried. 2009. Evidence for neurocognitive plasticity in at-risk older adults: The Experience Corps program. *Journal of Gerontology: Medical Sciences* 64A(12):1275–82.

Carlson, M. C., J. S. Saczynski, G. W. Rebok, T. Seeman, T. A. Glass, S. McGill, J. Tielsch, K. D. Frick, J. Hill, and L. P. Fried. 2008. Exploring the effects of an "everyday" activity program on executive function and memory in older adults: Experience Corps. *Gerontologist* 48(6):793–801.

Carlton-LaNey, I. 2007. Doing the Lord's work. *Generations* 30(4):47–50.

Chaplin, T. M., K. Hong, K. Bergquist, and R. Sinha. 2008. Gender differences in response to emotional stress: An assessment across subjective, behavioral, and physiological domains and relations to alcohol craving. *Alcohol Clinical and Experimental Research* 23(7):1242–50.

Cohen, G. 2003. The social portfolio: The place of activity in mental wellness as people age. In *Mental Wellness in Aging: Strength Based Approaches*, ed. J. L. Ronch and J. Goldfield, pp. 113–22. Baltimore: Health Professions Press.

Croezen, S., A. Haveman-Neis, V. J. Alvarado, P. van't Veer, and C. P. G. M. De Groot. 2009. Characterization of different groups of elderly according to social engagement activity patterns. *Journal of Nutrition, Health & Aging* 13(9):776–81.

Dupuis-Blanchard, S., A. Neufeld, and V. R. Strang. 2009. The significance of social engagement in relocated older adults. *Qualitative Health Research* 19(9):1186–95.

Ellaway, A., and S. Macintyre. 2007. Is social participation associated with cardiovascular disease risk factors? *Social Science & Medicine* 64:1384–91.

Everard, K. M., H. W. Lach, E. B. Fisher, and M. C. Baum. 2000. Relationship of activity and social support to the functional health of older adults. *Journal of Gerontology: Social Sciences* 55B(4):S208–12.

Gilleard, C., M. Hyde, and P. Higgs. 2007. Community and communication in the third age: The impact of internet and cell phone use on attachment to place in later life in England. *Journal of Gerontology: Social Sciences* 62(4):276–83.

Glass, T., and J. Balfour. 2003. Neighborhoods, aging, and functional limitations. In *Neighborhoods and Health*, ed. I. Kawachi and L. Berkman, pp. 303–34. New York: Oxford University Press.

Glass, T., C. Mendes de Leon, S. Bass, and L. Berkman. 2006. Social engagement and depressive symptoms in later life: Longitudinal findings. *Journal of Aging and Health* 18(4):604–28.

Glei, D. A., D. A. Landau, N. Goldman, Y. L. Chuang, G. Rodróguez, and M. Weinstein. 2005. Participating in social activities helps preserve cognitive function: An analysis of a longitudinal, population-based study of the elderly. *International Journal of Epidemiology* 34(4):864–71.

Greenfield, E. A. 2009. Felt obligation to help others as a protective factor against losses in psychological well-being following functional decline in middle and later life. *Journal of Gerontology: Social Sciences* 64B(6):723–32.

Greenfield, E. A., and N. F. Marks. 2004. Formal volunteering as a protective factor for older adults' psychological well-being. *Journal of Gerontology: Social Sciences* 59B(5):S258–64.

Greiner, K. A., C. Li, I. Kawachi, D. C. Hunt, and J. S. Ahluwalia. 2004. The relationships of social participation and community rating to health and health behaviors in areas with high and low population density. *Social Science & Medicine* 59(11):2303–12.

Hao, Y. 2008. Productive activities and psychological well-being among older adults. *Journal of Gerontology: Social Sciences* 63B(2):S64–72.

Harlow, R. E., and N. Cantor. 1996. Still participating after all these years: A study of life task participation in later life. *Journal of Personality and Social Psychology* 71:1235–49.

Harwood, R., P. Pound, and S. Ebrahim. 2000. Determinants of social engagement in older men. *Psychology, Health, and Medicine* 5(1):75–85.

Hermes, G. L., L. Rosenthal, A. Montag, and M. K. McClintock. 2005. Social isolation and the inflammatory response: Sex differences in the enduring effects of a prior stressor. *American Journal of Physiology—Regulatory, Integrative and Comparative Physiology* 290:R273–82.

House, J., K. Landis, and D. Umberson. 1988. Social relationship and health. *Science* 241(4865):540–45.

Independent Sector. 2000. *America's Senior Volunteers*. Washington, DC: Independent Sector.

Jang, Y., J. A. Mortimer, W. E. Haley, and A. R. Borenstein Graves. 2004. The role of social engagement in life satisfaction: Its significance among older individuals with disease and disability. *Journal of Applied Gerontology* 23(3):266–78.

Kahana, J., and L. Force. 2008. Toward inclusion: A public-centered approach to promote civic engagement by the elderly. *Public Policy & Aging Report* 18(3):30–35.

Kajantie, E., and D. I. Phillips. 2006. The effect of sex and hormonal status on the physiological response to acute psychosocial stress. *Psychoneuroendocrinology* 31(2):151–78.

Kawachi, I., and L. F. Berkman. 2000. Social cohesion, social capital, and health. In *Social Epidemiology*, ed. L. F. Berkman and I. Kawachi, pp. 174–90. New York: Oxford University Press.

Krause, N. 2006. Neighborhood deterioration, social skills, and social relationships in late life. *International Journal of Aging and Human Development* 62(3):185–207.

Krause, N. 2009. Meaning in life and mortality. *Journal of Gerontology: Social Sciences,* 64B(4):517–27.

Krueger, K. R., R. S. Wilson, J. M. Kamenetsky, L. L. Barnes, J. L. Bienias, and D. A. Bennett. 2009. Social engagement and cognitive function in old age. *Experimental Aging Research* 35(1):45–60.

Lee, H. Y., S. N. Jang, S. Lee, S. I. Cho, and E. O. Park. 2008. The relationship between social participation and self-rated health by sex and age: A cross-sectional survey. *International Journal of Nursing Studies* 45(7):1042–54.

Lefrançois, R., G. Leclerc, and N. Poulin. 1998. Predictors of activity involvement among older adults. *Activities, Adaptation, & Aging* 22(4):15–29.

Lennartsson, C., and M. Silverstein. 2001. Does engagement with life enhance survival of elderly people in Sweden? The role of social and leisure activities. *Journals of Gerontology Series B: Psychological Sciences and Social Sciences* 56(6): S335–42.

Li, Y. 2007. Recovering from spousal bereavement in later life: Does volunteer participation play a role? *Journals of Gerontology Series B: Psychological Sciences and Social Sciences* 62B:S257–66.

Lindström, M., B. S. Hanson, and P. O. Östergren. 2001. Socioeconomic differences in leisure time physical activity: The role of social participation and social capital in shaping health related behavior. *Social Science & Medicine* 52(3):441–51.

Lövdén, M., P. Ghisletta, and U. Lindenberger. 2005. Social participation attenuates decline in perceptual speed in old and very old age. *Psychology and Aging* 20(3):423–34.

Lutgendorf, S. K., A. K. Sood, B. Anderson, S. McGinn, H. Maiseri, M. Dao, J. I. Sorosky, K. De Geest, J. Ritchie, and D. M. Lubaroff. 2005. Social support, psychological distress, and natural killer cell activity in ovarian cancer. *Journal of Clinical Oncology* 23(28):7105–13.

Maier, H., and P. L. Klumb. 2005. Social participation and survival at older ages: Is the effect driven by activity content or context? *European Journal of Ageing* 2(1):31–39.

Marottoli, R., C. Mendes de Leon, T. Glass, C. Williams, L. Cooney, and L. Berkman. 2000. Consequences of driving cessation: Decreased out-of-home activity levels. *Journal of Gerontology: Social Sciences* 55B(6):S334–40.

Mars, G., G. Kempen, M. Post, I. Proot, I. Mesters, and J. van Eijk. 2009. The Maastricht social participation profile: Development and clinimetric properties in older adults with a chronic physical illness. *Quality of Life Research* 18(9):1207–18.

Martinson, M., and M. Minkler. 2006. Civic engagement and older adults: A critical perspective. *Gerontologist* 46(3):318–24.

McBride, A. 2007. Civic engagement, older adults, and inclusion. *Generations* 30(4):66–71.

Mendes de Leon, C. F., T. A. Glass, and L. F. Berkman. 2003. Social engagement and disability in a community population of older adults. *American Journal of Epidemiology* 157:633–42.

Michael, Y. L., L. F. Berkman, G. A. Colditz, and I. Kawachi. 2001. Living arrangements, social integration, and change in functional health status. *American Journal of Epidemiology* 153(2):123–31.

Miller, R., S. Ballew, M. Shardell, G. Hicks, W. Hawkes, B. Resnick, and J. Magaziner. 2009. Repeat falls and the recovery of social participation in the year posthip fracture. *Age and Ageing* 38(5):570–75.

Morrow-Howell, N., S. Hong, and F. Tang. 2009. Who benefits from volunteering? Variations in perceived benefits. *Gerontologist* 49(1):91–102.

Morrow-Howell, N., G. O'Neill, and J. Greenfield. 2010. Civic engagement: Policies and programs to support a resilient aging society. In *The Handbook of Resilience in Aging*, ed. B. Resnick, K. Roberto, and L. Gwyther. New York: Springer.

Musick, M. A., A. R. Herzog, and J. S. House. 1999. Volunteering and mortality among older adults: Findings from a national sample. *Journal of Gerontology: Social Sciences* 56:769–84.

Musick, M. A., and J. Wilson. 2008. *Volunteers: A Social Profile.* Bloomington: Indiana University Press.

Musick, M. A., J. Wilson, and W. B. Bynum. 2000. Race and formal volunteering: The differential effects of class and religion. *Social Forces* 78(4):1539–71.

National Governors Association. 2008. *Increasing Volunteerism among Older Adults: Benefits and Strategies for States.* Washington, DC: NGA Center for Best Practices.

Newall, N. E., J. G. Chipperfield, R. A. Clifton, R. P. Perry, A. U. Swift, and J .C. Ruthig. 2009. Causal beliefs, social participation, and loneliness among older adults: A longitudinal study. *Journal of Social and Personal Relationships* 26(2–3):273.

Nonogaki, K., K. Nozue, and Y. Oka. 2007. Social isolation affects the development of obesity and type 2 diabetes in mice. *Endocrinology* 148(10):4658–66.

Nummela, O., T. Sulander, O. Rahkonen, A. Karisto, and A. Uutela. 2008. Social participation, trust and self-rated health: A study among ageing people in urban, semi-urban and rural settings. *Health & Place* 14(2):243–53.

Piliavin, J. A., and E. Siegl. 2007. Health benefits of volunteering in the Wisconsin Longitudinal Study. *Journal of Health and Social Behavior* 48(4):450–64.

Public Law 111–13—Apr. 21, 2009. Retrieved October 7, 2010, from http://frwebgate .access.gpo.gov/cgi-bin/getdoc.cgi?dbname=111_cong_public_laws&docid=f:pub l013.111.pdf.

Putnam, R. 2004. Commentary: "Health by association": Some comments. *International Journal of Epidemiology* 33:667–71.

Ramsay, S., S. Ebrahim, P. Whincup, O. Papacosta, R. Morris, L. Lennon, and S. G. Wannamethee. 2008. Social engagement and the risk of cardiovascular disease mortality: Results of a prospective population-based study of older men. *Annual Epidemiology* 18(6):476–83.

Resnick, H. E., B. E. Fries, and L. M. Verbrugge. 1997. Windows to their world: The effect of sensory impairments on social engagement and activity time in nursing home residents. *Journal of Gerontology: Social Sciences* 52B(3):S135–44.

Rohe, W. 2004. Building social capital through community development. *Journal of the American Planning Association* 70(3):158–64.

Rohleder, N., N. C. Schommer, D. H. Hellhammer, R. Engel, and C. Kirschbaum. 2001. Sex differences in glucocorticoid sensitivity of proinflammatory cytokine production after psychosocial stress. *Psychosomatic Medicine* 63(6):966–72.

Rowe, J. W., and R. Kahn. 1998. *Successful Aging.* New York: Random House.

Saczynski, J. S., L. A. Pfeider, K. Masaki, E. S. C. Korf, D. Laurin, L. White, and L. J. Launder. 2006. The effect of social engagement on incident dementia: The Honolulu-Asia aging study. *American Journal of Epidemiology* 163(5):433–40.

Scharlach, A. 2009. Creating aging-friendly communities. *Generations* 33(2):5–11.

Sirven, N., and T. Debrand. 2008. Social participation and healthy ageing: An international comparison using SHARE data. *Social Science & Medicine* 67(12):2017–26.

Sørensen, L. V., U. Axelsen, and K. Avlund. 2002. Social participation and functional ability from age 75 to age 80. *Scandinavian Journal of Occupational Therapy* 9(2): 71–78.

Sundquist, K., M. Lindstrom, M. Malmstrom, S. Johansson, and J. Sundquist. 2004. Social participation and coronary heart disease. *Social Science & Medicine* 58(3): 615–22.

Tan, E. J., G. W. Rebok, Q. Yu, C. E. Frangakis, M. C. Carlson, T. Wang, M. Ricks, E. K. Tanner, S. McGill, and L. P. Fried. 2009. The long-term relationship between high-intensity volunteering and physical activity in older African American women. *Journal of Gerontology: Social Sciences* 64B(2):304–11.

Tan, E. J., E. K. Tanner, T. E. Seeman, Q.-L. Xue, G. W. Rebok, K. D. Frick, M. C. Carlson, T. Wang, R. L. Piferi, S. McGill, K. E. Whitfield, and L. P. Fried. 2010. Marketing public health through older adult volunteering. *American Journal of Public Health* 100(4):727–34.

Tan, E. J., Q. Xue, T. Li, M. C. Carlson, and L. P. Fried. 2006. Volunteering: A physical activity intervention for older adults: The Experience Corps program in Baltimore. *Journal of Urban Health: Bulletin of the New York Academy of Medicine* 83(5):954–69.

Thoits, P. A., and L. N. Hewitt. 2001. Volunteer work and well-being. *Journal of Health and Social Behavior* 42(2):115–31.

Tomaka, J. 2006. The relation of social isolation, loneliness, and support to disease outcomes among the elderly. *Journal of Aging and Health* 18(3):359–84.

Uslaner, E. M. 2004. Trust, civic engagement, and the internet. *Political Communication* 21(2):223–42.

Utz, R., D. Carr, R. Nesse, and C. Wortman. 2002. The effect of widowhood on older adults' social participation: An evaluation of activity, disengagement and continuity theories. *Gerontologist* 42(4):522–33.

Vail, J. 2008. Virtual volunteering widens opportunity. *Philanthropy Journal* (Nov. 12), www.philanthropyjournal.org/resources/special-reports/volunteers-boards/virtual-volunteering-widens-opportunity (accessed 12 Jan. 2010).

Wen, M., L. Hawkley, and J. Cacioppo. 2006. Objective and perceived neighborhood environment, individual SES and psychosocial factors, and self-rated health. *Social Science & Medicine* 63(10):2575–90.

Wilson, L., and S. Simon. 2006. *Civic Engagement and the Baby Boomer Generation.* New York: Haworth Press.

World Health Organization (WHO). 2002. *Active Ageing: A Policy Framework.* Geneva: World Health Organization.

World Health Organization (WHO). 2007. *Global Age-Friendly Cities Project.* Geneva: World Health Organization.

Zunzunegui, M. V., B. W. Alvarado, T. Del Ser, and A. Otero. 2003. Social networks, social integration, and social engagement determine cognitive decline in community-dwelling Spanish older adults. *Journal of Gerontology: Social Sciences* 54B(2): S93–100.

CHAPTER 11

Public Health Policy Successes

David M. Buchner, MD, MPH

Over the past 50 years, the life expectancy of older Americans has steadily increased, and age-specific rates of disability have decreased. This is a major accomplishment for public health. As explained in other chapters in this book, we now know a great deal about what can be done to promote healthy aging. In particular, we know that prevention works in older adults and is essential for healthy aging. Vaccinations in older adults prevent infectious diseases such as influenza and herpes zoster (shingles). Older adults benefit from clinical preventive services, such as screening for high blood pressure. Aspirin can reduce risk of myocardial infarction and ischemic stroke. Regular physical activity reduces the risk of many chronic diseases, including dementia. And so on.

A basic model that guides public health approaches to prevention is the social-ecological model (fig. 11.1). The model indicates that successful solutions to complex health problems require coordinated interventions at intrapersonal (or individual), interpersonal, institutional (or organizational), community, and public policy (or societal) levels (McLeroy, Bibeau, Steckler, and

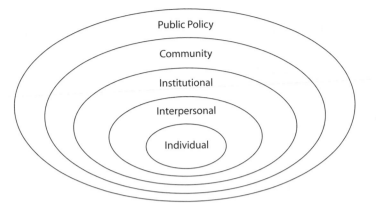

Fig. 11.1. The social-ecological model. The nested ovals indicate that interventions at one level influence factors affecting health at that level and lower levels. *Source*: Adapted from McLeroy et al., 1988

Glanz, 1988). Policy interventions are fundamental to the social-ecological approach. While policy interventions can occur at any level of the model, they are more relevant to organization and community levels and essential to societal-level approaches. The model provides a starting point for understanding the role of policy interventions, while other models (discussed below) further characterize the role of policy in prevention and healthy aging.

The purpose of this chapter is to discuss the role of policy in the prevention of disease, chronic conditions, and disability in older adults. We limit the scope of the chapter primarily to policy and prevention issues of major importance to older adults and that are relatively specific to older adults. This subset of topics does not include many important issues. For example, seatbelt laws are policies that effectively reduce risk of injury from motor vehicle collisions in all age groups. The federal law that mandates the publication of *Dietary Guidelines for Americans* every 5 years results in dietary recommendations for all age groups above 2 years of age.

Unlike many articles about health policy, this chapter does not focus on controversial policies, on policy failures, or on current "hot topics" in health policy. Rather, the focus is mainly on successful policies implemented over the past several decades, so as to demonstrate how policy approaches can and have contributed to healthy aging. Finally, it is beyond the scope of this single chapter to focus on policies that drive the social determinants of health (see chap. 5). These complex and extensive policies deal with issues such as poverty, education, and social class. Social Security, for example, is a key policy in this area for older adults.

The chapter begins with general background information about the roles of public health policy in prevention. Next, it provides two concrete examples of how policies have contributed to success stories in public health: tobacco control, and population-wide increases in rates of influenza vaccination in older adults. The discussion then focuses on specific policies of importance to prevention in older adults. Finally, the chapter considers the future of policy interventions in prevention, especially those called for by the Patient Protection and Affordable Care Act of 2010.

PUBLIC HEALTH POLICY AND PREVENTION
Prevention Policies and Their Implementation

Definitions of *policy* in public health are usually broad. Public health policy comprises laws, regulations, and judicial decrees. Guidelines and recommendations from public health agencies are policies, as are the funding decisions allocating resources to initiatives dealing with prevention. The scope of policies can be national, regional, statewide, or local. Community-level and organization-level interventions may have policy components. Businesses have policies related to worksite health promotion, such as a policy to provide financial incentives to participate in health promotion programs. Health plans have policies related to providing preventive care, such as clinical practice guidelines.

The development and implementation of policies are essential to public health practice and to the prevention of disease. Along with "assessment" and "assurance," "policy development" is one of the three core functions of public health. Policy development links scientific knowledge to societal values in an inclusive, consensus-building process that seeks shared ownership of policy decisions (Scutchfield and Keck, 2009). Also, one of the 10 essential public health services is to "develop policies and plans that support individual and community health efforts" (Scutchfield and Keck, 2009, p. 8). In 1999, the Centers for Disease Control and Prevention (CDC) identified 10 great public health achievements of the twentieth century: vaccination, motor vehicle safety, safer workplaces, control of infectious diseases, decline in deaths from coronary heart disease and stroke, safer and healthier foods, healthier mothers and babies, family planning, fluoridation of drinking water, and recognition of tobacco use as a health hazard (Centers for Disease Control and Prevention, 1999a). Policy changes played a major role in each achievement.

Because health is influenced by a complicated, interconnected set of determinants, policies outside the health sector also play an important role in promoting health. School policies about physical education influence physical activity and obesity in children. Farm policies affect the nutritional quality of food we eat. Environmental policies affect air and water quality. Transportation policies that create infrastructure for walking and bicycling affect health-enhancing physical activity. Broadly speaking, these are public health policies.

Models of the Impact of Policy Approaches in Public Health

In addition to the social-ecological model, several other frameworks have been proposed to characterize the use and potential impact of health policy interventions, including those focused on prevention. A well-known framework classifies prevention into primary, secondary, and tertiary prevention. Population-based, primary intervention has the most impact. This approach prevents the development of risk factors for disease ("primordial prevention"), for example, the onset of smoking in youth. Primary prevention also involves risk factor modification, e.g., smoking cessation programs. Other frameworks have been proposed, which include a number of factors related to the impact of public health interventions: policy change, environmental change, social capital, community partnerships, biology and genetics, working conditions, social support, infrastructure support (e.g., surveillance and training), population-based screening, case management, and prevention of complications of disease through medical care interventions (Frieden, 2010).

A framework developed by Frieden (2010) called "the health impact pyramid" builds upon these previous frameworks (fig. 11.2). Historically, there has been an emphasis on clinical interventions in discussions about the health impact of policy and other approaches. Frieden's framework reverses this emphasis. The first tier (base of the pyramid) is "socioeconomic factors" that indicate the relatively large impact of interventions that address social determinants of health. Counseling and education interventions (the fifth tier) and clinical interventions (the fourth tier) are positioned at the narrow top of the pyramid, indicating that they have relatively small impact. Interventions in the middle two tiers of the model are regarded as having intermediate amounts of impact on health. "Changing the context to make individual's default decisions healthy" is the second tier. This tier embodies the concept of making the healthy choice the easy choice. For example, in the Netherlands, bicycle infrastructure is a major part of the transportation system, with separate bike lanes and large bicycle parking lots. It is relatively easy and inexpensive to commute by bicycle. Bicycle commuting involves

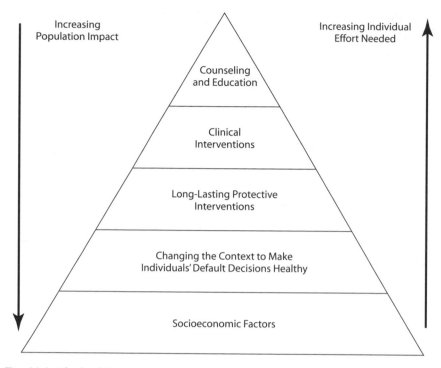

Increasing
Population Impact

Increasing Individual
Effort Needed

Counseling
and Education

Clinical
Interventions

Long-Lasting Protective
Interventions

Changing the Context to Make
Individuals' Default Decisions Healthy

Socioeconomic Factors

Fig. 11.2. The health impact pyramid. *Source*: Frieden, 2010, by permission of
Sheridan Press

regular physical activity, which causes substantial health benefits. This context makes a healthy choice (physically active commuting) a much easier choice. The middle level of the model (third tier) is "long-lasting protective interventions." An example is immunization, which provides long-term benefits without the need for ongoing clinical care.

In terms of understanding the impact of policy interventions per se, the social-ecological model indicates that the impact of the policy depends on its scope, with policy interventions at the highest level (public policy or societal level) having greatest potential for impact. The health impact pyramid indicates that the impact of the policy depends on the health determinants addressed. For example, consider two interventions that are both at the societal level of the social-ecologic model: a national policy that funds clinical counseling for tobacco use, and a national policy increasing cigarette taxes. The latter intervention would have more impact as it operates at a more fundamental (lower) tier of the health impact pyramid. However, both the social-ecological model and the health impact pyramid frameworks embody the idea that a comprehensive approach to a health problem involves intervention at all levels. Interventions at multiple levels can be synergistic and can increase the reach of a comprehensive approach in the target population.

The Role of Evidence

Another important factor in understanding the impact of health policies is the quality and amount of evidence regarding the impact of the policy. An *evidence-based public health policy* is based on research and public health science. Generally speaking, evidence-based policies are identified by systematic reviews of the literature such as those performed by the Task Force on Community Preventive Services, as described below. Policies with intermediate levels of evidence regarding effectiveness are sometimes referred to as "best practices" or "promising practices." It can be appropriate to implement such policies, using reasoning along the line of "we don't know everything, but we know enough to act."

Another important group of policies are those that drive evidence-based interventions. These policies can be considered evidence-based if they are successful in leading to implementation of evidence-based interventions. For example, there are several evidence-based programs for improving physical activity in older adults. Suppose a Medicare Advantage health plan adds a benefit (i.e., a new policy) to its coverage, subsidizing the cost of an evidence-based exercise program. If evaluations of this benefit policy demonstrate that it increases enrollment in the exercise-based program, the benefit becomes an evidence-based approach to promoting physical activity in older adults.

However, the ability of scientific evidence to influence actual policy decisions varies (see discussion of Medicare preventive benefits below as an example). There are a number of barriers to implementing effective public health policy, including the power of vested interests and the complexity of policy making (Brownson, Chriqui, and Stamatakis, 2009), resulting in a gap between what the evidence shows and the policies that are developed and implemented. Reviews of existing policies have documented this gap (Hartsfield, Moulton, and McKie, 2007; Moulton et al., 2009). A systematic review of public health laws and policies located 107 "model" laws and policies covering 16 topics, including tobacco control, injury prevention, and school health. Only 13 of these laws and policies (12%) included a discussion of their evidence basis (Moulton et al., 2009).

Brownson et al. (2009) recently identified three domains of public health policy to address when working on evidence-based policies. *Process* deals with increasing the likelihood that evidence-based policies are adopted. *Con-*

tent addresses the specific policy elements that influence effectiveness of the policy. *Outcome* documents the potential effects of the policy.

Longevity, Cost-Effectiveness, and Personal Choice

Although preventive care is usually cost-effective with respect to population health, only a few preventive interventions are cost savings in terms of medical care expenditures (Cohen, Neumann, and Weinstein, 2008). Debates about whether prevention policies provide cost savings are misguided. We pay for gains in health due to medical treatment. We should also pay for gains in health due to prevention.

Some have argued that prevention only postpones death and, by doing so, increases the burden of disease and medical expenditures in the final years of life. Evidence disputes this conclusion (Goetzel, 2009). An analysis of Medicare data reported that healthy older adults at age 70 live longer than those in poorer health, yet their cumulative Medicare expenditures prior to death were similar to those who died earlier (Lubitz, Kramarow, and Lentzner, 2003). Also, the findings of this study supported the hypothesis of "compression of morbidity." In brief, this hypothesis states that, assuming that individuals have a genetically determined life span, it is possible to compress morbidity into a relatively short period during the end of life (Fries, 1980). The study reported that individuals projected to live the longest as a result of having better health at baseline also had the fewest absolute number of years living with functional impairments and disability.

In summary, it is not a foregone conclusion that preventive interventions in older adults will increase burden of disease and medical expenditures. Further, there is a plausible biologic model involving compression of morbidity that can explain how preventive interventions can improve health and quality of life without major impact on medical expenditures.

Debates about prevention policy also commonly involve the issue of personal responsibility for health, particularly discussions dealing with reducing behavioral risk factors for disease such as tobacco use, unhealthy diets, and lack of physical activity. While an extended discussion of this issue of personal responsibility is beyond the scope of this chapter, the public health viewpoint is that personal responsibility for health is obviously important. However, social and physical environments that support healthy choices are also important (Brownell et al., 2010). The health impact pyramid (fig. 11.2) specifically regards interventions that "change the social context" to provide such support. As noted by Frieden, "The defining characteristic of this tier of interventions is that individuals would have to expend significant effort not to benefit from them" (Frieden, 2010, p. 591).

CASE STUDIES OF PUBLIC HEALTH ACHIEVEMENT
Tobacco

Over the past decades, tobacco use has been the leading cause of preventable death and disease in adults in the United States. Cigarette smoking causes about 438,000 deaths annually, and another 20 people suffer from a tobacco-related illness for every person who dies from tobacco use (Centers for Disease Control and Prevention, 2007). Exposure to secondhand smoke causes additional premature death and disease in people who do not use tobacco.

As noted earlier, policy interventions to change behavior and promote healthy lifestyles historically first emphasized clinical approaches. This is the case with tobacco control. Tobacco control began with approaches that sought to influence the individual smoker directly, including public education and clinical counseling (Green et al., 2006). Policies that utilized these approaches were easier to implement in a culture emphasizing the role of individual choice in smoking. These policies are regarded to have relatively small effects. A recent analysis reported that clinic-based smoking cessation counseling did not have a major effect on preventable deaths, particularly relative to the effects of such interventions as screening and treatment of hypertension (Farley, Dalal, Mostashari, and Frieden, 2010).

Then the practices of the tobacco industry, such as aggressive marketing of cigarettes to youth, began to incite public outrage. The result was public support for more effective policies operating at the more influential levels of the health impact pyramid. These policies included enforcement of laws restricting youth access, increasing taxes on tobacco products, and clean indoor air laws that banned indoor smoking, thereby preventing exposure of nonsmoking adults and children to secondhand tobacco smoke. Today, comprehensive tobacco control programs include interventions at all levels of the health impact pyramid.

Since the early 1970s, rates of tobacco use have declined (fig. 11.3). This public health success is mainly the result of successful evidence-based policy initiatives. Based on systematic evidence reviews, the Task Force on Community Preventive Services currently recommends several evidence-based interventions to reduce tobacco use (table 11.1). Together, the interventions constitute the core of an evidence-based approach to prevention and control the epidemic of chronic disease due to tobacco use. As noted by CDC, "We

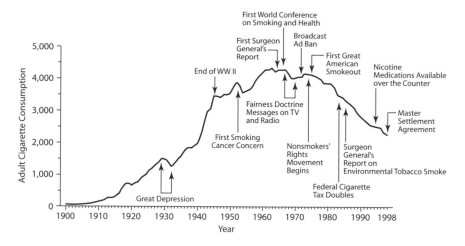

Fig. 11.3. Annual adult (per capita) cigarette consumption and major events related to smoking and tobacco control, 1900-1998. *Source*: Centers for Disease Control and Prevention, 1999b

know how to end the epidemic. Evidence-based, statewide tobacco control programs that are comprehensive, sustained, and accountable have been shown to reduce smoking rates, tobacco-related deaths, and diseases caused by smoking" (Centers for Disease Control and Prevention, 2007, p. 7).

Policies to reduce tobacco use drive interventions at all levels of the social-ecological model. Tobacco taxes to increase the unit cost of tobacco products and smoking bans in public spaces exemplify societal-level policy interventions to reduce tobacco use. Counter-marketing campaigns operate at the community level to influence the media and social environment and are driven by funding (budget) policies of both government and not-for-profit organizations. At the organizational level, worksites implement smoke-free policies, and health plans implement systems that remind health care providers to address tobacco use with their patients. Smoking cessation programs are individual-level interventions that are promoted by policies that reduce the client's out-of-pocket costs.

While reduction in smoking rates is a major public health success, tobacco use remains a major public health issue. Accordingly, CDC continues to provide funding for tobacco control to communities that emphasize policy, systems, and environmental changes (Centers for Disease Control and Prevention, 2010a). For example, a community in New York used this funding to facilitate the adoption of a city ordinance reducing exposure to secondhand smoke and banning smoking in all city parks and playgrounds.

TABLE 11.1

Evidence-based interventions to reduce use of tobacco recommended by the Task Force on Community Preventive Services in the Community Guide

Interventions to reduce tobacco use initiation
    Increasing the unit price for tobacco products
    Mass media education campaigns combined with other interventions

Interventions to increase tobacco use cessation
    Provider reminder systems when used alone
    Provider reminder systems with provider education
    Reducing client out-of-pocket costs for cessation therapies
    Multicomponent interventions that include telephone support

Interventions to reduce exposure to environmental tobacco smoke
    Smoking bans and restrictions

Interventions to restrict youth access to tobacco products
    Community mobilization with additional interventions

Interventions to decrease tobacco use in worksite settings
    Smoke-free policies to reduce tobacco use among workers
    Incentives and competitions when combined with additional interventions

Source: Task Force on Community Preventive Services, *Tobacco Use*, 2010a

Influenza Immunization

Influenza is a contagious viral infection that causes substantial morbidity and mortality, particularly in older adults. Seasonal influenza epidemics occur each year in the winter. (Seasonal influenza is distinct from the novel H1N1 influenza that emerged in 2008.) In the 1990s, the number of deaths attributed to seasonal influenza varied from a low of about 16,000 deaths in the mildest flu season to over 52,000 deaths in the worst flu season (Thompson et al., 2003). During a typical flu season, about 90% of deaths due to influenza occur in people aged 65 and older.

Influenza immunization (flu shots) effectively reduces the risk of contracting influenza. A recent study estimated that influenza vaccines in community-dwelling elderly reduce the risk of hospitalization for pneumonia or influenza by 27% and the risk of death by 48% (Nichol, Nordin, Nelson, Mullooly, and Hak, 2007). As shown in figure 11.4, rates of influenza immunization in older adults have increased over time. In the 1970s, only about 15%–20% of older adults received vaccinations each year; by 1993, vaccination rates approached 50% (Centers for Disease Control and Prevention, 1996). By 2003, vaccination rates reached the level of 65%–70% (Centers for Disease Control and Prevention, 2005).

Public health policy is largely responsible for this success. National re-

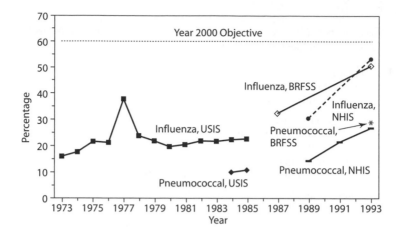

Fig. 11.4. Estimated vaccination levels for influenza and pneumococcal vaccines in adults aged 65 and older, by year, as assessed by self-report on national surveys, 1973–93. *Source*: Centers for Disease Control and Prevention, 1996 *Note*: The Healthy People Year 2000 Objective 20.11 was to increase pneumococcal and influenza vaccination levels to ≥60% for persons at high risk for complications from influenza and pneumococcal diseases, including adults aged 65 and older. By 2003, influenza vaccination levels exceeded the year 2000 objective (Centers for Disease Control and Prevention, 2005). BRFSS = Behavioral Risk Factor Surveillance System; NHIS = National Health Interview Survey; USIS = U.S. Immunization Survey.

search funding has been devoted to developing and testing vaccines and to developing interventions to promote use of vaccines. Government policies drive the work of the Advisory Committee on Immunization Practices, which issues evidence-based recommendations for influenza immunization. The Community Guide recommends 11 strategies to promote vaccination of preventable diseases generally, including increasing access to flu shots by offering immunization in multiple community sites (Task Force on Community Preventive Services, 2010b). Medicare policy allows reimbursement to clinics for providing flu shots. Many health plans now use "standing orders" to reduce barriers to immunization of patients and issue reminders to clinicians and to plan participants regarding annual flu shots. CDC policy has resulted in a sophisticated surveillance system to monitor influenza activity, involving surveillance of laboratory tests for influenza viruses, outpatient illnesses, mortality, hospitalizations, and geographic spread of influenza (Centers for Disease Control and Prevention, 2010b).

Policy innovation continues in the area of promotion of influenza vaccinations. Immunizations are now available in a variety of community settings, including airports, grocery stores, and pharmacies. An innovative program funded by the Robert Wood Johnson Foundation took advantage of the fact that Election Day in November is during the fall season when influenza immunizations are most appropriate. The program provided modest funding to public health agencies to make arrangements for influenza immunization to be provided at polling places. An evaluation of the program indicated that 80% of adult vaccine recipients were in high-priority groups and 28% were new influenza vaccination recipients (Shenson and Adams, 2008). This "Vote and Vax" intervention can be regarded as an evidence-based policy intervention, because an evaluation of the policy shows that it effectively promoted the evidence-based intervention of influenza immunization. The potential for impact is very good, as the intervention is in the middle tier of both the social-ecological model (at the institutional level) and the health impact pyramid (long-lasting protective intervention).

FEDERAL INITIATIVES RELATED TO PREVENTION POLICY IN OLDER ADULTS

As described in the first chapter of this volume, there are many federal health-related agencies and initiatives that promote healthy aging and prevention in older adults. In addition to agencies established through legislation, there are other federal structures that engage in initiating prevention efforts.

Healthy People Initiative

By the late 1980s, a process for setting U.S. national health objectives evolved into the Healthy People initiative. The Healthy People policy initiative emphasizes prevention and sets comprehensive national health objectives for a wide variety of health indicators. Healthy People objectives specify targets for improving U.S. health indicators. Progress toward meeting targets is monitored using data from a variety of public health surveillance systems. Healthy People 2010 included two cross-cutting goals, 467 specific objectives organized into 28 focus areas, and 10 leading health indicators (U.S. Department of Health and Human Services, 2010b). Health objectives have been updated every 10 years, as Healthy People 2000, Healthy People 2010, and Healthy People 2020.

Healthy People facilitates collaboration among federal agencies and partners to align resources, strategies, and research so as to achieve objectives. Many state health agencies use Healthy People as a resource in setting state-level objectives. A preliminary analysis of Healthy People 2010 showed that for 71% of the objectives and sub-objectives (with at least two data points over the decade), the United States either progressed toward (52%) or met (19%) the target (Koh, 2010). These data demonstrate broad improvements on many diseases, risk factors, and behaviors of importance to health in older adults.

Health objectives in most areas of Healthy People apply to older adults, including objectives related to risk factors (e.g., physical activity) and chronic disease burden (e.g., heart disease and stroke). Importantly, the draft of Healthy People 2020 includes a chapter and set of objectives focused just on older adults. These objectives emphasize prevention of functional limitations and disability with aging, including (for the first time) an objective related to prevention of cognitive impairment.

U.S. Preventive Services Task Force (USPSTF)

The USPSTF was first convened by the Public Health Service in 1984. Since 1998, the USPSTF has been sponsored by the Agency for Healthcare Research and Quality (AHRQ). Federal law mandates that AHRQ convene the USPSTF to develop recommendations for the use of clinical preventive services, based on reviews of the scientific evidence (Agency for Healthcare Research and Quality, 2010). The work of USPSTF has been essential to establishing a major role for prevention in the health care system and to building consensus on effective preventive services. From the standpoint of the social-ecological model, the USPSTF operates at the societal level. From the standpoint of the health impact pyramid, the recommendations operate at one of the top three levels of the model, indicating good impact overall on health. Optimal use of major preventive care recommendations could prevent 50,000–100,000 deaths annually in adults under the age of 80 (Farley et al., 2010).

Several policy aspects of the USPSTF are worth noting. First, the Task Force was set up as an independent federal advisory committee and issues recommendations without the need for approval or review by federal agencies. Second, the Task Force seeks public comment on drafts of recommendations. That is, primary care physicians, health plans, and other stakeholders in the recommendations have an opportunity to provide input on draft recommendations and to suggest topics for new systematic reviews. Third, systematic reviews of the evidence are updated as new evidence emerges, so that recommendations are current and evolve over time. Fourth, the Task Force considers both the risks and benefits of a preventive intervention, so that it can issue a recommendation against a preventive service on the grounds that it is likely to do more harm than good. This system has led to a truly comprehensive approach to evidence-based prevention. Currently, about 45 clinical preventive interventions are recommended based on scientific evidence.

Medicare Policy

Coverage for clinical preventive services by Medicare is a major policy success for prevention in older adults. Medicare is the primary health insurance for virtually all Americans aged 65 and older, so it is an excellent vehicle for providing coverage for prevention. Preventive benefits currently covered by Medicare as of May 2010 are shown in table 11.2. The "Welcome to Medicare" visit listed in table 11.2 is a one-time examination that focuses on prevention. The visit provides education, counseling, and referral for modifiable risk factors (e.g., tobacco use or inactivity), and the visit is used to develop a plan for getting appropriate preventive services.

Medicare policy regarding prevention provides an example of how policy making can be complicated and use inefficient mechanisms. Before 2010, the core statute for Medicare had not delegated regulatory authority to establish coverage for preventive services. Coverage for each preventive service has been authorized by Congress. Scientific evidence is constantly emerging, and this structure has made it difficult for Medicare preventive benefits to be updated in a timely manner. For example, in 2008 the Advisory Committee on Immunization Practices recommended that adults aged 60 and older routinely receive a new vaccine that prevents herpes zoster (shingles) (Centers for Disease Control and Prevention, 2008). (Zoster can cause a serious chronic pain syndrome in older adults.) Medicare does not currently cover this vaccine.

Medicare policy illustrates the problem of gaps between evidence-based recommendations and actual policies. The legislative process allows for special interests and other factors besides scientific evidence to influence Medicare benefits. Medicare has covered annual prostate screening for men, though this screening is not recommended by the U.S. Preventive Services Task Force (Agency for Healthcare Research and Quality, 2010). The USP-STF recommends routine colonoscopy for colon cancer screening in older adults no more often than every 10 years, while Medicare covers more frequent screening.

The Patient Protection and Affordable Care Act of 2010 (commonly known as the health reform bill) includes provisions that affect Medicare preventive

TABLE 11.2
Medicare preventive benefits as of May 2010

"Welcome to Medicare" visit (includes a referral for an ultrasound screening for
   abdominal aortic aneurysm for eligible beneficiaries)
Adult immunization—influenza immunization, pneumococcal vaccination, hepatitis
   B vaccination
Colorectal cancer screening
Mammography screening
Pap test and pelvic examination screening
Prostate cancer screening
Cardiovascular disease screening
Diabetes screening
Glaucoma screening
Bone mass measurement
Diabetes self-management, supplies, and services
Medical nutrition therapy
Smoking cessation support

Source: Centers for Medicare and Medicaid Services, 2010

services that are not yet reflected in table 11.2. The act removes most co-payments and deductibles for preventive services. It authorizes an annual wellness visit for personalized prevention plans. It provides the Secretary of Health and Human Services the authority to modify existing preventive services, so they can be consistent with USPSTF recommendations.

Medicare has funded evidence-based reviews to identify effective interventions to increase use of preventive services (RAND Corporation, 2003), and it implements such interventions. It can track use of preventive services using both claims data and surveys of Medicare beneficiaries. Medicare also provides educational materials for both older adults and health care providers (Centers for Medicare and Medicaid Services, 2010).

Policies to Increase Use of Clinical Preventive Services

Despite progress in promoting preventive care, much remains to be done. Less than half of older adults are up-to-date with routinely recommended vaccinations and cancer screening (Shenson, Bolen, Adams, Seeff, and Blackman, 2005). From a public health perspective, too large a responsibility for clinical prevention has been placed on the medical care system, which is focused primarily on treatment and has been preoccupied with the problems of inadequate quality of care (Chassin, Galvin, and the National Roundtable on Health Care Quality, 1998) and rapidly increasing medical care expenditures.

Several policy changes could address this problem. One group of potential policy changes would operate at the organizational level of the social-ecological model and could be used in an attempt to improve the performance of health plans. For example, one could pursue policies to increase the number of primary care providers who are most involved in preventive care of older adults. The relatively low compensation of primary care providers has led to a marked decline in the number of these providers and in the number of medical residents planning a career in primary care (Garibaldi, 2005). It can be difficult to squeeze preventive care into office visits that already address multiple issues. Some have suggested models of primary care with lower daily volume of patients (Casalino, 2010). Others argue that new policies are necessary to foster better collaboration between public health and medical care (McGinnis, 2006).

Policies that operate at the community level of the social-ecological model are also possible and potentially could have a broader reach and impact. An example of a policy that encourages collaboration between public health and medicine is funding for community-based (as opposed to clinic-based) systems for promoting preventive care in older adults. An example of this approach is Sickness Prevention Achieved through Regional Collaboration (SPARC) (Shenson, 2006). In the SPARC model, a medical clinic is just one element of a coordinated set of locations and activities to promote preventive care. The SPARC model involves an outreach campaign using local partners to reach community residents that either provides preventive services in the community (e.g., vaccinations) or schedules referrals to a clinic (e.g., appointments for mammography).

An international survey of adults of all ages reported that the percentage of U.S. adults receiving preventive care compares favorably with that of adults in Australia, Canada, New Zealand, and the United Kingdom (Schoen et al., 2004). For example, Americans were most likely to receive reminders for preventive care and most likely to receive advice on weight, nutrition, and exercise.

Task Force on Community Preventive Services

The Task Force on Community Preventive Services was established in 1996 by the U.S. Department of Health and Human Services. The Task Force uses systematic reviews of evidence to identify effective community-level interventions. CDC provides logistical support for the work of the Task Force.

Several policy aspects of the Task Force's Community Guide are worth noting. First, the guide had to devise its own methodology for systematic review that set evidence standards in a different manner from those of the USP-

TABLE 11.3

Seven high-priority actions to prevent chronic disease identified by
the Partnership for Prevention

1. Enhance in-school physical education
2. Increase access to places for physical activity
3. Promote healthy foods in schools
4. Increase access to healthy foods in communities
5. Make public places and worksites smoke-free
6. Increase the price of tobacco products
7. Ensure access to clinical preventive services

Source: Partnership for Prevention, 2010
Note: Each action involves community-level approaches to prevention.

STF (Briss et al, 2000). Second, the recommendations of the Community Guide are inherently at the most influential levels of both the social-ecological model (focus on organization, community, and society levels) and the health impact pyramid (focus on the bottom three tiers of social determinants, context of health decisions, and long-lasting protective interventions). In particular, the Community Guide makes recommendations about interventions affecting social determinants of health. For example, it recommends tenant-based rental assistance programs and recommends against policies facilitating transfer of juveniles to adult justice systems. Third, when there is sufficient evidence, the Community Guide provides economic recommendations such as the cost-effectiveness of implementing a recommendation. Finally, the Community Guide process is structured to obtain regular input from stakeholders, with a system of formal liaison to numerous agencies and organizations that are stakeholders in implementing recommendations.

The Task Force on Community Preventive Services currently recommends numerous evidence-based, community-level interventions, and policies play a role in promoting the implementation of each of them. However, policies that promote interventions specific to older adults are unusual. Seven priority community interventions identified by the Partnership for Prevention are not specific to older adults (table 11.3). Of course, all are justifiable, and it is desirable for a community intervention to have inclusive effects and prevent disease in many or all subgroups of the population.

Policies that focus on promoting community-level prevention specifically in older adults are an evolving area of health policy. By considering policies that promote healthy retirement communities, one gains insight into what such policies might encompass. Retirement communities can be established under the provisions of the Fair Housing Act, which provides an exemption

TABLE 11.4

Policy initiatives to promote healthy aging in retirement communities

---

Keep sidewalks well maintained, lighted, and clear of snow.

Look for ways to make streets and intersections more pedestrian-friendly and safe.

Increase the duration of time for yellow and green periods of traffic lights and increase the size of street signs.

Implement measures that decrease the speed and frequency of automobile traffic.

Evaluate, develop, and implement active community environment policies.

Add walking and bicycle paths that include points of interest (destination points).

Add new parks, maintain existing parks, and increase the number of park benches or tables.

Improve children's play facilities.

Add bicycle lanes and allow nonlicensed, personal electronic vehicles or golf carts to use these lanes.

Change residential zoning restrictions to allow seniors walking distance access to needed goods and services (e.g., health clinics, pubs, supermarkets, and shops).

Evaluate public transportation and consider shuttle buses to points of interest or facilities, such as malls or hospitals.

Lobby state or provincial governments for step-down driving license laws that permit elderly seniors to drive longer (e.g., licenses restricted to daytime or local driving).

Implement a policy that supports private sector involvement and ability to address senior needs.

Implement property tax concessions for seniors.

Provide incentives for private sector investment (e.g., relaxation of urban planning restrictions).

Support community-based nongovernmental organizations that address seniors' interests.

Facilitate senior participation in municipal government activities (i.e., look to seniors as a new source of part-time civil servants). This includes both creating employment opportunities for seniors and looking to seniors as a source of knowledge and labor.

Promote senior-led volunteerism.

Increase the perception of security by making police presence a part of the community.

Source: Masotti et al., 2006

Note: The list was originally developed for "naturally occurring" retirement communities, but policies apply more broadly to creating healthy communities for older adults.

for senior housing, so this housing can exclude families with children (U.S. Department of Housing and Urban Development, 2010). There are also so-called naturally occurring retirement communities.

A study of "naturally occurring" retirement communities (Masotti, Fick, Johnson-Masotti, and MacLeod, 2006) identified a list of policies related to prevention that are fairly specific to older adults (table 11.4). The study listed these policies as supporting the development of healthy "naturally occurring" retirement communities—defined as communities with a high concentration of older residents. The study concluded that municipal governments can use policies to stimulate the development of healthy environments for older adults. The policies in table 11.4 provide a perspective on policies to promote community-level preventive interventions in older adults. The policies have a local focus and have broad effects across a number of areas. They vary in the amount of evidence supporting their use. A healthy environment for older adults is produced by the total effect of all the policies, and policies can have synergistic effects.

FUTURE POLICY INITIATIVES

Policy development is a core function of public health and is essential to prevention of disease. Over the past several decades, the United States has established substantial public health capacity in the development and implementation of policies related to prevention in older adults. Public health practice in tobacco control and promotion of influenza immunization demonstrate the use of such policies.

Older adults commonly benefit from prevention policies that promote health in all age groups. Prevention policies have also been implemented to primarily influence the health of older adults. Medicare policies regarding coverage of clinical prevention services are a key set of such policies. There are also examples of policies emphasizing community-based prevention in older adults, but this area of policy is less well developed. A range of policies is necessary to create social and physical environments that support healthy aging. Though not discussed in this chapter, policies that address social determinants of health theoretically have great potential to prevent disease and disability in older adults (see chap. 5).

Substantial progress has been made on the policies related to clinical preventive care in older adults. The current need is for similar progress in the area of policies related to community-level approaches to prevention. As indicated in the section above, policies related to retirement communities are a logical and appropriate focus of this work.

The passage of the 2010 Patient Protection and Affordable Care Act (PPACA) provides an opportunity for moving forward on community-level policies and interventions specific to older adults. The act authorizes grants to health departments to develop and evaluate pilot programs for public health community interventions to promote the health of Medicare beneficiaries (U.S. Department of Health and Human Services, 2010a). The act also requires evaluations of prevention initiatives in older adults, undertaken by the Centers for Medicare and Medicaid Services and the Administration on Aging. Further, the PPACA creates a council within the Department of Health and Human Services to provide leadership and coordination among federal agencies and departments in activities related to prevention. The council is directed to develop a national strategy for improving health through federally supported prevention. A prevention and public health fund is also established to provide expanded and sustained investment in prevention. These and future policy initiatives may play a major role in enhancing the health of the American older population.

REFERENCES

Agency for Healthcare Research and Quality. 2010. *U.S. Preventive Services Task Force. About the USPSTF*. Retrieved November 1, 2010, from www.uspreventive servicestaskforce.org/about.htm.
Briss, P. A., S. Zaza, M. Pappaioanou, J. Fielding, L. Wright-De Agüero, B. I. Truman, D. P. Hopkins, P. D. Mullen, R. S. Thompson, S. H. Woolf, V. G. Carande-Kulis, L. Anderson, A. R. Hinman, D. V. McQueen, S. M. Teutsch, and J. R. Harris. 2000. Developing an evidence-based Guide to Community Preventive Services—methods. *American Journal of Preventive Medicine* 18(Suppl. 1):35–43.
Brownell, K. D., R. Kersh, D. S. Ludwig, R. C. Post, R. M. Puhl, M. B. Schwartz, and W. C. Willett. 2010. Personal responsibility and obesity: A constructive approach to a controversial issue. *Health Affairs* 29:379–87.
Brownson, R. C., J. F. Chriqui, and K. A. Stamatakis. 2009. Understanding evidence-based public health policy. *American Journal of Public Health* 99:1576–83.
Casalino, L. P. 2010. A Martian's prescription for primary care: Overhaul the physician's workday. *Health Affairs* 29:785–90.
Centers for Disease Control and Prevention. 1996. Pneumococcal and influenza vaccination levels among adults aged >65 years—United States, 1993. *Morbidity and Mortality Weekly Report* 45:1853–59.
Centers for Disease Control and Prevention. 1999a. Ten great public health achievements—United States, 1900–1999. *Morbidity and Mortality Weekly Report* 48:241–43.
Centers for Disease Control and Prevention. 1999b. Tobacco Use—United States, 1900–1999. *Morbidity and Mortality Weekly Report* 48:986–93.
Centers for Disease Control and Prevention. 2005. Influenza vaccination levels among persons aged ≥65 years and among persons aged 18–64 years with high risk conditions—United States, 2003. *Morbidity and Mortality Weekly Report* 54: 1045–49.
Centers for Disease Control and Prevention. 2007. *Best Practices for Comprehensive Tobacco Control Programs—2007*. Atlanta: U.S. Department of Health and Human Services, Centers for Disease Control and Prevention, Office on Smoking and Health.
Centers for Disease Control and Prevention. 2008. Prevention of herpes zoster. *Morbidity and Mortality Weekly Report* 57:1–30.
Centers for Disease Control and Prevention. 2010a. *Communities Putting Prevention to Work. Policy, Systems, and Environmental Change*. Retrieved November 1, 2010, from www.cdc.gov/CommunitiesPuttingPreventiontoWork/policy/index.htm.
Centers for Disease Control and Prevention. 2010b. *Flu Activity and Surveillance. Reports and Surveillance Methods in the United States*. Retrieved November 1, 2010, from www.cdc.gov/flu/weekly/fluactivity.htm.

Centers for Medicare and Medicaid Services. 2010. *Prevention—General Information*. Retrieved June 15, 2010, from www.cms.gov/PrevntionGenInfo/.

Chassin, M. R., R. W. Galvin, and the National Roundtable on Health Care Quality. 1998. The urgent need to improve health care quality. *Journal of the American Medical Association* 280:1000–1005.

Cohen, J. T., P. J. Neumann, and M. C. Weinstein. 2008. Does preventive care save money? Health economics and the presidential candidates. *New England Journal of Medicine* 358:661–63.

Farley, T. A., M. A. Dalal, F. Mostashari, and T. R. Frieden. 2010. Deaths preventable in the U.S. by improvements in use of clinical preventive services. *American Journal of Preventive Medicine* 38:600–609.

Frieden, T. R. 2010. A framework for public health action: The health impact pyramid. *American Journal of Public Health* 100:590–95.

Fries, J. F. 1980. Aging, natural death and the compression of morbidity. *New England Journal of Medicine* 303:130–36.

Garibaldi, R. A. 2005. Career plans for trainees in internal medicine residency programs. *Academic Medicine* 80:507–12.

Goetzel, R. Z. 2009. Do prevention or treatment services save money? The wrong debate. *Health Affairs* 28:37–41.

Green, L. W., C. T. Orleans, J. M. Ottoson, R. Camerson, J. P. Pierce, and E. P. Begginhaus. 2006. Inferring strategies for disseminating physical activity policies, programs, and practices from the successes of tobacco control. *American Journal of Preventive Medicine* 31:S66–81.

Hartsfield, D., A. D. Moulton, and K. L. McKie. 2007. A review of model public health laws. *American Journal of Public Health* 97:S56–61.

Koh, H. K. 2010. A 2020 vision for Healthy People. *New England Journal of Medicine* 362:1653–56.

Lubitz, J., L. Cia, E. Kramarow, and H. Lentzner. 2003. Health, life expectancy, and health care spending among the elderly. *New England Journal of Medicine* 349:1048–55.

Masotti, P. J., R. Fick, A. Johnson-Masotti, and S. MacLeod. 2006. Healthy naturally occurring retirement communities: A low-cost approach to facilitate healthy aging. *American Journal of Public Health* 96:1164–70.

McGinnis, J. M. 2006. Can public health and medicine partner in the public interest? *Health Affairs* 25:1044–52.

McLeroy, K. R., D. Bibeau, A. Steckler, and K. Glanz. 1988. An ecological perspective on health promotion programs. *Health Education Quarterly* 15:351–77.

Moulton, A. D., S. L. Mercer, T. Popovic, P. A. Briss, R. A. Goodman, M. L. Thombley, R. A. Hahn, and D. M. Fox. 2009. The scientific basis for law as a public health tool. *American Journal of Public Health* 99:17–24.

Nichol, K. L., J. D. Nordin, D. B. Nelson, J. P. Mullooly, and E. Hak. 2007. Effectiveness of influenza vaccine in the community-dwelling elderly. *New England Journal of Medicine* 357:1373–81.

Partnership for Prevention. 2010. *Take Action to Prevent Chronic Diseases*. Retrieved June 15, 2010, from www.prevent.org/content/view/12/6/.

RAND Corporation. 2003. *Interventions That Increase the Utilization of Medicare-Funded Preventive Services for Persons Age 65 and Older.* Retrieved November 1, 2010, from www.rand.org/pubs/reprints/2007/RAND_RP1229.part1.pdf.

Schoen, C., R. Osborn, P. T. Huynh, M. Doty, K. Davis, K. Zapert, and J. Peugh. 2004. Primary care and health system performance: Adults' experiences in five countries. *Health Affairs* W4:487–503.

Scutchfield, F. D., and C. W. Keck. 2009. Concepts and definitions of public health practice. In *Principles of Public Health Practice*, 3rd ed., ed. F. D. Scutchfield and C. W. Keck, pp. 2–11. Clifton Park, NY: Delmar.

Shenson, D. 2006. Putting prevention in its place: The shift from clinic to community. *Health Affairs* 25:1012–15.

Shenson, D., and M. Adams. 2008. The Vote and Vax Program. Public health at polling places. *Journal of Public Health Management and Practice* 14:1–5.

Shenson, D., J. Bolen, M. Adams, L. Seeff, and D. Blackman. 2005. Are older adults up-to-date with cancer screening and vaccinations? *Preventing Chronic Disease* 2:1–21. Retrieved November 1, 2010, from www.cdc.gov/pcd/issues/2005/jul/05_0021.htm.

Task Force on Community Preventive Services. 2010a. *Tobacco Use.* Retrieved November 1, 2010, from www.thecommunityguide.org/tobacco/index.html.

Task Force on Community Preventive Services. 2010b. *Vaccinations to Prevent Diseases.* Retrieved November 1, 2010, from http://thecommunityguide.org/vaccines/index.html.

Thompson, W. W., D. K. Shay, E. Weintraub, L. Brammer, N. Cox, L. J. Anderson, and K. Fukuda. 2003. Mortality associated with influenza and respiratory syncytial virus in the United States. *Journal of the American Medical Association* 289:179–86.

U.S. Department of Health and Human Services. 2010a. *Health Reform and the Department of Health and Human Services.* Retrieved November 1, 2010, from http://healthreform.gov/health_reform_and_hhs.html.

U.S. Department of Health and Human Services. 2010b. *Healthy People.* Retrieved November 1, 2010, from http://healthypeople.gov/.

U.S. Department of Housing and Urban Development. 2010. *Senior Housing: What You Should Know . . .* Retrieved November 1, 2010, from www.hud.gov/offices/fheo/seniors/index.cfm.

PART IV

Public Health Infrastructure
for an Aging Society

CHAPTER 12

Technology and Aging

David Lindeman, PhD

The capacity of the U.S. health care system is rapidly being tested by the demands of a growing aging and disabled population, with significant ramifications for public health. As indicated in other chapters throughout this volume, the challenges posed by the shear increase in population aging— combined with the disproportionate level of chronic illness among older adults, projected shortages in the long-term care workforce, pressures on family caregivers, and rapid increases in the costs of health care—require significant changes in the way health providers address the needs of older adults. Fortunately, several emerging technologies already address these challenges or have the potential to do so and also improve the well-being of older people on both an individual and a systems level.

Technology can be an enabler for improving the health system through better integration and efficiency of care and for improving access to and quality of care. Historically, technology has significantly improved the health of older adults through such areas as diagnostics, imaging, communications, surveillance, and health informatics. In the second decade of the twenty-first century, however, we are witnessing an unprecedented change in the way technology can and will improve the well-being of older adults. Advances in technologies are reframing how health care will be delivered; how older adults, family caregivers, and service providers communicate; how the health care workforce is trained; and how older adults obtain access to care and services. These new technologies will not only improve the quality of aging services and care but also enhance the daily lives of older adults and significantly contribute to their independence.

Technology encompasses a broad array of communication, monitoring, data, and analytic tools. This chapter reviews several of the prominent emerging technologies for aging services that have potential for significant impact, including remote monitoring and telehealth, health information technology (i.e., electronic health records), technologies for aging safely in place, mobile health, and workforce training technologies. Forthcoming advances and trends in each respective emerging technology are considered. Operational and socioeconomic-political barriers that may limit these technologies from reaching their full potential are addressed. Finally, strategies are recommended for encouraging the broader adoption of technologies that will clearly have an ever-increasing role in improving health in an aging society.

ALIGNMENT OF OLDER ADULTS AND TECHNOLOGY

Concurrent with the socioeconomic trends associated with population aging (briefly summarized at the beginning of this chapter), there have been rapid changes and a proliferation in many forms of technology. This is evidenced by enhancements in communications, sensors, automation, and data analytics technologies. The confluence of these factors has led to significant alterations in how health care is provided to older adults and how older adults are able to manage their own health. Taken together, they are creating a paradigm shift in the role technology can and does play in aging and public health. As advances in technology expand the capacity of health care delivery to meet the needs and challenges of an aging population through innovative service delivery redesign, care management processes that support evidence-based and coordinated care, patient-provider communications, and self-management will emerge to provide care solutions at many levels and across settings and conditions. While the landscape of health care and aging is rapidly changing, older adults are increasingly using technology in their daily lives, with mobile phones, the Internet, social media, monitoring, and personal health records becoming ever more commonplace among them. Because of their wide reach, these technologies can be used to support older adults in their homes and communities, greatly bolstering public health efforts to improve the health of the aging population.

IMPROVING THE DELIVERY OF CARE OF OLDER ADULTS THROUGH TECHNOLOGY

Technology has become integrally bound with the health care delivery system for older adults in home-based, community-based, and residential settings. Five specific technology areas will be discussed: remote monitoring and telehealth, health information technology (i.e., electronic health records), technologies for aging safely in place, mobile health, and workforce training technologies. Although this is not an exhaustive list of relevant technologies, these are the ones that collectively are creating systemic changes in public health and aging.

Remote Monitoring and Telehealth

The use of remote technologies and telehealth is one of the central means through which technology benefits older adults in the delivery and improvement of care for chronic disease. Remote patient monitoring (RPM) refers to a wide variety of technologies designed to manage and monitor a range of health conditions. Remote technologies primarily support chronic care through RPM of physiological characteristics, optimization of medication management (i.e., medication monitoring, adherence, and reconciliation), and behaviors related to cognitive impairment. Many chronic conditions that drive health care utilization respond to remote technologies by becoming less debilitating or requiring less personal care. They also maintain older adults' independent functioning through less-resource-intensive care. These remote technologies allow older adults and persons with disabilities to be cared for in less intensive health care settings with lower-acuity services. RPM technologies can facilitate six components of chronic disease management: (1) early intervention—to detect deterioration and intervene before unscheduled and preventable services are needed; (2) integration of care—exchange of data and communication across multiple comorbidities, multiple providers, and complex disease states; (3) coaching—motivational interviewing and other techniques to encourage patient behavioral change and self-care; (4) increased trust—patients' satisfaction and feelings of "connectedness" with providers; (5) workforce changes—shifts to lower-cost and more plentiful health care workers, including medical assistants, community health workers, and social workers; and (6) increased workforce productivity because of decreased home visit travel time and automated documentation (Coye, Haselkorn, and DeMello, 2009).

Remote technologies can also help shift care to a progressively lower acuity care setting or to personnel with lower skill levels. Non-clinicians can incorporate limited clinician responsibility. Unlicensed caregivers can take on narrow responsibilities usually undertaken by licensed direct-care workers. And older adults can take on work formerly conducted by family members and unlicensed caregivers.

A number of studies have found that RPM platforms contribute to better health outcomes and decreased health care costs and utilization for chronic diseases such as congestive heart failure, respiratory illness, and diabetes (Stachura and Khasanshina, 2007). Such platforms traditionally involve in-home monitoring devices and sometimes adjacent technologies (such as an online or mobile interface) and are linked to clinician management and feedback.

Point-of-care monitoring devices, such as weight scales, glucometers, implantable cardioverter-defibrillators, and blood pressure monitors, may individually collect and report health data. They may also become part of a fully integrated health data collection, analysis, and reporting system that communicates to multiple nodes of the health system. Such integrated systems provide alerts when health conditions decline, allowing patients, caregivers, and clinicians to intervene and modify treatment plans as needed. Monitoring technologies are becoming increasingly smaller and less obtrusive, as well as more personalized and portable. With portability, remote monitoring will not only reduce time and distance between patients and providers but also allow both patients and providers to have more freedom of movement.

Some of the strongest evidence of the potential effectiveness of remote technologies has been found by studies conducted by the New England Healthcare Institute (NEHI) and the Veterans Health Administration (VHA). NEHI looked at using RPM with persons with heart failure compared with disease management and standard care in terms of cost and reduction in hospital readmissions. The study identified a 60 percent reduction in hospital readmissions when RPM was compared with standard care, as well as a 50 percent reduction in readmissions compared with disease management programs. NEHI found that RPM could prevent between 460,000 and 627,000 heart failure–related hospital readmissions each year, with an estimated annual national cost savings of up to $6.4 billion (New England Healthcare Institute, 2009).

The VHA has pioneered the use of home-based technologies for chronic disease management in both urban and rural settings through its Care Coordination/Home Telehealth (CCHT) program. The CCHT intervention was designed to help manage the care of chronically ill veterans in noninstitutionalized settings. Darkins et al. (2008) found that the CCHT program resulted in significantly lower costs of care, as well as decreased health care utilization and high patient satisfaction for thousands of veterans. Older adults enrolled in the CCHT program in 2006 and 2007 showed a 25% reduction in bed days of care, a 20% reduction in numbers of admissions, and a mean patient satisfaction score rating of 86%. The cost of the program was $1,600 per patient per annum, compared with the direct cost of VHA home-based primary care services of $13,121 per patient per annum and market nursing home care rates that averaged $77,745 per patient per annum.

Technologies that help improve medication use in older adults are also promising. Because medication adherence is considered an instrumental activity of daily living, the ability to manage medications successfully is an important factor in maintaining independence in the older adult population (Hayes, Klein-Schwartz, and Gonzales, 2009). Suboptimal medication adherence can have negative consequences for individuals, families, and society, and medication nonadherence significantly increases the cost and burden of illness (Kocurek, 2009). The New England Healthcare Institute (2009) estimates that $290 billion of health care expenditures could be avoided each year if medication adherence were improved. Medication nonadherence is considered responsible for 33%–69% of medication-related hospital admissions; 23% of all nursing home admissions; increased use of expensive, specialized medical resources; unneeded medication changes; unexplained treatment failures; and repeat office visits (Kocurek, 2009).

Sophisticated in-home medication dispensers can significantly improve medication adherence. Such devices can be programmed and prefilled to dispense the right medications in the right quantities at the right time to individuals in their homes and allow caregivers to remotely monitor whether the medications were taken appropriately or not. One study (Buckwalter, Wakefield, Hanna, and Lehmann, 2004) demonstrated that use of a sophisticated medication dispenser was associated with significantly lower hospital and emergency department visits compared with use of a simple, plastic medication organizer.

Telehealth, more broadly, defines remote technologies as the incorporation of telecommunications, health information, videoconferencing, and "store-and-forward" technologies to deliver health care and health education.

Telehealth, including telemedicine, encompasses assessment, diagnosis, treatment, monitoring, and health education. Telehealth includes such programs as tele–Intensive Care Unit, telestroke, and telepharmacy and enables a small number of highly skilled practitioners to support the care of large numbers of older adults across wide geographic areas, removing the barriers of time, distance, and provider scarcity.

Videoconferencing technologies enable two-way discussions between and among patients and providers. Studies have demonstrated that use of videoconferencing to deliver health services is associated with positive health outcomes that at times exceed the performance of non-telehealth treatment (Center for Connected Health Policy, 2010). Store-and-forward technologies electronically transmit prerecorded videos and digital images between providers and medical specialists using encrypted Internet connections, major broadband networks, high-speed telecommunications lines, and private point-to-point broadband connections (Center for Connected Health Policy, 2010). These telehealth technologies provide many benefits, including reduced clinical wait times, eliminating the need to travel from one site to another for both patients and providers, increased patient access to care, improved quality of care and safety, and reductions in costs of care.

It is widely recognized that effective use of videoconferencing and store-and-forward technologies will depend on having adequate telecommunications bandwidth, often referred to as "broadband." The American Recovery and Reinvestment Act of 2009 (ARRA) established the National Purposes mandate to improve broadband infrastructure and services for health care delivery, as well as several other national priorities. The Federal Communications Commission estimates that the United States could achieve $700 billion in net savings in the next 15–25 years by better enabling efficient health information delivery and RPM (Federal Communications Commission, 2010).

Health Information Technology (HIT)

With the passage of the American Recovery and Reinvestment Act of 2009, over $22 billion in funding was allocated for the implementation of electronic health records (EHRs) through the introduction of the Health Information Technology for Economic and Clinical Health (HITECH) Act, bringing EHRs to the forefront of public health and aging discussions (Blumenthal and Tavenner, 2010). The HITECH Act includes $27 billion over 10 years for EHR adoption incentives. EHRs have the potential to improve health care outcomes through reducing medical errors, enhancing communication around patient diagnosis and treatment, improving early identification of at-risk patients, increasing workforce productivity, and allowing patients to have an active role in managing their own care (Blumenthal and Tavenner, 2010). EHR utilization has also demonstrated the ability to reduce medical errors and health care utilization, promote patient-centered care and greater administrative efficiency, and share and aggregate health information for clinical and public health–related purposes (Chen, Garrido, Chock, Okawa, and Liang, 2009; Kramer, Richard, Epstein, Winn, and May, 2009).

The activities facilitated by EHRs are especially relevant to older adults, many of whom suffer from chronic conditions that benefit from significant care coordination. Older adults are also more likely to have an extensive medication regimen and to receive care from multiple providers and across multiple sites (including the home, community, and inpatient settings) (Centers for Disease Control and the Merck Company Foundation, 2007). Despite their many benefits, the adoption of EHRs across the entire United States has not surpassed 50% and lags behind several other countries (Davis, Doty, Shea, and Stremikis, 2009). Commonly cited barriers to the widespread adoption of EHRs in the United States include a lack of financial incentives for providers, as well as workflow, awareness, and resource barriers (particularly for small physician practices and hospitals) (Poon et al., 2006).

As a result, initiatives such as the HITECH Act have emerged to accelerate the deployment of EHRs in order to fill these gaps. HITECH has earmarked up to $44,000 (through Medicare) and $63,750 (through Medicaid) per clinician in incentive payments to providers who incorporate EHR systems that follow "meaningful use" guidelines. These guidelines are designed to make sure that EHRs are able to support core functionalities that can enhance patient care, such as demographic and clinical information, computerized order entry, decision support for clinicians, e-prescribing, and information sharing. Hospitals are also eligible for incentive payments, as well as penalties for non-adoption, starting in 2016 from the Centers for Medicare and Medicaid Services (CMS) (OmniMD, 2010).

Besides these financial incentives, other resources to support providers in their implementation of EHRs have been created, including regional extension centers (RECs) to provide training, guidance, and technical support to providers (U.S. Department of Health and Human Services, 2010a). The U.S. government's goal is that such programs will lead to each person utilizing an EHR in the United States by 2014, with total spending on EHR systems projected to increase from $850 million in 2009 to $1.85 billion by 2014 (Healthcare Informatics, 2009; INPUT, 2009). At present, less attention has been given to increasing the usage rates of EHRs in long-term care (LTC) settings compared with inpatient and ambulatory settings, resulting in lower adoption rates for EHR and related technologies for skilled nursing facilities, rehabilitation hospitals, and home health settings compared with other health care settings (Poon et al., 2006).

Several organizations have successfully adopted and utilized EHRs, including Kaiser Permanente's My Health Manager EHR, which is currently used by over 3 million patients (Kaiser Permanente, 2009). Chen et al. (2009) found that Kaiser's EHR use reduced primary and specialty office visits by over 20% in its Hawaii region while increasing secure e-mail messaging and scheduled telephone visits, leading to more efficient and patient-centered care. Another example of highly successful EHR implementation has occurred within the Veterans Administration (VA) through its Veterans Health Administration Systems and Technology Architecture (VistA) EHR system, which is of particular relevance for older adults owing to demographics of the veteran population. More than 5.3 million VistA records have been created, and the system has been noted for helping facilitate the organization's My HealtheVet (appointment scheduling and prescription refilling) and CCHT programs (Naditz, 2008).

In addition to EHRs, a number of related HIT initiatives were created in the HITECH Act in an effort to build a Nationwide Health Information Network (NHIN) that will connect providers, consumers, and others to support health and health care. Some of these initiatives include the State Health Information Exchange Cooperative Agreement Program (statewide or regional entities to facilitate health information sharing across hospitals and health providers), the Beacon Community Program (a grant program for communities to strengthen their HIT capabilities by connecting multiple community entities through IT infrastructure), the Strategic Health IT Advanced Research Projects (SHARP) Program (a grant program that funds research to overcome well-documented HIT adoption barriers), and four Health IT Workforce programs to increase the number of trained health IT professionals. Many of these programs are particularly relevant for older adults; for example, many of the Beacon communities are targeting chronic conditions such as diabetes, heart disease, pulmonary disease, and cancer (U.S. Department of Health and Human Services, 2010b, 2010c).

The widespread use of EHRs and other HIT tools can help achieve healthier, safer, and better coordinated care outcomes for older adults given the large number of older adults served by Medicare and, to a lesser extent, Medicaid. Current incentives for providers to adopt EHRs are driving rapid acceleration of their adoption. The continued implementation of HIT will provide tools to improve the health care and public health systems at large by increasing efficiency and sustainability; improving health outcomes; expanding access to affordable care; and providing patients, providers, and other entities with timely access to health-promoting information.

Technologies for Aging Safely in Place

Technology plays a central role in supporting older adults' preference to remain at home in the least restrictive environment possible, for as long as possible. Home- and community-based technologies that prolong older adults' ability to live independently in their homes and communities are extensive. Some of the most common examples include patient-safety monitoring technologies (which encompass fall detection and prevention and location tracking), assistive devices, and modifications in the home or residential environment. These technologies address or ameliorate major areas of functional and cognitive impairment, which are strong contributors to morbidity and mortality for older adults. The number of older adults with disabilities (sensory, physical, mental, and other) in the United States is significant, with 45% of adults aged 65–69, 47% of adults aged 70–74, 58% of adults aged 75–79, and 74% of adults aged 80 years and older having some form of disability (Administration on Aging, 2010).

Evidence demonstrates the efficacy of such technologies in supporting the independence of older adults. In a randomized controlled trial, the use of assistive and environmental technologies resulted in slower functional decline than traditional care and reduced paid caregiver costs (Mann, Ottenbacher, Fraas, Tomita, and Granger, 1999). As the population ages, the need for technologies to facilitate aging in place will become even more pressing. Though significant barriers to adopting these technologies currently exist, the market for them is nonetheless rapidly expanding. Policies such as the Assistive Technology Act of 1998 and the Improving Access to Assistive Technology for Individuals with Disabilities Act of 2004 are helping drive more rapid uptake of these technologies.

Patient safety monitoring technologies include fall detection, fall prevention, and location-tracking devices that monitor patients in terms of their location, balance, and gait. They allow caregivers and other parties to assess patient mobility and safety. Additional patient safety monitoring technologies include stove-use detectors, smoke and temperature monitors, and door locks. Falls are the major focus of patient safety monitoring technologies, as they are a costly and prevalent issue for older adults. Falls are the leading cause of injury in older adults over the age of 65 (Ontario Medical Association, 1992), and over one-third of this population suffers falls each year in the United States (Hausdorff, Rios, and Edelberg, 2001). Falls are a major cause of hospitalizations and nursing home admissions (Curtin, 2005), and fear of falls can create negative effects such as decreased physical activity and social interaction and increased dependence (Ontario Public Health Association, 1998).

Fall detection technologies actively or passively identify whether a fall has taken place and alert others that an individual has fallen. These technologies include personal emergency response systems (PERS) and passive sensors. PERS have been widely adopted by older adults, with currently 1.3 million installed devices in the United States and a projected market of $1 billion (L. Orlov, pers. comm., 2010). Fall prevention technologies, many of which are still in the developmental stage, measure gait and balance to predict the likelihood of falls via pressure and other types of sensors embedded in the user's shoe, cane, or other assistive technology.

Location-tracking technologies enable caregivers and others to locate older adults who are prone to wandering. These technologies employ numerous tracking techniques, including Wi-Fi, GPS, cellular networks, and radio frequency located in a device worn or occupied by the user. Tracking devices vary by tracking technique, signal activation, involvement of third parties, and level of acuity for device activation. The key to these safety technologies' success is generally attributed to patient-specific alert mechanisms being used in conjunction with support services (Associated Press, 2010).

Assistive technologies support the safety and independence of older adults by maintaining or improving a person's ability to perform daily activities. These technologies span a wide range of functions, helping compensate for physical, sensory, and cognitive disabilities in order to facilitate independent living. Examples of assistive technologies include mobility aids (such as a lighted cane to prevent falls in the dark or a walker with an electronic component), visual aids (such as screen readers or video magnifiers), listening aids (such as infrared systems to enhance the volume of television sets or one-to-one communicators that can amplify and deliver sound to a hearing aid), and technologies designed to address cognitive impairments. The U.S. assistive technology market was estimated at $38.2 billion in 2008, having increased from $36.4 billion in 2007, and is expected to reach $49.3 billion by 2013 (McWilliams, 2008). Vision and reading aids currently make up the greatest portion of assistive technologies by far, followed by communication aids, daily living aids, mobility aids, and access and other aids.

Technology applied to the physical environment, as is seen in "smart homes," is increasingly expanding. Smart homes apply complex technologies that improve older adults' ease of using household fixtures and appliances while also improving their safety and prolonging independent living (Chan, Campo, Esteve, and Fourniols, 1999). These homes are embedded with sensors and other technological devices to create a physical environment that can be tailored to older adults' needs, including preventing falls, facilitating visits, and communicating with caregivers in an emergency. Such homes create an assistive environment for older adults, harnessing the potential of using many technologies simultaneously to improve their independence. The global smart home market is currently undergoing rapid growth and is estimated to reach $13.4 billion by 2014, primarily driven by the needs of the aging population (Markets and Markets, 2010).

Mobile Health Technologies

Mobile health (mHealth) is one of the most rapidly expanding, as well as rapidly changing, technologies that impact older adults and public health. mHealth generally refers to the delivery of health-related services to patients, clinicians, and caregivers through mobile technology platforms on cellular or wireless networks. Mobile technologies can include cell phones, smartphones, portable tablets, and mobile-enabled diagnostic devices. As cell phones have become a primary application-development platform, the number of health-related mobile technologies has increased significantly, providing new forms of access to health information and services to promote personal wellness, preventive care, behavior change, and chronic disease management. Some of these applications focus on the integration of mobile technologies with the workflow of more formal health care practices. Exemplifying the rapid expansion of mHealth, physicians' use of smartphones, estimated at around 64% in 2010, is expected to top 80% by 2012 (Fierce Mobil Healthcare, 2010). Smartphones give physicians an alternative means to stay updated on health information, medications, and patient data, as well as perform administrative functions that support patient care. mHealth offers significant opportunities to promote better patient adherence behaviors, reduce health care utilization and costs, engage patients and caregivers, and increase access to health services and education (Mechael et al., 2010). mHealth can also improve communications between older adults and providers, between older adults and informal caregivers, and among older adults themselves.

Mobile phone–based disease management systems and text-based programs for chronic disease management and medication adherence and monitoring are rapidly expanding (Cole-Lewis and Kershaw, 2010). An estimated 98% of cell phones worldwide have basic text message capabilities (Terry, 2008). Text messaging is a communication protocol that allows written messages to be delivered between phones or portable devices over a network. Different types of technology standards allow delivery of written messages (e.g., Short Message Service [SMS]) and multimedia messages like images, audio, rich text, or video (e.g., Multimedia Messaging Service [MMS]).

Patients, caregivers, and clinicians can utilize mHealth technologies to access health information, and clinicians can provide interventions in a patient's home by remotely accessing health information and utilizing decision support tools. The Visiting Nurse Service of New York (VNSNY) has instituted a treatment protocol for visiting nurses in home health care using decision support tools via portable tablet devices. The nursing staff uses personal computers (tablet computers) that run a secure EHR that regularly updates referrals and continuing patients and wirelessly communicates between the tablet and VNSNY's mainframe. The VNSNY IT intervention identifies patients at risk of a potentially serious medication problem, prioritizes cases needing immediate attention, and identifies nurse care protocols to efficiently focus time and attention (Center for Technology and Aging, 2010).

The application of mobile technologies to health care delivery can contribute to improved coordination within the health care system. At present, mHealth interventions have mostly been detached, stand-alone health care solutions as opposed to integrated within systems of care. mHealth has the potential to provide a wider sphere of influence and more targeted applications than the Internet as an instrument of health care delivery. Effective deployment of mobile health care applications will require a scalable, flexible, and configurable approach with extensive coordination between the telecommunications industry and health experts. To rapidly expand, mHealth services will require a transition from silos to systems, improved documentation on the costs and benefits of these interventions, and stakeholders submerging their own self-interests for the public good of improved health (Mechael et al., 2010).

Workforce Training Technologies

As the health care workforce shortage in general and the long-term care workforce shortage in particular have become more acute, a growing need has arisen for innovations in teaching and training methods for professionals and paraprofessionals. Remote training/simulation technologies and remote supervision offer a partial but increasingly important contribution to solving this challenge. In their basic form, remote training and simulation technologies are systems that support the training of professional and direct-care workers who may not be physically colocated with their educator. The training can occur synchronously in real time or asynchronously in the manner of an online education course. Remote training is exemplified by Web-based technologies that range from basic e-learning courses to collaborative Web conferencing platforms and immersive virtual environments.

Training is of crucial importance in preparing the health care field in general, but particularly when developing new and innovative technology programs. Technology-based training is an efficient means of providing staff with the skills and competencies to be able to deliver care to older adults. The VHA has established a virtual training center that serves as the core for its national training center for home telehealth. New clinicians receive three weeks of virtual training via the virtual training center. With the development of master preceptors, who assist with training and solve programmatic issues at the local level, the center has the capacity to train hundreds of staff each year.

Medical simulation centers in university, military, and public health settings around the United States are actively training professionals using a variety of technologies, including interactive mannequins, virtual environments, team scenario training, and hybrid systems that combine physical and virtual environments. Results from these remote and virtual training initiatives are contributing to advances in geriatric curricula. Within U.S. medical training the medical licensing exam process requires health care professionals to pass test components based in simulated settings, using actors as "standardized patients." In the future, simulation techniques may be utilized much more within all fields of medical specialty training and become ubiquitous in continuing medical education and recertification.

Virtual and Web-based environments are increasingly being used to train professionals and paraprofessionals in home or long-term care settings. Remote training and supervision can be accomplished using existing video-conferencing technologies that utilize analog or digital communication systems. E-learning programs can significantly expand the abilities and knowledge of informal caregivers and the formal workforce. E-learning initiatives such as the Savvy Caregiver Program from the Rosalynn Carter Institute for Caregiving have demonstrated positive outcomes in improving the quality of life for older adults who are under the care of a family caregiver (Smith and Bell, 2005). Multimedia courses, such as Cornell University's Environmental Geriatrics Program, are actively conducting training across care roles specifically focused on geriatric care. This Web-based course enables students to make a virtual home visit with an older patient with multiple sensory and cognitive impairments and experience challenges that an impaired elder may face in the home (Environmental Geriatrics, 2008).

PUBLIC HEALTH 2.0: TECHNOLOGY AND SOCIAL INNOVATION

The technology and public health landscape is much broader than the five areas discussed above. Technologies as diffuse as mapping, cognitive training programs, persuasive gaming, and robotics are already influencing public health by creating new methods for conducting public health surveillance, delivering memory training, providing health education and promotion programs, and supporting staff in common tasks, respectively. The emergent field of urban informatics may lead to the next generation of healthy cities. Technology is being used more extensively in home automation and car safety, two critical areas that influence older adult autonomy, independence, and the ability to remain in one's own home.

It is important to mention social networking or social media, the technology that is rapidly growing and portends a significant contribution to improving the health and well-being of older adults. Social media can contribute to older adults' social connectedness and mental well-being by improving their access to health information and care management and improving communication between older adults and their formal and informal caregivers. Also, the creation of hubs or commons and open source systems will lead to new methods of aggregating and accessing health-related data. Collectively, these trends demonstrate the potential for technology to make the health sector more consumer focused, while emphasizing the consumer responsibility of older adults to contribute to their own health and independence through networks such as www.patientslikeme.com. The advances in both technology infrastructure and technology processes will enable health care providers to reach older adults on an even wider platform than ever before for public health purposes.

BARRIERS TO ADOPTING EMERGING TECHNOLOGIES

Although the advantages of using technology to improve both the health and independence of older adults and the capacity of the health care workforce become increasingly apparent, significant gaps still remain to its adoption and diffusion as a result of cost and lack of reimbursement, low awareness, workflow issues, and the usability and design of these technologies (Mallenius, Rossi, and Tuunainen, 2010). Both operational and socioeconomic-political barriers impede the spread of technology into health and social services, even for technologies that are already commonly used for other purposes, such as mobile phones and the Internet. Among the greater operational or programmatic barriers to the wider adoption and diffusion of technology are the lack of access to technology for both older adults and the public health workforce, limitations in workforce training in technology use, health care information privacy concerns, and a limited evidence base supporting the added value of technologies.

Older adults have been much slower to gain access to technology than younger population cohorts, with variation by technology. Adults living with chronic disease are significantly less likely than healthy adults to have access to the Internet (62% vs. 81%) (Lenhart, Purcell, Smith, and Zickuhr, 2010). Similarly, much of the long-term care workforce, especially staff in home care, assisted living, skilled care, and other residential care settings, generally has limited access to the Internet/broadband, in part owing to economics. While technology is rapidly becoming more affordable and accessible, it is often still beyond the resources of many community-based and residential care providers, much less the means of many older adults.

Even though technology provides new avenues for addressing the historical scarcity of geriatric educators and training programs for the workforce through remote training, simulations, and telehealth, there is only limited evidence so far that technology-based geriatric training has made a significant improvement in the number of staff being trained. Further, training programs for professionals and paraprofessionals do not yet sufficiently address the use of new technologies, either at the time of initial training or through continuing education. Remote training, simulation, and telehealth add value through scalability and efficiency, yet the additional costs of development, updating, and adapting education programs via technology are significant.

Emerging technologies, in particular those involved in transmitting personal health information, raise concerns regarding confidentiality and privacy risks. Although emerging technologies in and of themselves do not directly create problems in health care privacy, addressing confidentiality and meeting regulatory guidelines for protecting clinical information require considerable time for training staff and program implementation. Confidentiality is of particular issue in meeting the needs of the cognitively impaired and their family caregivers.

The evidence base to support clinical outcomes, return on investment, and patient and provider satisfaction for many potentially beneficial technologies is limited. Despite the robust body of research on pilot programs for new technologies, few studies document the benefits of technology-supported care compared with standard care or have conducted comparative effectiveness research between similar technologies. Randomized controlled trials or longitudinal studies of emerging technologies are difficult to undertake because of rapidly changing technologies, morbidity and mortality of the population, limited clinical and utilization data, and the cost of conducting such rigorous studies. Where the evidence of improved clinical outcomes and reduced costs is strong, such as that provided through the VHA CCHT study of RPM and telehealth, it has not been sufficient to convince either the broader provider community or policy makers to widely adopt or expand the use of those technologies in aging services in other systems or settings.

Key socioeconomic-political impediments to the rapid expansion of emerging technologies are lack of consumer awareness, workforce resistance to technology, and lack of payer alignment and/or a strong business case for technology. Older adults' basic awareness of an available technology is necessary for that technology to be effectively utilized. The current cohort of older adults requiring long-term care is steadily becoming more comfortable with technology through the use of cellular phones and the Internet, but older adults still have a limited awareness of the array of technologies that can improve their independence and connectedness (Lenhart et al., 2010). In addition, many older adults are reluctant to pay out of pocket for technologies. Regardless of cost, there is still significant resistance among older people to certain technologies, such as robotics, and to the stigma of using some technologies, such as assistive devices or obtrusive remote technologies. On the other hand, it is important to note that awareness of and the willingness to pay for technologies such as remote monitoring and cognitive training continues to increase among family caregivers and baby boomers.

The professional and paraprofessional workforce may resist the incorporation of technology into care practices. Concerns on the part of the workforce regarding the introduction of new technologies are due to a real or perceived threat that technologies could require changes in accepted practice standards, require additional training, result in more rather than less work, or even threaten livelihoods altogether. The greatest obstacle to expanding the use of beneficial technologies for aging and long-term care, however, relates to the lack of payer alignment to and adequate business models for emerging technologies. Public and private payers will often cover the costs of technology hardware, but more often than not they do not cover the costs for its effective use. Few business models exist for successfully implementing new technologies in aging. We lack business models that effectively address return on investment, care processes, or marketing strategies to the satisfaction of providers or policy makers.

FUTURE DIRECTIONS FOR IMPROVING THE HEALTH AND WELL-BEING OF OLDER ADULTS

For technologies to successfully serve as a transformative force for aging services and long-term care, several recommendations can be advanced.

Scalability and Sustainability

To date, many emerging technologies that can improve the public health of older adults, such as remote monitoring, have been introduced as demonstration projects or pilots. CMS is currently testing the effectiveness of stand-alone and integrated technologies for managing chronic care. Historically, except for demonstration projects undertaken by large systems such as the VHA or Kaiser Permanente, demonstration projects have rarely been sustained, much less replicated. Similarly, remote training programs for geriatrics currently make up a relatively limited proportion of training efforts by long-term care organizations or by state and/or federal governments. Demonstration projects using technologies to improve chronic care or geriatric training should be designed from the outset with the intent to ensure sustainability, replicability, and scalability.

Comparative Effectiveness Research

The adoption of beneficial technologies for older adult health care, the long-term care workforce, and remote training needs to be supported by successful evidence-based research that addresses technology in applied settings. Providers, payers, and policy makers require strong evidence before implementing work process redesign and changes in workforce training. Studies that incorporate assessments of technology-enabled care models, advances in training, and the testing of new business models need to be conducted in a full range of service settings. These evaluation studies need to focus on the use of technology in improving prevention and care processes, such as care transition interventions and reducing post-acute care hospitalizations, as well as on new forms of care delivery such as accountable care organizations and the patient-centered medical home. The Center for Medicare and Medicaid Innovation (CMMI) provides an excellent means for conducting comparative effectiveness studies of promising technology-based care programs. The findings from this work will need systematic dissemination, not only to providers and workforce educators but also to policy makers and regulators who can ultimately translate them into changes in reimbursement and practice guidelines.

Training Requirements, Curricula, and Implementation

Geriatric training programs for all persons who deliver care to older adults, including paraprofessionals, social workers, pharmacists, nurses, physicians, and other health care providers, should include technology as a core component of primary geriatric curricula. Given the rapid advances in technology and applications of technology to care processes, technology training also needs to be included in all continuing education curricula. In some cases, this will require working with professional associations to modify their national training standards (e.g., Nurse Practice Act/Nurse Delegation Act). Applying remote training and simulation technologies offers a significant, cost-effective means of supplementing or substituting for on-site education and training and should be widely adopted as a means of addressing workforce shortages.

Reimbursement and Business Models

The ultimate driver for maximizing the benefits of information, communication, and other emerging technologies and achieving their more rapid and widespread deployment among aging and public health services will be through building the business case for technology adoption and realigning payment mechanisms. Remote monitoring and medication management technologies exemplify how many emerging technologies are not yet supported by strong business models. In general, these technologies are paid for out of pocket by patients and their caregivers, and for the most part only by health care providers in capitated programs. In the case of remote monitors and assistive devices, reimbursement practices will pay for some technology devices but not for others. Similarly, the cost of training staff in the use of technology is generally not paid for. Without sufficient understanding of how emerging technologies improve care outcomes, return on investment, the efficiency of the workforce, and the satisfaction of older adults and providers, it will be very challenging to convince providers and policy makers of their utility and impact. In essence, the development of a strong business case for the use of various technologies is critically needed to inform the decisions of both providers and policy makers.

CONCLUSIONS

As the United States struggles to improve health care in general, and for older adults in particular, technology offers a means to significantly have an impact in improving older adults' well-being from a public health perspective. The United States is facing a critical juncture in public health and aging. Health spending is continuing to climb, quality of care and access to care for older adults are often inadequate, and the delivery of health promotion and long-term care is uneven and often delivered in a disjointed, poorly coordinated fashion. Even though further research is needed to determine how the power of technology can be fully harnessed as a means of improving the health of older adults, a number of technologies are already sufficiently advanced to offer immediate impact.

Over the coming decade, technology will be a transformative agent for both older adults and the health care workforce. New technologies, many of which have not even been envisioned, will have a far-ranging impact on access to care, the cost of care, and, most importantly, the quality of care. Emerging technologies will not only improve the efficiency, productivity, and capacity of the health care workforce in the management of chronic disease and delivery of aging services but also provide changes in the way care providers work and how older adults, their family caregivers, and providers interact, enabling a more patient-centric approach to health care and empowering older adults to manage their own health. Whether it is through enabling new care processes or creating more powerful health analytics, these technologies will significantly change how care is designed and delivered. Technology will change where care is provided, taking health and social services to older adults, whether they are at home, in the community, or in residential settings. Ultimately, technology offers more than the promise of successfully improving care processes and workforce capacity while reducing health care costs. It will be a transformative agent to create sustainable improvements in the health and well-being of older adults.

REFERENCES

Administration on Aging. 2010. *Assistive Technology.* Retrieved on March 5, 2010, from www.aoa.gov/AoAroot/Press_Room/Products_Materials/fact/pdf/Assistive_Tech nology.pdf.

Associated Press. 2010. *At-Home Technology Can Monitor Seniors for Safety.* Retrieved on January 9, 2010, from http://bostonherald.com/business/healthcare/view.bg?articleid=1221632.

Blumenthal, D., and M. Tavenner. 2010. The "Meaningful Use" regulation for electronic health records. *New England Journal of Medicine* 363:501–4.

Buckwalter, K. C., B. J. Wakefield, B. Hanna, and J. Lehmann. 2004. New technology for medication adherence: Electronically managed medication dispensing system. *Journal of Gerontological Nursing* 30(7):5–8.

Center for Connected Health Policy. 2010. *What is Telehealth/Remote Patient Monitoring?* Retrieved on November 4, 2010, from www.connectedhealthca.org/what-is-telehealth/patient-monitoring/.

Center for Technology and Aging. 2010. *IMPACT-CI: Improving Medication Management Practices and Care Transitions through Technology.* Retrieved on July 7, 2010, from www.techandaging.org/grants_VNSNY.html.

Centers for Disease Control and Prevention and the Merck Company Foundation. 2007. *The State of Aging and Health in America 2007.* Whitehouse Station, NJ: Merck Company Foundation.

Chan, M., E. Campo, D. Esteve, and J. Fourniols. 1999. Smart homes—current features and future perspectives. *Maturitas* 64:90–97.

Chen, C., T. Garrido, D. Chock, G. Okawa, and L. Liang. 2009. The Kaiser Permanente electronic health record: Transforming and streamlining modalities of care. *Health Affairs* 28:323–33.

Cole-Lewis, H., and T. Kershaw. 2010. Text messaging as a tool for behavior change in disease prevention and management. *Epidemiologic Reviews* 32:56–69.

Coye, M. J., A. Haselkorn, and S. DeMello. 2009. Remote patient management: Technology enabled innovation and evolving business models for chronic disease care. *Health Affairs* 28:126–35.

Curtin, A. J. 2005. Prevention of falls in older adults. *Medicine & Health Rhode Island* 88:22–25.

Darkins, A., P. Ryan, R. Kobb, L. Foster, E. Edmonson, and B. Wakefield. 2008. Care coordination/home telehealth: The systematic implementation of health informatics, home telehealth, and disease management to support the care of veteran patients with chronic conditions. *Telemedicine Journal & E-Health* 14:1118–26.

Davis, K., M. Doty, K. Shea, and K. Stremikis. 2009. Health information technology and physician perceptions of quality of care and satisfaction. *Health Policy* 90:239–46.

Environmental Geriatrics. 2010. *Multimedia Course: 3D Animated Virtual Home.* Retrieved September 8, 2010, from www.environmentalgeriatrics.com/.

Federal Communications Commission. 2010. *Connecting America: The National*

Broadband Plan. Retrieved on December 10, 2010, from www.broadband.gov/plan/.

Fierce Mobile Healthcare. 2010. *Physician Smartphone Adoption Said to Top 80 Percent by 2012.* Retrieved March 17, 2010, from www.fiercemobilehealthcare.com/story/physician-smartphone-adoption-said-top-80–percent-2012/2010–03–09#ixzz0iSlCQ2qa.

Hausdorff, J., D. Rios, and H. Edelberg. 2001. Gait variability and fall risk in community-living older adults: A 1–year prospective study. *Archives of Physical Medicine & Rehabilitation* 82:1050–56.

Hayes, B. D., W. Klein-Schwartz, and L. F. Gonzales. 2009. Causes of therapeutic errors in older adults: Evaluation of National Poison Center data. *Journal of American Geriatrics Society* 57:653–58.

Healthcare Informatics. 2009. *The State of EHR Adoption: On the Road to Improving Patient Safety.* Retrieved on September 28, 2010, from www.thebreakawaygroup.com/publications/2010%20–%20Health%20Care%20Informatics%20–%20The%20State%20Of%20EHR%20Adoption%20–%20White%20Paper.pdf.

INPUT. 2009. *Health IT Transformation: FY2009–FY2014 State and Local Market Forecast.* Retrieved on November 11, 2010, from www.input.com/corp/library/detail.cfm?ItemID=9153.

Kaiser Permanente. 2009. *Three Million People Now Using Kaiser Permanente's Personal Health Record.* Retrieved on October 20, 2010, from http://xnet.kp.org/newscenter/pressreleases/nat/2009/042209myhealthmgr.html.

Kocurek, B. 2009. Promoting medication adherence in older adults . . . and the rest of us. *Diabetes Spectrum* 22(2):80–85.

Kramer, A., A. A. Richard, A. Epstein, D. Winn, and K. May. 2009. *Understanding the Costs and Benefits of Health Information Technology in Nursing Homes and Home Health Agencies: Case Study Findings.* Washington, DC: Office of Disability, Aging and Long-Term Care Policy, Assistant Secretary for Planning and Evaluation, U.S. Department of Health and Human Services.

Lenhart, A., K. Purcell, A. Smith, and K. Zickuhr. 2010. *Pew Internet. Social Media and Young Adults.* Retrieved June 6, 2010, from http://pewinternet.org/Reports/2010/Social-Media-and-Young-Adults/Summary-of-Findings.aspx.

Mallenius, S., M. Rossi, and V. Tuunainen. 2010. *Factors Affecting the Adoption and Use of Mobile Devices and Services by Elderly People—Results from a Pilot Study.* Retrieved March 15, 2010, from http://citeseerx.ist.psu.edu/viewdoc/download?doi=10.1.1.130.2463&rep=rep1&type=pdf.

Mann, W., K. Ottenbacher, L. Fraas, M. Tomita, and C. Granger. 1999. Effectiveness of assistive technology and environmental interventions in maintaining independence and reducing home care costs for the frail elderly. A randomized controlled trial. *Archives of Family Medicine* 8:210–17.

Markets and Markets. 2010. *Global Smart Homes Market.* Retrieved on November 11, 2010, from www.marketsandmarkets.com/Market-Reports/smart-homes-and-assisted-living-advanced-technologie-and-global-market-121.html.

McWilliams, A. 2008. *Disabled and Elderly Assistive Technologies in the U.S. October*

2008. BCC Research. Retrieved on November 11, 2010, from www.bccresearch.com/report/HLC047B.html.

Mechael, P., N. Hima, S. Kaonga, A. Searle, L. Kwan, L. Goldberger, L. Fu, and J. Ossman. 2010. *Barriers and Gaps Affecting mHealth in Low and Middle Income Countries: Policy White Paper*. New York: Center for Global Health and Economic Development, Earth Institute, Columbia University.

Naditz, A. 2008. Telemedicine at the VA: VistA, MyHealtheVet, and other VA programs. *Telemedicine and e-Health* 14:330–32.

New England Healthcare Institute. 2009. *Remote Physiological Monitoring Report: Research Update*. Retrieved on July 7, 2010, from www.nehi.net/publications/36/remote_physiological_monitoring_research_update.

OmniMD. 2010. *Has Government Set EHR Goals Too High?* Retrieved September 21, 2010, from www.myemrstimulus.com/government-set-ehr-goals-high/.

Ontario Medical Association. 1992. *Falls in the Elderly: A Report of the OMA Committee on Accidental Injuries*. Toronto: OMA, November 1992, p. 1.

Ontario Public Health Association. 1998. *Prevention of Falls in the Elderly Population*. Retrieved on December 10, 2010, from www.opha.on.ca/resources/docs/falls.pdf.

Poon, E., A. Jha, M. Christino, M. Honour, R. Fernandopulle, B. Middleton, J. Newhouse, L. Leape, D. Bates, D. Blumenthal, and R. Kausal. 2006. Assessing the level of healthcare information technology adoption in the United States: A snapshot. *BMC Medical Informatics and Decision Making* 6.

Smith, S., and P. Bell. 2005. Examining the effectiveness of the Savvy Caregiver Program among rural Colorado residents. *Rural and Remote Health* 5:466.

Stachura, M., and E. Khasanshina. 2007. *Telehomecare and Remote Monitoring: An Outcomes Overview*. Retrieved on October 31, 2010, from www.advamed.org/NR/rdonlyres/2250724C-5005–45CD-A3C9–0EC0CD3132A1/0/TelehomecarereportFNL103107.pdf.

Terry, M. 2008. Text messaging in healthcare: The elephant knocking at the door. *Telemedicine and e-Health* 14:520–24.

U.S. Department of Health and Human Services. 2010a. *HealthIT, REC Program*. Retrieved on August 14, 2010, from www.healthit.hhs.gov/portal/server.pt?open=512&objID=1495&mode=2.

U.S. Department of Health and Human Services. 2010b. *HITECH Programs*. Retrieved on November 11, 2010, from http://healthit.hhs.gov/portal/server.pt?open=512&objID=1487&mode=2.

U.S. Department of Health and Human Services. 2010c. *ONC Beacon Community Program: Improving Health through Health IT*. Retrieved on June 12, 2010, from http://healthit.hhs.gov/portal/server.pt/community/healthit_hhs_gov_onc_beacon_communities_program_improving_health_through_health_it/1805.

Public Health Workforce

Preparing for an Aging Society

Janet C. Frank, DrPH
Joan Weiss, PhD, RN, CRNP

This chapter focuses on preparing the public health workforce with the skills, knowledge, and abilities for its role in protecting and promoting the health of older adults. Public health, for all of the varied types of professionals working in the field, has not addressed the preparation of its workforce for the "aging boom." Schools of public health do not have any requirement concerning aging, even though adults aged 65 years and older will soon be close to 20% of the total U.S. population (Prohaska and Wallace, 1997; Wallace, Levin, Villa, and Beck, 1998; Molina and Wallace, 2007). The increased size and proportion of the older adult population will place disproportionate demands on our public health systems and services. Health care reform legislation enacted in 2010 offers opportunities to refine the roles for public health and aging professionals to more adequately address the needs of older Americans.

There are a number of integral public health workforce professionals who are trained outside of schools and programs in public health. The curriculum provided to these groups, such as physicians, social workers, and nurses, also has minimal focus on aging content (Berkman, Silverstone, Simmons,

Volland, and Howe, 2000; Berman et al., 2005; Eleazer, Doshi, Wieland, Boland, and Hirth, 2005; Center for Health Workforce Studies, 2006). For example, in many schools of medicine, physicians graduate with only a one-month required in-service hospital rotation that includes some exposure to caring for older adults (Bragg and Warshaw, 2005).

The Institute of Medicine (IOM) report "Retooling for an Aging America" (2008) sets forth a key recommendation to improve the competencies of all members of the health care workforce in providing care and services to older adults. Several professions, including medicine, nursing, social work, and pharmacy, have developed competencies specific to the care of older adults (Wendt, Peterson, and Douglass, 1993; AACN and John A. Hartford Foundation Institute for Geriatric Nursing, 2000; CalSWEC Aging Initiative, 2006; American Society of Consultant Pharmacists, 2007; AAMC and John A. Hartford Foundation, 2008). Public health currently does not have competencies specific to caring for older adults. Consensus-driven professional competency development is seen as a necessary early step to bring the need for required specialized curricula to the attention of professional public health programs and schools.

The content covered in this chapter is threefold. It begins with a description of the demographics of public health personnel and their key roles related to older adults. Second, it examines the current academic preparation of public health and related professions' students and trainees. It concludes with future directions and recommendations, including the development of key competencies for public health personnel relating to older adults. Although the focus is on public health schools and programs, the recommendations are applicable to other professional groups that often have a major role in developing policies and programs, as well as providing clinical health care and services to older adults.

DEFINITIONS AND DEMOGRAPHICS OF PUBLIC HEALTH PERSONNEL

The public health workforce is large, diverse, and growing older. The number of full-time-equivalent public health professionals working for federal, state, and local public health agencies was estimated to be over 550,000 in 2004 (Gebbie and Turnock, 2006). This count does not include many professionals working in community agencies and other nonfederal organizations that focus on the health of populations. As defined by the IOM, "A public health professional is a person educated in public health or a related discipline who is employed to improve health through a population focus" (IOM, 2003, p. 4). This description is consistent with that of the U.S. Department of Health and Human Services, which describes the public health workforce to include all personnel providing essential public health services, regardless of the agency or organization where they work (U.S. Department of Health and Human Services, 1997).

Public health professionals are themselves growing older. By 2012, approximately 100,000 government-based public health workers will be eligible to retire—almost 20% of the public sector workforce (ASPH, 2008). The Association of State and Territorial Health Officials (ASTHO) conducted a State Public Health Workforce Survey in 2007 and noted the "graying workforce" as a major area of concern (ASTHO, 2008). This study also documented that the average age of a public health worker in state government is 47, and the average age of new hires in state health agencies is 40. Among the reporting states, approximately one-third (29%) of the public health workforce will be eligible to retire by 2012, with several states projecting rates as high as 56% (ASTHO, 2008).

The aging of the public health workforce and commensurate retirement eligibility have a critical impact on public health organizations' leadership. Nationally, around 65% of local health agency top executives are aged 50 or older, according to the National Association of County and City Health Officials (NACCHO) 2005 National Profile of Local Health Departments. Many leaders and managers in public health agencies have been in their positions for years. When their leaders retire, many agencies, especially smaller ones, are left without suitable replacements and often without a viable succession plan. Workforce planning is critical given the data on retirement eligibility. The benefits of workforce planning include the ability to strategically align workforce and organizational needs, develop strategies to address gaps in workforce supply and demand, and determine key human resource functional needs or competencies for the organization's strategic direction (ASTHO, 2008).

A major aspect of workforce planning is succession planning. Succession planning consists of the arrangements an organization makes to ensure that its leadership is continuous, and it includes identifying how executive positions will be filled in the event of turnover. Succession plans may include preparing talent from within an organization or planning recruitment activities for external candidates. These plans are particularly important to ensure that public health agencies minimize risk to the populations they serve and have a reliably strong response in the case of emergencies. Succession plans have added importance in a job market in which agencies will be increasingly competing for experienced leaders. That a field as important as public health might be left without sufficient leadership in the next 5 years should be a wake-up call at all levels.

PUBLIC HEALTH PERSONNEL: KEY ROLES AND FUNCTIONS

The overarching role for public health professionals is to protect and promote the public's health. It is useful to conceptualize key roles and functions of public health personnel within a social-ecological public health framework. The Framework for Public Health Action, as described by Frieden (2010), proposes a five-level pyramid utilizing a social-ecological approach based on a public health intervention's impact potential. It is a framework for improving the public's health. Applying this framework, interventions that focus on social-economic determinants are at its base, and the four levels above the base represent interventions that change the context for health (e.g., safe water), long-term protective interventions (e.g., immunizations), direct clinical care, and, at the top, counseling and education. The bottom tiers have the most potential for improving the public's health, and as the layers ascend the pyramid, the interventions require more focus on a person-centered individual level, such as behavior change (see chap. 8 for application of this framework to research translation). Having well-trained public health professionals to perform the tasks required for each level within the social-ecological framework is important for all population groups, including older adults.

Public health professionals serve a number of different functions within each level of the Framework for Public Health Action. The Public Health Workforce Enumeration 2000 report classified public health personnel into four broad categories: administrative, technical, professional, and clerical support (Center for Health Policy, 2000). Public health administrative personnel include health planners, managers, and policy analysts at the national, state, and local levels, as well as midlevel managers such as program directors. This category of personnel is relevant for all levels in the social-ecological framework, but most importantly at the sociodemographic and contextual change levels. Technical personnel working in laboratories across the nation have increasingly important roles in systems development, data management, and reporting. Technical personnel are required for all levels of the framework but have a critical role in the contextual change level of the pyramid. The professional category includes the myriad of licensed health care personnel who provide long-term protective interventions (e.g., immuniza-

TABLE 13.1
*Public health professionals critical to the
older population*

Administrative
    Health planner
    Licensure/inspection/regulatory specialist
    Policy or program analyst
    Program manager
    Public relations/media specialist
    Researcher
Technical
    Computer programmer
    Epidemiologist
    Infection control/disease investigator
    Laboratory scientist
    Laboratory technician
    Occupation safety and health specialist
Professional
    Marriage and family therapist
    Medical and public health social worker
    Mental health/substance abuse social worker
    Mental health counselor
    PH dental worker
    PH educator
    PH nurse
    PH nutritionist
    PH optometrist
    PH pharmacist
    PH physical therapist
    PH physician
    PH program specialist
    PH student
    Psychiatric nurse
    Psychiatrist
    Psychologist
    Substance abuse and behavioral disorders counselor

---

tions), direct care, and/or counseling and education to older people. This chapter does not address clerical support. Table 13.1 lists examples of administrative, technical, and professional roles for public health professionals with a major role in planning and providing services for the older population (Center for Health Policy, 2000).

PUBLIC HEALTH AND AGING EDUCATION AND TRAINING

The following section summarizes what is known about public health and aging curricula at schools and programs in public health and related professions. Ad-

ditionally, a summary of available training programs for public health professionals that may include content on aging or working with older adults is provided.

Accredited Schools and Programs in Public Health

There have been no studies in the past 5 years on curricula or student enrollment in aging-related coursework in public health schools and programs. In
the mid-1990s, there were two such published reports. Prohaska (1992) found
that the majority of public health schools had a documented listing in their
published catalogs that included at least one course referencing aging. A
more comprehensive study that queried schools of public health and other
professional schools was conducted in 1994 by the California Geriatric Education Center (CGEC) with funding from the Health Resources and Services Administration's Bureau of Health Professions (Wallace et al., 1998).
This study found that almost three-quarters (72%) of the schools of public
health had at least one course that included a topic related to aging, compared
with 33% of other master of public health degree granting departments. Findings from the survey also showed that enrollment was modest. For all aging-
related courses offered during a year, it was estimated that 6% of graduates had
taken one or more courses on any health and aging topic (Wallace et al., 1998).

The seminal work by the Health Resources and Services Administration's
Bureau of Health Professions (HRSA BHPr), entitled "A National Agenda for
Geriatric Education: White Papers," first documented the lack of training
and preparedness for the many needed health and social service professions,
the concerns for major service delivery systems (e.g., long-term care), and
mechanisms for delivery of services and education (e.g., case management)
(U.S. Department of Health and Human Services, 1995). One chapter devoted to public health summarized the state of training in schools of public
health. That chapter also provided some key recommendations in three
broad areas to improve the preparedness of professionals and public health
programs for older adults, which are summarized in table 13.2.

In 2005, the HRSA BHPr assessed the progress made in accomplishing the
recommendations from the 1995 White Papers. There were minimal achievements made in addressing the 10 recommendations concerning public
health. Also in 2005, a second survey was conducted as a part of a report to
the Aging Council of the Association of Schools of Public Health. This survey was administered to 36 schools of public health (response rate 92%) and
62 public health programs (response rate 61%). This Web-based survey was
modeled after the 1994 public health and aging curriculum study (Wallace

TABLE 13.2

Bureau of Health Professions 1995 White Paper recommendations for public health and aging

---

Educational issues

1. Increase linkages between public health and aging networks through education, training, and collaboration
2. Expand continuing education in public health and aging; improve opportunities for lifelong learning
3. Develop methods and standards for timely information dissemination of advances in public health and aging to practitioners in aging and the general public
4. Implement new technologies that facilitate learning and communication between aging programs in schools of public health and public health practitioners in aging

Attitudes and perceptions of the older adult population

5. Improve the knowledge and attitudes of public health students about older persons
6. Increase the attention of public health education and practice to issues of diversity among older adults

Strategic plans and other administrative issues and evaluation

7. Promote interdisciplinary practice through interdisciplinary role socialization in accredited public health programs
8. Stabilize public health education funding

Source: Wallace, Prohaska, Silverman, and Cary, 1995

et al., 1998). The findings reinforce that there was a limited amount of aging content in schools of public health and public health programs and a paucity of faculty with aging-related interests. In the 2004–5 academic year, respondents estimated a total of just fewer than 500 students enrolled in at least one course with aging content. This is less than 3% of the approximately 19,000 public health students enrolled in schools across the country (Molina and Wallace, 2007).

In 2010, Frank and Wallace (under development) examined the available data on doctorally prepared professionals in the field of public health and aging. To gain insight into "current leadership" in public health and aging, the types of degrees for Gerontological Health Section membership of the American Public Health Association were tallied. Out of a total of 524 section members, 235 of them had doctorate-level degrees. Nine listed doctorates in public health (DrPH); 158 listed doctor of philosophy, including PhDs in public health; 48 listed medical degrees; and 20 listed other types of doctorates. These individuals are the current research, policy, and program leaders for the field of public health and aging.

To examine the contributions from academic centers, Wallace reviewed the Proquest Digital Dissertations database (http://proquest.umi.com/login) and looked for dissertations in the past 5 years within the subject "public health" and title words "elderly, older, or aging," and he found 296. One-third were for master's degree dissertations, and two-thirds ($n = 195$) were doctoral dissertations. Based on these findings, there are approximately 40 public health doctoral graduates with dissertations in aging being "produced" each year, on average, for the past 5 years nationwide (J. C. Frank and S. P. Wallace, unpublished data collected for the CGEC).

This research on aging curricula within accredited schools and programs documents that the scope and quantity of public health and aging training are currently inadequate (Molina and Wallace, 2007). Overall, the narrow scope of aging curricula and the relatively small numbers of students enrolled in courses using these curricula have led to the conclusion that the potential supply of public health professionals with training in aging issues does not meet the workforce demand for such trained individuals.

Public Health–Related Professions: Preparation and Production
Medicine

Almost all (98%) medical schools now require some type of exposure to geriatrics; however, it is often inadequate and focused on hospital care of older adults (IOM, 2008). The necessary preparation of physicians has two goals: to create a cadre of geriatric specialists and geriatric academicians while providing adequate training opportunities in the continuum of care to all physicians. Schools of medicine are falling short in meeting both of these goals, in spite of major philanthropic investment in programs and consistent federal funding for geriatric education.

Currently, there are about 7,000 physicians certified in geriatric medicine and almost 1,600 certified in geriatric psychiatry, and these numbers are decreasing over time (IOM, 2008). For advanced training of physicians there are 1– to 3–year fellowships. In addition, the HRSA BHPr Geriatric Academic Career Awards Program provides career advancement support for physicians, nurses, dentists, psychologists, social workers, pharmacists, and allied health junior faculty who are working as clinician educators in academia. Of physicians specially trained in public health who hold both medical and master of public health degrees, 154 are members of the American Geriatrics Society (AGS), which represents less than 3% of its total membership of 5,503 physicians (E. Lois of AGS, pers. comm., Aug. 6, 2010).

Nursing

Nurses are one of the largest health professions working in public health systems, typically health departments or home health agencies. Two-thirds of baccalaureate programs in schools of nursing do not require even one course on geriatrics in spite of having nationally ratified geriatric competencies for nurses (IOM, 2008). Over 40% of nurses receive their education in 2–year associate degree programs at community colleges, and the amount of geriatrics content in their programs is unknown (IOM, 2008). There is a geriatrics certification available for nurses, but only 1% of registered nurses and less than 3% of advanced practice nurses are certified in geriatrics.

A major barrier to providing more geriatric content in curricula is well-trained nursing faculty to teach the courses. A number of private and publicly funded programs have addressed and continue to promote geriatric nursing faculty development and curriculum expansion. Given the small and uneven exposure to geriatrics in formal training programs for nurses, it is relatively safe to conclude that practicing nurses do not receive adequate preparation in geriatrics. Furthermore, there are no data available on the numbers of public health nurses with a geriatric specialty or the amount of geriatrics content that is included in courses in nursing programs.

Pharmacy

Less than half (43%) of schools of pharmacy have a specific course on geriatrics, although all schools provide the opportunity for advanced training in geriatrics or long-term care (IOM, 2008). The accrediting body of 4–year doctor of pharmacy degree programs recommends that geriatrics be included in the curricula but does not require it (IOM, 2008). The American Society of Health-Systems Pharmacists currently accredits 351 second-year residency training programs, 8 of which are in geriatric pharmacy (IOM, 2008). There is a geriatric certification available for pharmacists; however, less than 1% (1,297) are certified. With the exception of HRSA's Geriatric Education Centers program, little funding has been targeted to geriatric pharmacy faculty or curriculum development in schools of pharmacy. There are no data on the preparation of public health pharmacists in geriatrics or aging.

Social Work

There are 471 baccalaureate and 201 master of social work programs accredited by the Council on Social Work Education (www.cswe.org) that graduate approximately 31,000 students annually (ASPE, 2006). The most recent data on aging curricula available in baccalaureate programs are from 1988 and suggest that 80% of these programs do not have specific courses on the aging population (Lubben, Damron-Rodriguez, and Beck, 1992).

A more recent survey of master's-level programs indicated that almost one-third offered some type of aging specialization or concentration but only 5% of students complete such programs (www.cswe.org). Major philanthropic support has been provided to increase the production of geriatric social workers, most notably by the John A. Hartford Foundation and Atlantic Philanthropies. These projects have supported comprehensive competency development, faculty development, practicum partnerships for fieldwork training, and development of model curricula (IOM, 2008).

Unlike other professions working in public health service delivery, there are some data on the preparedness of social workers currently employed in public welfare programs and community-based aging service organizations. For example, data from the state of California reveal that in county welfare agencies and aging service organizations about 60% of all agencies had no staff who had even taken one academic course with geriatrics or aging content (CalSWEC Aging Initiative, 2006). For the 40% of the county welfare group that did have at least one staff with academic training, 21% had only one staff and 18% had two or more staff with formal training. Of the aging service organizations that had staff trained in aging, 12% had one, 10% had two, and 17% had three or more staff with formal training. Of note, all agencies reported a deficit in several social work and aging competencies that they identified as important for their workforce (CalSWEC Aging Initiative, 2006).

Overall, based on the available data, it is clear that schools and programs in public health and the related health professions do not offer adequate training to students in aging content areas. In addition, compared to other professional schools, public health is lagging far behind other disciplines that have roles in public health. Many current health and social service agency personnel delivering services do not have adequate preparation to meet the needs of older adults. Academic programs need to increase the availability of and requirements to include courses on aging and gerontology in public health programming, so that future service providers will be better prepared than those currently in these positions.

Public Health and Aging Traineeships and Training Programs

There are a number of public agencies that provide traineeships and training programs in public health or aging to help prepare the public health workforce for an aging society. The primary agencies at the national level include the HRSA, the Centers for Disease Control and Prevention (CDC), the National Institute on Aging (NIA), and the Veterans Administration. An overview of selected programs sponsored by these agencies, which either explicitly promote training in aging and public health or have the potential to include aging and/or public health and aging within their training programs, is given in the appendix.

Health Resources and Services Administration

HRSA sponsors a number of training programs that focus on geriatrics and gerontology that either include or could include public health. Of the eight programs identified in the appendix, the Geriatric Education Center (GEC) program has provided much of the public health and aging training on a national level. In addition, GECs have provided a significant amount of the information that is known about the availability of courses on aging topics in schools and programs in public health.

HRSA's BHPr offers a number of opportunities for training in public health and aging. Most notable is the Public Health Training Center (PHTC) program. A review of the PHTC websites reflected that currently one PHTC, the Heartland Public Health Education and Training Center, has an aging-related organization listed as a practice partner, and three PHTCs each list one aging-related training/education topic. This program has the potential to expand its focus on public health and aging.

Centers for Disease Control and Prevention

CDC is another federal agency that offers training initiatives for students, faculty, and public health practitioners. CDC sponsors four programs to promote aging expertise within the current and future public health workforce as shown in the appendix. For example, the Prevention Research Center (PRC) program identifies a number of training programs for students. The CDC-PRC Minority Fellowship focused on doctoral-level students of ethnic or racial minority origin, providing 2 years of training and guided research at a PRC, including the Healthy Aging Research Network (more information can be found at www.cdc.gov/prc/training/students/cdc-prc-minority-fellowship .htm).

National Institute on Aging

NIA sponsors five programs, with each funding the operation of centers. Each center provides pilot grants or career development grants to assistant professor–level faculty, including faculty from schools of public health. There are 30 Alzheimer's Disease Research Centers, 13 Edward R. Roybal Centers, 14 Demography and Economics of Aging Centers, 11 Claude D. Pepper Older Americans Independence Centers, and 6 Resource Centers for Minority

Aging Research (RCMAR). In addition, there are four fellowship or trainee-ship opportunities that can include public health faculty.

Pilot grants and career development awards to faculty in schools of public health have only been available relatively recently through the RCMAR pro-gram. Of the 131 minority faculty who had received RCMAR pilot awards, 12 were from schools of public health (unpublished data, UCLA National RCMAR Coordinating Center). There are increasing opportunities to ad-dress public health and aging through the NIA programs, especially through the RCMAR programs and the Roybal Centers.

Veterans Administration

The Veterans Administration's Geriatric Research Education and Clinical Center (GRECC) program aims to attract scientists and health science stu-dents to the field of geriatrics in order to help increase the basic knowledge of aging, transmit this knowledge to health care providers, and improve the quality of care delivered to elders. Currently there are 20 GRECCs funded, with the three in Baltimore, Palo Alto, and Greater Los Angeles addressing public health and aging.

There are many opportunities for federal programs to attend to the unique public health needs of older adults. For example, older adults are more sus-ceptible to changes in the water supply, air quality, and the environment. Additionally, older adults may be faced with limited mobility, and public health is poised to address these needs through initiatives to promote the built environment. Thus, public health can play a role in coordinating across sec-tors such as transportation, housing, food safety, agriculture, commerce, legal, and education for the public health workforce to ensure the health of the nation's older adults. In addition, public health prevention and early de-tection activities starting early in life can result in a healthier older genera-tion with fewer disabilities. Public health workforce training programs can be effective catalysts to promote healthy aging by preparing a proactive work-force that promotes population health and healthy communities. Although federal investment in programs to improve the care of older adults is expand-ing, as documented in the appendix, there is an urgent need for data from both national and regional perspectives across all programs. Longitudinal data are needed to help define determinants of healthy aging and local plan-ning efforts. Data are also needed to determine healthy behaviors in older adults and for providers to develop communication skills (see chap. 4).

FUTURE DIRECTIONS AND RECOMMENDATIONS
Recommendation 1

Increase the recognition of the importance of public health and aging training. Societal challenges have shaped the focus and priorities in the field of public health from its earliest beginnings. Recently, crisis-driven issues such as environmental pollution and bioterrorism have captured significant public health attention and resources, yet health issues related to our rapidly aging population have lagged behind. There is a tremendous unmet need for public health and aging training programs, and strengthening these programs could have a significant impact on our nation's ability to care for our aging population.

Recommendation 2

Improve the types of data and data collection to document participation of public health students, professionals, and faculty in training on aging. There needs to be new comprehensive research that provides data on what is being taught in schools and programs in public health, the availability of faculty, and the number of students electing to take classes. Also, additional research is needed to determine how much exposure professional staff have had to aging coursework and continuing education training programs.

Progress in achieving the 1995 White Paper recommendations for public health and aging should be monitored given the current state of aging and public health. A compendium of resources, syllabi, course materials, and teaching tools from existing public health and aging courses should be developed as a centralized resource to promote course development and offerings within schools and programs of public health, gerontology, and related academic programs. To facilitate distribution of existing course materials and resources, the development of an online database would be useful.

Recommendation 3

Involve older adults as members of the public health workforce. Older people, owing to the myriad of chronic illnesses they may have, often need to play key roles in their own care. Health care reform legislation supported "patient-centered care" and activating patients to become more central to the care processes they are involved in. For several years, the evidence has demonstrated that patients who are engaged in chronic disease self-management programs have better health outcomes (Lorig et al., 1999). As part of the American Recovery and Reinvestment Act of 2009, five initiatives were funded as part of "Communities Putting Prevention to Work." One of these programs focuses on creating sustainable systems that combine the public health delivery system with aging service organizations. Forty-five grants were made to states and territories to deliver the Chronic Disease Self-Management Program (CDSMP) to older adults (www.healthyagingprograms.org/index .asp). These national programs make community-based programs in self-management accessible to older adults and provide the practical "how to" side of self-management activities often lacking in traditional patient education (Cleland and Ekman, 2010). The public health workforce could be trained to assist in these efforts to reinforce the older person's self-management skills that are gained through these programs. Older adults can and do have important roles in managing their health, and future public health training programs should support these efforts since public health providers have a unique opportunity to influence behaviors on a large scale.

Recommendation 4

Create special leadership academies to address the aging of the public health workforce, with an emphasis on inclusion of public health and aging content. Given the aging of the public health workforce, it is clear that new leadership must be developed to replace those who are retiring. There will need to be multiple strategies deployed, including a focus on adequate succession planning within public health agencies and organizations. In addition, it would be extremely timely to develop several model programs funded by federal agencies or foundations that would address both the impending leadership vacuum and the lack of training about public health and older adults. There are currently several established programs in geriatric medicine (Association of Directors of Geriatric Academic Programs Leadership Scholars) and leadership programs for geriatric nursing and social work funded by the John A. Hartford Foundation (www.jhartfound.org/).

Recommendation 5

Develop aging-specific public health educational competencies. The IOM report "Retooling for an Aging America" (2008) makes very specific recommendations regarding improving the competencies of the health care workforce to ready it to provide needed care for older adults. Yet unlike other disciplines, including medicine, nursing, social work, and pharmacy, public health has yet to develop geriatric or aging-related competencies (Wendt et al., 1993; AACN and John A. Hartford Foundation Institute for Geriatric Nursing, 2000; CalSWEC Aging Initiative, 2006; American Society of Consultant Pharmacists, 2007; AAMC and John A. Hartford Foundation, 2008). These national competencies guide the curricula in professional schools and serve as a benchmark for professional practice. Public health has developed core competencies for master of public health programs (ASPH, 2006). The 119 competencies are embedded within five disciplinary areas and seven cross-cutting interdisciplinary themes. They are an excellent global set of competencies for the field.

There are also very specific competencies for the field of public health, such as those in bioterrorism and disaster preparedness (Calhoun, Rowney, Eng, and Hoffman, 2005). Public health is an important discipline in addressing the needs of the older population and has a strong role in health promotion, prevention, and care delivery to older persons and their families (Wallace, 2005). Public health, as a profession, needs to be included in "retooling" for an aging America and develop aging-related competencies that can create a base upon which to build.

Developing competencies for the field of public health is important to accomplish now for several reasons. First, it will gain the national attention of the public health academic programs and engage their leadership and faculty in the competency development process. Second, it will produce the criteria for public health curriculum development that can be used for schools and other training centers, like the PHTCs and the GECs. In addition, because schools of public health are just now being required to document how they fulfill the basic competencies, they are particularly attuned to the need for competencies across all major topics. Finally, it will document that aging is an important area for public health to address.

Public health, as a field, is far behind other disciplines in addressing the geriatric preparation needs of its faculty and professionals. Yet the field has so much to offer through prevention and health promotion to optimize healthy aging. The national public health care delivery system has a critical role to play in designing new models of care and providing comprehensive health care to older adults.

CONCLUSION

This chapter has focused on the preparation of the public health workforce to address the needs of the burgeoning older population. There are special skills, knowledge, and abilities required by public health professionals in order to fulfill their roles in protecting and promoting the health of older adults. Public health has not addressed the preparation of its workforce for the "aging boom." Federal program support has attempted to provide programmatic opportunities for the bridge between aging and public health, but these programs are not often maximized for this purpose. There is much that needs to be done, and we have provided five major recommendations to address the issues we have identified and to improve the qualifications and readiness of the diverse public health workforce for an aging society.

APPENDIX

Public Health Training and Traineeships

Agency / Title of program	Purpose of program	Current activities
Health Resources and Services Administration (http://bhpr.hrsa.gov/)		
Comprehensive Geriatric Education Programs (CGEP)	Provides support to (1) train and educate individuals who will provide geriatric care to older adults, (2) develop and disseminate curricula relating to the treatment of the health problems of older individuals, (3) train faculty members in geriatrics, and (4) provide continuing education to individuals who provide geriatric care.	In 2010, 27 grants were funded. Of these, six grantees (22%) provide education and training in public health and aging (http://bhpr.hrsa .gov/grants/geriatrics .htm).
Geriatric Education Centers (GECs)	Funds are used to (1) improve the education and training of health professionals in geriatrics, (2) develop and disseminate curricula relating to the treatment of the health problems of the elderly, (3) train and retrain faculty to provide instruction in geriatrics, (4) support continuing education of health professionals who provide geriatric care, and (5) provide students with clinical training in geriatrics in nursing homes, chronic and acute disease hospitals, and ambulatory care.	In 2010, 45 grants were funded. Fifteen (33%) of these grantees include public health faculty and public health organizations (http:// bhpr.hrsa.gov/grants/ geriatrics.htm).

APPENDIX *continued*

Agency/Title of program	Purpose of program	Current activities
Geriatric Training for Physicians, Dentists, and Behavioral and Mental Health Professionals Program	Provides support to accredited schools of medicine, schools of osteopathic medicine, teaching hospitals, and graduate medical education programs for geriatric training projects to train physicians, dentists, and behavioral and mental health professionals who plan to teach geriatric medicine, geriatric dentistry, or geriatric behavioral or mental health.	In 2010, 13 grants were funded. Five (38%) of these grantees provide training in public health and aging (http://bhpr.hrsa.gov/grants/geriatrics.htm).
Geriatric Academic Career Awards Program	Promote career development of health professions faculty as clinician educators in the disciplines of allopathic medicine, osteopathic medicine, dentistry, nursing, psychology, social work, pharmacy, and allied health.	In 2010, 68 awards were made. None focus on public health and aging (http://bhpr.hrsa.gov/grants/geriatrics.htm).
Public Health Training Centers Program	Provides graduate or specialized training in public health to expand and enhance training opportunities that focus on the technical, scientific, managerial, and leadership competencies and capabilities of the current and future public health workforce.	In 2010, 33 grants were funded. One grantee addresses public health and aging (http://bhpr.hrsa.gov/grants/public.htm).
Public Health Traineeship Program	Provides traineeships to individuals enrolled in graduate or specialized training programs in public health.	In 2010, 30 grants were funded. Grantees have not reported any training experiences that focus on aging (http://bhpr.hrsa.gov/grants/public.htm).
Preventive Medicine Residency Program	Provides support for the planning of, development of, operation of, or participation (including financial assistance to residents) in preventive medicine and public health.	In 2010, 17 grants were funded. None address public health and aging (http://bhpr.hrsa.gov/grants/public.htm).
Residency Training in Dental Public Health Program	Provides support to plan and develop new dental public health residency training programs or maintain or improve existing dental public health residency training programs, and provides financial assistance to residents in dental public health residency training programs.	In 2010, six grants were funded. None address public health and aging (http://bhpr.hrsa.gov/grants/public.htm).

continued

APPENDIX *continued*

Agency/Title of program	Purpose of program	Current activities

Centers for Disease Control and Prevention (www.cdc.gov/fellowships)

Prevention Research Centers (PRC) Minority Fellowship	Provides support for doctoral-level students of ethnic or racial minority origin for 2 years of training and guided research at a Prevention Research Center. The 2-year fellowship began in 2002 and provides training in prevention research and community-based participatory research and the opportunity to gain practical, first-hand experience in prevention research.	Fellows participate in projects under the direction of leading experts in public health and prevention research. Fellows work on current PRC projects and are encouraged to propose their own projects related to PRC activities. There are four new 2010 fellows and three continuing fellows. Several are working on aging-related topics (e.g., diabetes), and one past fellow focused on healthy aging. The program has supported 38 fellows since its inception (www.cdc.gov/prc/about-prc-program/minority-fellowship.htm).
CDC Healthy Aging Research Network (CDC HAN)	Works nationally to understand the determinants of healthy aging, identify interventions that promote healthy aging, and translate those interventions into sustainable community-based programs.	Develops and provides training programs, often as Web-based modules and online distance learning programs (www.prc-han.org). CDC's Healthy Aging Program also supports a nonresidential fellow as part of the Health and Aging Policy Fellowships (www.healthand agingpolicy.org).
Public Health Prevention Service (PHPS) Program	Provides 3 years of training and service for master's-level public health professionals. Focuses on public health program management and provides experience in program planning, implementation, and evaluation through specialized hands-on training and mentorship at CDC and in state and local health organizations.	The program sponsors approximately 20 individuals each year. CDC's Healthy Aging Program offers rotations for the PHPS program, and four PHPS graduates are current members of that program (www.cdc.gov/PHPS/index.html).

APPENDIX *continued*

Agency/Title of program	Purpose of program	Current activities
Public Health Residency/Fellowship Program	Accredited by the Accreditation Council for Graduate Medical Education. It meets the residency requirement of the American Board of Preventive Medicine, in the specialty of Public Health and General Preventive Medicine. Combined class size ranges from 6 to 14 persons per year. The PMR/F practicum provides a balance between service and supervised on-the-job learning in public health and preventive medicine practice.	Practicum assignments include mentoring by experienced public health practitioners, hands-on experience in public health and preventive medicine practice, and classroom training (www.cdc.gov/prev med/).

National Institute on Aging (www.nia.nih.gov/GrantsAndTraining/TrainingSupport.htm)

Alzheimer's Disease Research Centers (ADRCs)	Located at major medical institutions across the nation, researchers work to translate research advances into improved diagnosis and care for Alzheimer's disease patients while, at the same time, focusing on the program's long-term goal—finding a way to cure and possibly prevent AD.	In 2010, 30 centers and one coordinating center were funded. Each center offers pilot research awards and mentored training to junior faculty involved in developing careers in Alzheimer's disease and related disorders research. The ADEAR Center does not collect specific information that addresses public health (www.nia .nih.gov/Alzheimers/ ResearchInformation/ ResearchCenters/ #what)
Edward R. Roybal Centers	Designed to move promising social and behavioral research findings out of the laboratory and into programs and practices that will improve the lives of older people and help society adapt to an aging population. The centers focus on a range of projects, including maintaining mobility and physical function, enhancing driving performance, understanding financial and medical decision making, and sharpening cognitive function.	In 2010, 13 centers were funded. The Roybal Centers do not collect information specifically on public health faculty involvement. One center is addressing the gap between available evidence-based health promotion programs and their use by minority older adults (www.nia .nih.gov/ResearchInfor mation/ExtramuralPro grams/BehavioralAnd SocialResearch/roybals .htm).

continued

APPENDIX *continued*

Agency/Title of program	Purpose of program	Current activities
Centers on Demography and Economics of Aging	Designed to investigate aspects of health and health care, the societal impact of population aging, and the economic and social circumstances of older people. Each center has its own set of disciplinary specializations, although research conducted at the different centers is often interrelated. Many centers also conduct research on global aging and cross-national comparisons, and several are pioneering work on the biodemography of aging, investigating the relationships among biology and genetics, health and mortality, and life expectancy.	In 2010, 14 centers were funded. Each center provides pilot research support to junior faculty and training opportunities such as lecture series and short courses. These centers do not collect data on public health faculty involvement and training (www.nia.nih.gov/ ResearchInformation/ ExtramuralPrograms/ BehavioralAndSocial Research/demogcenters .htm).
Claude D. Pepper Older Americans Independence Centers	Designed to develop or strengthen institutions' programs that focus and sustain progress on a key area in aging research. Each area of focus is one in which progress could contribute to greater independence for older persons and offer opportunities for training and career development in aging research.	In 2010, 11 centers and one coordinating center were funded. Each center offers pilot awards to faculty and career development awards to faculty from many disciplines including public health. The focus of the centers is largely on research, not education, and they do not collect data on the number of public health faculty involved (www.nia.nih .gov/NewsAndEvents/ Links/2010Spring.htm).
Resource Centers for Minority Aging Research	The mission is to decrease health disparities by increasing the number of researchers who focus on the health of minority elders, enhancing the diversity in the professional workforce by mentoring minority academic researchers for careers in minority elders health research, improving recruitment and retention methods used to enlist minority elders in research studies, creating culturally sensitive health measures	In 2010, six centers and one coordinating center were funded (www .rcmar.ucla.edu).

APPENDIX *continued*

Agency / Title of program	Purpose of program	Current activities
	that assess the health status of minority elders with greater precision, and increasing the effectiveness of interventions designed to improve their health and well-being.	
Institutional Training Grants	Offers T32, T34, and T35 grant opportunities to institutions for fellowships and training awards for predoctoral, postdoctoral, and junior faculty to be trained as investigators in aging research or for health professions doctorate. There are also special program initiatives for training minority individuals and to support minority-serving institutions.	In fiscal year 2009, 3,200 T type (institutional) grants were awarded; however, no information was available on public health involvement (http://grants.nih .gov/training/outcomes .htm).
Individual Fellowships	Offers the Ruth L. Kirschstein National Research Service Award and individual fellowship grants at the predoctoral, postdoctoral, and senior fellow levels.	In fiscal year 2009, 3,200 F type (institutional and individual) grants were awarded; however, no information was available on public health involvement (www.nia .nih.gov/GrantsAnd Training/Individual FellowshipsAwards.htm).
Research Career Development Awards	Provides individual career development opportunities to develop research and clinical scientist careers in aging at the early and middle career stages. The K07 Academic Career award is for established senior researchers to build aging research into their institutions.	In fiscal year 2009, 4,300 K type (institutional and individual) grants were awarded; however, no information was available on public health involvement (www.nia .nih.gov/GrantsAnd Training/CareerDevel opment.htm).
Summer Institute on Aging Research	Includes lectures, seminars, and small-group discussions in research design relative to aging, including issues relevant to aging of ethnic and racial minorities. Discussion sessions will focus on methodological approaches and interventions. The program also includes consultation on the development of research interests and advice on preparing and submitting research grant applications to NIA.	This program is offered annually (http://grants .nih.gov/training/out comes.htm). The Summer Institute is part of the T type (T35) program captured above (www.nia.nih.gov/News AndEvents/Calendar/ SummerInstitute2010 .htm).

continued

APPENDIX *continued*

Agency/Title of program	Purpose of program	Current activities
Veterans Administration (www.va.gov/grecc/)		
Geriatric Research Education and Clinical Center	Provides support to attract scientists and health science students to the field of geriatrics in order to help increase the basic knowledge of aging, transmit this knowledge to health care providers, and improve the quality of care delivered to elders.	In 2010, there were 20 GRECCs (www.va.gov/grecc/).

ACKNOWLEDGMENTS

The findings and conclusions in this chapter are those of the authors and do not necessarily reflect the official position of the Health Resources and Services Administration.

REFERENCES

AACN and John A. Hartford Foundation Institute for Geriatric Nursing. 2000. *Older Adults: Recommended Baccalaureate Competencies and Curricular Guidelines for Geriatric Nursing Care.* Retrieved August 2, 2010, from www.aacn.nche.edu/education/gercomp.htm.

AAMC and John A. Hartford Foundation. 2008. Consensus Conference on Competencies in Geriatric Education. *Minimum Geriatric Competencies for Medical Students.* Retrieved August 1, 2010 from www.pogoe.org/Minimum_Geriatric_Competencies.

American Society of Consultant Pharmacists. 2007. *Geriatric Pharmacy Curriculum Guide,* 2nd ed. Retrieved August 10, 2010, from www.ascp.com/search/node/Geriatric%20Pharmacy%20Curriculum%20Guide.

Assistant Secretary for Planning and Evaluation (ASPE), U.S. Department of Health and Human Services. 2006. *The Supply and Demand of Professional Social Workers Providing Long-Term Care Services.* Washington, DC: ASPE Office of Disability, Aging and Long-Term Care Policy.

Association of Schools of Public Health (ASPH). 2006. *Master's of Public Health Core Competency Model.* Retrieved August 7, 2010, from www.asph.org/userfiles/version2.3.pdf.

Association of Schools of Public Health (ASPH). 2008. Policy Brief: *Confronting the Public Health Workforce Crisis.* Retrieved December 2, 2010, from www.asph.org.

Association of State and Territorial Health Officials (ASTHO). 2008. *2007 State Public Health Workforce Shortage Report.* Retrieved December 2, 2010, from biotech.law.lsu.edu/cdc/astho/WorkforceReport.pdf.

Berkman, B., B. Silverstone, W. J. Simmons, P. J. Volland, and J. L. Howe. 2000. Social work gerontological practice: The need for faculty development in the new millennium. *Journal of Gerontological Social Work* 34(1):5–23.

Berman, A., M. Mezey, M. Kobayashi, T. Fulmer, J. Stanley, D. Thornlow, and P. Rosenfeld. 2005. Gerontological nursing content in baccalaureate nursing programs: Comparison of findings from 1997 and 2003. *Journal of Professional Nursing* 21:268–75.

Bragg, E. J., and G. A. Warshaw. 2005. ACGME requirements for geriatrics medicine curricula in medical specialties: Progress made and progress needed. *Academic Medicine* 80:279–85.

Calhoun, J. G., R. Rowney, E. Eng, and Y. Hoffman. 2005. Competency mapping and analysis for public health preparedness training initiatives. *Public Health Reports* 120(Suppl. 1):91–99.

CalSWEC Aging Initiative. 2006. *California Social Work Education Center (CalSWEC) Aging Initiative: Aging Competencies*. Retrieved August 13, 2010, from http://calswec.berkeley.edu/CalSWEC/AgingCompetencies_All_Feb2006.pdf.

Center for Health Policy at the Columbia University School of Nursing, HRSA, Bureau of Health Professions, National Center for Health Workforce Information and Analysis. 2000. *The Public Health Workforce Enumeration 2000*. Retrieved August 24, 2010, from ftp://ftp.hrsa.gov//bhpr/nationalcenter/phworkforce2000.pdf.

Center for Health Workforce Studies, School of Public Health, University at Albany. 2006. *The Impact of the Aging Population on the Health Workforce in the United States: Summary of Key Findings*. Retrieved August 3, 2010, from www.albany.edu/news/pdf_files/impact_of_aging_excerpt.pdf.

Cleland, J. G. F, and I. Ekman, 2010. Enlisting the help of the largest health care workforce—patients. *Journal of the American Medical Association* 304:1383–84.

Eleazer, G. P., R. Doshi, D. Wieland, R. Boland, and V. A. Hirth. 2005. Geriatric content in medical school curricula: Results of a national survey. *Journal of the American Geriatrics Society* 53:136–40.

Frieden, T. R., 2010. A framework for public health action: The health impact pyramid. *American Journal of Public Health* 100:590–95.

Gebbie, K. M., and B. J. Turnock. 2006. The public health workforce, 2006: New challenges. *Health Affairs* 25:923–33. Retrieved August 13, 2010, from http://content.healthaffairs.org/cgi/reprint/25/4/923.

Institute of Medicine of the National Academies (IOM). 2003. *Who Will Keep the Public Healthy? Educating Public Health Professionals for the 21st Century*, ed. K. Gebbie, L. Rosenstock, and L. M. Hernandez. Washington, DC: National Academies Press.

Institute of Medicine of the National Academies (IOM). 2008. *Retooling for an Aging America*. Washington, DC: National Academies Press.

Lorig, K. R., D. S. Sobel, A. L. Stewart, B. W. Brown, Jr., A. Bandura, P. Ritter, V. M. Gonzalez, D. D. Laurent, and H. R. Holman. 1999. Evidence suggesting that a chronic disease self-management program can improve health status while reducing hospitalization: A randomized trial. *Medical Care* 37(1):5–14.

Lubben, L. E., J. A. Damron-Rodriguez, and J. C. Beck. 1992. A national survey of aging curriculum in schools of social work. In *Geriatric Social Work Education*, ed. J. Mellor and R. Solloman, pp. 157–73. Binghamton, NY: Haworth Press.

Molina, L. C., and S. P. Wallace. 2007. Health and aging education in accredited public health programs. Paper presented at the American Public Health Association Annual Meeting, Washington, DC.

Prohaska, T. R. 1992. The current status of training in aging and public health. In *Proceedings from the Aging and Public Health Curriculum Development Workshop*, ed. S. P. Wallace and T. R. Prohaska, pp. 1–12. Los Angeles: UCLA/California Geriatric Education Center.

Prohaska, T. R., and S. P. Wallace. 1997. Implications of an aging society for the preparation of public health professionals. In *Public Health and Aging*, ed. T. Hickey, M. A. Speers, and T. R. Prohaska, pp. 99–120. Baltimore: Johns Hopkins University Press.

U.S. Department of Health and Human Services, HRSA BHPr. 1995. *A National Agenda for Geriatric Education: White Papers*. Rockville, MD: Author.

U.S. Department of Health and Human Services, Public Health Service. 1997. *The Public Health Workforce: An Agenda for the 21st Century*. Report of the Public Health Functions Project. Washington, DC: U.S. Government Printing Office.

Wallace, S. P. 2005. A public health perspective on aging. *Generations* 29(2):5–10.

Wallace, S. P., J. Levin, V. Villa, and J. C. Beck. 1998. The need for an increased emphasis on health and aging in public health education. *Gerontology & Geriatrics Education* 18(4):45–62.

Wallace, S. P., T. R. Prohaska, M. Silverman, and A. Cary. 1995. The state of the art of geriatric public health education and training. In *National Forum on Geriatric Education & Training: White Papers*, pp. 191–212. Washington, DC: U.S. Department of Health and Human Services, HRSA, Bureau of Health Professions.

Wendt, P. F., D. A. Peterson, and E. B. Douglass. 1993. *Core Principles and Outcomes of Gerontology, Geriatrics and Aging Studies Instruction*. Washington, DC. Report published by the Association for Gerontology in Higher Education (AGHE) and the University of Southern California.

CHAPTER 14

Disaster Preparedness, Response, and Recovery

Kathryn Hyer, MPP, PhD
Lisa M. Brown, PhD

Since September 11, 2001, billions of dollars have been spent to build an infrastructure to prepare for, respond to, and recover from disasters. One result of the terrorist attacks was the creation of the U.S. Department of Homeland Security (U.S. DHS), an agency charged with a wide range of activities from responsibility for border protection to detection of bioterrorism. The agency within DHS most closely associated with disaster response is the Federal Emergency Management Agency (FEMA) with its charter to prepare for and respond to all hazards and disasters.

With the vast expenditures for equipment and infrastructure development, Americans expected that the United States was prepared to cope with disasters. However, after Hurricane Katrina flattened 150 miles of the heavily populated Gulf Coast area on August 29, 2005, the world realized how ill-prepared FEMA was to deal with a major hurricane. While America watched TV reports broadcasting first responders' attempts to help Mississippi and Alabama residents, the levees broke in New Orleans. The subsequent deaths resulting from the storm surge flooding dramatically highlighted the vulnerabilities of older adults; while only 15% of the population in pre-Katrina New Orleans was aged 60 and older, 74% of hurricane-related deaths were people 60 and older, and nearly half of those were older than age 75 (Simerman, Ott, and Mellnik, 2005). The particular vulnerability of older adults, as a population that warrants special recognition during all phases of disasters, is the focus of this chapter on disaster preparedness, response, and recovery.

DEFINITION OF DISASTER

The terms *emergency, disaster,* and *catastrophic event* are often used interchangeably because there are features within each that are shared by all. A *hazard* has the potential to cause harm to safety, health, life, or the environment and increases vulnerability for adverse outcomes, although it may not require rapid response. An *emergency* is an event that exceeds the potential threat of a hazard and requires an immediate response that can be adequately managed at the local level. In contrast to an *individual trauma* (i.e., car accidents or criminal acts), which affects one person and the people in their informal social network, the occurrence of a disaster adversely affects social structures and dynamics and threatens the existence and functioning of larger geographic areas (Fullerton, Ursano, Norwood, and Holloway, 2003; Institute of Medicine [IOM], 2003). The World Health Organization defines a *disaster* as an event involving 100 or more people, with 10 or more deaths, an official disaster declaration, or an appeal for assistance (Below, Wirtz, and Guha-Sapir, 2009). Most disasters require more resources than are available in the immediate geographic area. A *catastrophe* is a sudden and extreme disastrous event that causes an upheaval in the functioning of communities requiring an extensive recovery process that fundamentally changes the surrounding environment (U.S. DHS, 2008).

Disasters can strike anytime and anywhere. Data on the type and frequency of disasters reported by FEMA reveal that, on average, a disaster occurs weekly in the United States (FEMA, 2010). In contrast, a fire department responds, on average, every 22 seconds to an emergency in the United States (Karter, 2009). Disasters are events of greater magnitude than emergencies (Guha-Sapir, 2000). Generally speaking, emergencies are far more frequent than disasters. Historically, more funding has been made available for education, training, and resources for emergency response than for infrequent events like disasters. For the public health system to optimally function during a complex, demanding, and potentially enduring disaster (e.g., flu pandemic, oil spill), it is necessary for responders to possess basic knowledge of the structure that governs delivery of services and resources to affected populations prior to the occurrence of an actual event. To achieve this goal, there has been a steady move toward all-hazards planning for disasters.

Most all-hazards approaches address four disaster phases. The first phase, mitigation, seeks to minimize the effects of a potential disaster. For example, to reduce the threat of flood damage, a home could be purchased outside of the surge zone. The second phase, disaster preparedness, ranges from preparing a personal disaster kit to developing community disaster plans. The third phase, response, involves activities to minimize the adverse consequences of a disaster. If sufficient warning takes place, such as with hurricanes and floods, it may be possible to evacuate in advance of an event to a safe area. Recovery is the final phase. This post-disaster period can be divided into three phases: acute or short-term (1 month or less), intermediate (1–12 months), and chronic or long-term (12 months or longer).

No two disasters are alike. In general, the short- and long-term public health response to a disaster will vary based on the type (i.e., natural, human-made, or communicable disease outbreak) and features of the event in conjunction with the characteristics of the affected population. Unique differences exist among types of disasters (e.g., an earthquake is different from a heat wave), and variability exists within any specific type of disaster (e.g., some earthquakes are bigger and more damaging than others). Parameters used to define disasters include the type of disaster, predictability, advance warning, frequency or probability of recurrence, duration of the disaster, intensity, and scope. The risk for disaster-related mental or physical illness varies according to the parameters of the disaster. The psychological effects of a high death rate combined with a surge in those seeking assistance may easily overwhelm existing public health systems of care. Because major disasters typically require more assistance than is available in the immediate area, communities that have access to outside resources tend to fare better than areas with limited assets and services. The ability of disaster responders to quickly mobilize and make available essential resources, such as water, food, and shelter, affects the recovery of the surviving population. In essence, there is an interaction between the parameters of a disaster and the characteristics of the community, influencing well-being and need for disaster behavioral health services.

While many conceptualize disasters primarily as severe geological (e.g., earthquake, tsunami) or weather-caused (e.g., hurricanes, tornados) incidents or human-made events due to terrorist acts or industrial accidents (oil spills), management of extensive disease outbreaks or the spread of an infectious disease such as the H1N1 and H5N1 flu now fall within the purview of DHS. Acknowledging the potential for significant and prolonged social disruption resulting from a 1918 type of flu pandemic, President George W. Bush reassigned the overall coordination of the pandemic response from the Centers for Disease Control and Prevention (CDC) to the Secretary of the U.S. DHS. Regardless of the genesis of the event, disasters are frequent, are potentially very disruptive, and require a public health response.

THE STRUCTURE OF EMERGENCY RESPONSE
IN THE UNITED STATES

The U.S. system of government is based on the principle of federalism, or the sharing of power between national and state (and local) governments. As might be expected, the initial responsibility for public health protection is local, where the event or, in the language of emergency management personnel, the "incident" physically occurs. Thus, residents in a community expect the initial responders to a hazardous condition or an emergency to be local fire, police, emergency medical services, and emergency management personnel.

A principle in emergency management, consistent with federalism principles, is "tiered" response; the management of an incident remains a local issue unless a jurisdiction's capabilities have been decimated by the event and local officials request county or state assistance. If the event requires assistance from other localities or if state authorities recognize the need to supplement local resources, the state may activate its emergency centers. The goal of a regional or state activation is to coordinate with local authorities to ensure that they have the personnel, tools, and equipment necessary. Depending on the magnitude of the event and the capacity of the state to respond, the governor may declare a statewide emergency or disaster. Similarly, when the state's capabilities are strained or the disaster is expected to exceed the state's resources, its governor may request federal assistance under the Robert T. Stafford Disaster Relief and Emergency Assistance Act (Public Law 100-707) to receive federal resources to supplement state and local capacity to carry out disaster relief and recovery activities (Robert T. Stafford Disaster Relief and Emergency Assistance Act, 1988).

The emergency operations center (EOC) is the physical location for managing the incident. In larger communities, EOCs are permanent, well-fortified physical facilities with redundant communication systems, generators, and all supplies necessary to operate 24 hours a day, 7 days a week during the emergency. EOCs are directed by a manager, and the physical location is frequently placed with the police or 911 systems for enhanced coordination and efficiency of operations. However, in smaller localities, the EOC function can be established to meet short-term needs in any location, but when activated it is operational 24 hours a day until the incident is resolved. If the incident destroys the physical location or renders the communications systems inoperable, the EOC functions will be moved to another geographic location, generally in close physical proximity to the original site of the emergency to monitor conditions on the ground.

In 2008, U.S. DHS published *National Response Framework* (U.S. DHS, 2008), which provides all government, agency, and nongovernmental organizations with the processes of how the U.S. responds to disasters or catastrophes. The word "framework" is an evolution from the original document written after September 11, 2001, entitled *National Response Plan* (U.S. DHS, 2004). Acknowledging the inability of the federal government to implement a true operational "plan" during Hurricane Katrina, the *Framework* (U.S. DHS, 2008, p. 3) "commits the Federal Government, in partnership with local, tribal, and State governments and the private sector . . . to capture specific authorities and best practices for managing incidents that range from the serious but purely local, to large-scale terrorist attacks or catastrophic natural disasters." The latter language reflects the earlier discussion of the need to respond to many possible scenarios and is also known as "all-hazards" planning.

Another tenet in federal, state, and local emergency response is "unity of effort" supported by a standardized approach to managing incidents called the National Incident Management System (NIMS). Once an incident is recognized as requiring a coordinated effort by multiple departments, the emergency management functions begin. The standardized response requires a hierarchical chain-of-command structure called the Incident Command System (ICS). The ICS is actually a flexible management system that can expand or contract as the situation warrants, but it always contains five functions that are needed during emergency situations: command, operations, planning, logistics, and finance/administration (fig. 14.1). Within the ICS there is one incident commander, the individual responsible for "all response activities, including the development of strategies and tactics and the ordering and release of resources" (U.S. DHS, 2008, p. 50). Adherence to the structure enables all personnel to have a common language and standard protocols for behavior during a disaster. Emergency management officials and public health officials supporting emergency efforts must have basic training in both NIMS and ICS. The training allows those involved in man-

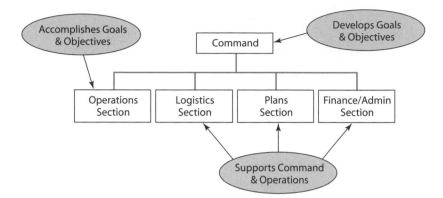

Fig. 14.1. Incident Command System (ICS) and roles for emergency response.

aging a disaster to understand the command reporting structures, common terminology, and roles and responsibilities inherent in a response operation.

A third tenet in disasters is a "systems" approach, because "unity of effort" requires the aging network service delivery systems to coordinate efforts with emergency management services for the common purpose of helping older adults during any phase of the disaster. The ICS management structure can be implemented at nongovernment agencies or organizations that support emergency planning efforts. Most hospitals have created their own ICS system. After Hurricane Katrina, the ICS was widely disseminated, especially to nongovernmental agencies, to encourage all organizations, such as hospitals, nursing homes, and aging network providers, to adapt the ICS framework to the organizations' functions during emergencies. The first nursing home ICS was developed by the Florida Health Care Association (FHCA) as part of its efforts to improve the development of comprehensive emergency plans in nursing homes (FHCA, 2008).

After Hurricane Katrina, the Administration on Aging (AoA), recognizing the special vulnerabilities of older adults during disasters, created the *Emergency Assistance Guide* (AoA, 2006), especially designed for aging service providers. This manual urges administrators of aging programs to forge partnerships with emergency managers at all levels of government and encourages providers to become familiar with the ICS and the structure of emergency management functions. Without knowledge of the emergency management functions, aging service providers will be hindered in their ability to advocate for their members and adequately assist communities and older adults with disaster preparation, response, and recovery.

The numbers and names of the 15 Emergency Support Functions (ESFs) that are within the unified management structure are shown in table 14.1. Two functions are particularly important to public health: mass care, emergency assistance, housing, and human services (ESF #6) and public health and medical services (ESF #8). The ESFs work together within the local or state operations centers during any incident, and these two functions are particularly relevant to older adults as a population during disasters. ESF #6 usually operates and monitors general shelters and any special needs shelters that may be established for older adults with medical needs or disabled individuals. ESF #8 is responsible for mortuary services after disasters, public health surveillance of quality of water and environment, and providing medical and mental health services to meet the needs of populations in the immediate aftermath of the disaster.

RISK AND RESILIENCE OF OLDER ADULTS DURING DISASTERS

Although most healthy older adults will be able to cope with the effects of a disaster, there are many who are at risk for short- and long-term adverse outcomes. Because every aspect of community life is disrupted during a disaster, the formal and informal support systems of older persons can quickly erode, resulting in a corresponding decline in health status. A person's informal social network is typically composed of family, friends, neighbors, and other close religious and social affiliations. After a disaster, a key role for public health response is to provide formal social support until informal support networks can be reestablished. To maximize the effectiveness of formal support networks (i.e., health care professionals, responders, relief workers) during all phases of a disaster, services should be coordinated and providers should possess basic knowledge about common social and health issues experienced by older adults. People who depend on others for assistance in performing activities of daily living because of limited mobility, physical disability, presence of medical or psychiatric illness, or cognitive impairment are at greater risk for adverse consequences at all phases of a disaster (Brown, Rothman, and Norris, 2007).

Older adults are at greater risk for health consequences after disasters because they are more likely to have multiple chronic conditions than other population groups. As Mokdad et al. (2005) pointed out after Katrina, existing or chronic conditions are often exacerbated by a disaster and become acute health concerns. The initial concern of public health officials after Katrina, as noted by Ford et al. (2006), was not chronic diseases but rather injuries, preventing outbreaks of infectious disease, and preserving life of survivors.

TABLE 14.1
Names, roles, and responsibilities of Emergency Support Functions (ESFs)

ESF #1: Transportation
ESF Coordinator: Department of Transportation
　Aviation/airspace management and control
　Transportation safety
　Restoration and recovery of transportation infrastructure
　Movement restrictions
　Damage and impact assessment
ESF #2: Communications
ESF Coordinator: DHS (National Communications System)
　Coordination with telecommunications and information technology industries
　Restoration and repair of telecommunications infrastructure
　Protection, restoration, and sustainment of national cyber and information technology
　　resources
　Oversight of communications within the federal incident management and response
　　structures
ESF #3: Public Works and Engineering
ESF Coordinator: Department of Defense (U.S. Army Corps of Engineers)
　Infrastructure protection and emergency repair
　Infrastructure restoration
　Engineering services and construction management
　Emergency contracting support for lifesaving and life-sustaining services
ESF #4: Firefighting
ESF Coordinator: Department of Agriculture (U.S. Forest Service)
　Coordination of federal firefighting activities
　Support to wildland, rural, and urban firefighting operations
ESF #5: Emergency Management
ESF Coordinator: DHS (FEMA)
　Coordination of incident management and response efforts
　Issuance of mission assignments
　Resource and human capital
　Incident action planning
　Financial management
ESF #6: Mass Care, Emergency Assistance, Housing, and Human Services
ESF Coordinator: DHS (FEMA)
　Mass care
　Emergency assistance
　Disaster housing
　Human services
ESF #7: Logistics Management and Resource Support
ESF Coordinator: General Services Administration and DHS (FEMA)
　Comprehensive, national incident logistics planning, management, and sustainment
　　capability
　Resource support (facility space, office equipment and supplies, contracting services, etc.)
ESF #8: Public Health and Medical Services
ESF Coordinator: Department of Health and Human Services
　Public health
　Medical
　Mental health services
　Mass fatality management
ESF #9: Search and Rescue

TABLE 14.1 *continued*

ESF Coordinator: DHS (FEMA)
  Lifesaving assistance
  Search and rescue operations
ESF #10: Oil and Hazardous Materials Response
ESF Coordinator: Environmental Protection Agency
  Oil and hazardous materials (chemical, biological, radiological, etc.) response
  Environmental short- and long-term cleanup
ESF #11: Agriculture and Natural Resources
ESF Coordinator: Department of Agriculture
  Nutrition assistance
  Animal and plant disease and pest response
  Food safety and security
  Natural and cultural resources and historic properties protection
  Safety and well-being of household pets
ESF #12: Energy
ESF Coordinator: Department of Energy
  Energy infrastructure assessment, repair, and restoration
  Energy industry utilities coordination
  Energy forecast
ESF #13: Public Safety and Security
ESF Coordinator: Department of Justice
  Facility and resource security
  Security planning and technical resource assistance
  Public safety and security support
  Support to access, traffic, and crowd control
ESF #14: Long-Term Community Recovery
ESF Coordinator: DHS (FEMA)
  Social and economic community impact assessment
  Long-term community recovery assistance to states, tribes, local governments, and the
    private sector
  Analysis and review of mitigation program implementation
ESF #15: External Affairs
ESF Coordinator: DHS
  Emergency public information and protective action guidance
  Media and community relations
  Congressional and international affairs
  Tribal and insular affairs

Within days, however, it became evident that the chronic care needs of the evacuees required attention. Mokdad et al. (2005) reported that 41% of Hurricane Katrina evacuees had at least one chronic health condition and required medication for diabetes, hypertension, and/or cardiovascular disease. There is agreement that CDC, along with its community public health partners, needs to include chronic disease management issues when planning for disasters (Mensah et al., 2004; Ford et al., 2006).

Beyond access to routine health care, many older adults with chronic medical conditions successfully live independently in the community with the assistance of many home and community services. Disruption of services like Meals on Wheels, loss of electrical power, or inability of a home health aide to continue to provide crucial services can rapidly lead to declines in an older person's health. Older adults with weaker social networks or who are socially isolated are more susceptible to a range of negative geriatric outcomes during a disaster. A person's functional status or level of disability *before* a disaster defines their vulnerability *during* a disaster and influences their ability to recover *after* a disaster (Ford et al., 2006; Brown, Cohen, and Kohlmaier, 2007). Loss of formal support systems accompanied by any new condition that hinders a person's ability to perform activities of daily living can result in illness, hospitalization, or death if not quickly recognized and appropriately addressed. Vulnerable older adults are more likely to experience dehydration, malnutrition, delirium, pressure sores, or medication side effects as a result of a disaster (Rothman and Brown, 2007). Evaluation of functional status and steps to enhance formal and informal support for older adult disaster casualties is crucial for reducing suffering, avoiding life-threatening complications, and improving outcomes during all phases of a disaster.

Persons without a familiar caregiver can become confused or delirious in a new environment after being evacuated. Disruptions in care and daily routines that can occur when responding to a disaster can be life threatening if they lead to dehydration, injury, or lack of self-care. Safeguards should be in place to evaluate high-risk older adults for cognitive status (Inouye, 2006). People with cognitive impairment may not ask for help or be able to make their needs known to responders or shelter staff when in distress. During disasters, older adults with dementia are at risk for isolation, delirium, and death (Huus, 2005). Moreover, without adequate training it can be difficult to distinguish between dementia and delirium. The ability to recognize and distinguish dementia and delirium should be mandatory for all first responders, humanitarian relief workers, and shelter personnel responsible for providing care to vulnerable older adults.

Members of the Medical Reserve Corps and the American Red Cross routinely receive psychological first aid training. Psychological first aid is a brief evidence-informed intervention that can be used by public health responders to reduce distress and to foster adaptive functioning in older adults after a disaster (Brown et al., 2009). Like medical first aid, anyone can be trained to use psychological first aid to treat people who have experienced a traumatic event. Psychological first aid training should include basic information about commonly occurring health problems among frail older adults (www.ahcancal
.org/facility_operations/disaster_planning/Documents/PsychologicalFirstAid

.pdf). This training may be the only opportunity for responders to receive education about geriatric health issues. Those who require more than psychological first aid are referred to a mental health provider for further assessment and treatment if necessary. Given the limited mental health services available in nursing homes after disasters (Brown et al., 2010), psychological first aid is an important resource for staff.

It is normal for a disaster to elicit powerful reactions in adults of all ages. Feelings of shock, horror, disbelief, anxiety, apprehension, fear, and anger are common responses to an uncommon event. While the type and parameters of a disaster influence psychological outcomes, premorbid existence of psychiatric symptoms or emotional distress is the best overall predictor of long-term impaired psychological functioning (Phifer and Norris, 1989; Kessler et al., 1999; Knight, Gatz, Heller, and Bengston, 2000). Low-level chronic stressors may be more important than the experience of a previous trauma in predicting post-disaster distress and speed of recovery (Norris, Friedman, and Watson, 2002). Older adults are at higher risk if they are experiencing ongoing family conflict, financial problems, neighborhood stress (e.g., crime), social isolation, or weak social networks. However, for the majority of older adults, most untreated disaster-related psychological distress will abate in time (Raphael, 2003). Nevertheless, even without the presence of preexisting psychiatric disorders or post-disaster psychological problems, many older adults will require assistance in preparing for, responding to, and recovering from disasters.

WHY ELDERS' RESIDENTIAL SETTING MATTERS FOR DISASTER RESPONSE

It is not the age of a person that creates vulnerability, but rather a constellation of factors that places people at higher risk for experiencing health and psychological problems. The demographic characteristics of the community, including the cultural and socioeconomic factors, influence the disaster preparedness and response. For example, a 71-year-old adult residing in a nursing home will have a different response to a disaster than their 71-year-old counterpart who lives in the community. In some instances, the 71-year-old nursing home resident may fare far better than an older adult living independently in the community who may be overlooked in a public shelter and not receive needed assistance. Furthermore, public health responders do not generally recognize that the unique needs of older adults vary depending on setting, the regulations governing disaster planning and response, the existing formal and informal social support network, and the premorbid health status of the population. Older adults may resist asking for help for a variety of reasons. Uncertainty about how to access services, stigma related to accepting assistance, pride, and belief that others have fared far worse are common barriers to treatment that have been described in research studies (Brown et al., 2007). Outreach activities, prior to and after a disaster, should be targeted to this population.

This section reviews current community and disaster preparedness and response standards in a range of community and health care settings where older adults are more likely to reside. Because older adults, as a population, are more vulnerable for adverse outcomes owing to the complex interplay of health, cognitive, and functional issues that have been described, the ability of community and health care providers to plan and then minimize the risk for adverse consequences is critical to maintaining older adults during and after disasters. This section begins with older adults living in the community and identifies a range of housing options across the continuum of care. We move to community living with support services and discuss assisted living facilities as a special case of community living with support. Finally, we provide information on disaster preparedness in nursing homes because this residential environment, considered institutional living, is also the most heavily regulated during disasters. Despite the regulations, persons living in nursing homes are at great risk during disasters.

As Mokdad et al. (2005) pointed out after Katrina, existing or chronic conditions are often exacerbated by a disaster and become acute health concerns. Access to adequate medication supply prior to a disaster is a key policy issue. During declared emergencies, public health departments may want to urge their state to adopt regulations that allow emergency prescription refills for community-dwelling older adults who are members of managed care organizations. Because 80% of older adults have at least one chronic condition and access to ongoing medications is vital, older adults need to have an adequate supply of medication to avoid adverse health consequences during disasters (Mokdad et al., 2005; Aldrich and Benson, 2008). Hurricane Katrina taught public health agencies that older adults with only a 3-day supply ran out of medications, and this exacerbated the poor outcomes during the disaster. By adopting regulations that allow managed care members to refill prescriptions during declared emergencies, people with chronic conditions are better prepared to cope with interruptions in services.

An underlying theme in this section is the need for the aging services network—providers of adult day care, Meals on Wheels, and case management services—to work with and through their Area Agency on Aging (AAA) or Aging and Disability Resource Center (ADRC) to identify older adults living in the community who are at risk during disasters. As suggested in the section on emergency management structure, aging service providers play a critical role in supporting older adults and enabling them to remain in noninstitutional settings. However, the frailty of segments of this population suggests that AAAs and ADRCs need to forge a strong relationship with local emergency management operations centers and public health departments to develop mechanisms to help older adults prepare for, respond to, and recover from natural and man-made disasters. As Mokdad et al. (2005) recommended, it is critical that public health offices work to help communities plan for disasters by recognizing the growing numbers of elders with chronic disease and disabled and other vulnerable populations requiring support before, during, and after disasters.

Older Adults Living in the Community

Over 93% of adults aged 65 years and older live independently in traditional community settings; 2% live in community housing settings, and 4% live in nursing homes (Federal Interagency Forum on Aging-Related Statistics, 2010). Increasing age is a risk factor for moving to community settings with more services such as meal preparation and laundry services. Even for those aged 85 and over, the vast majority (78%) live in traditional community settings, 7% live in community housing with services, and 15% live in nursing homes (Federal Interagency Forum on Aging-Related Statistics, 2010).

Although healthy older adults who are living in the community are at lower risk for adverse physical and mental outcomes than a nursing home resident, they assume a greater degree of personal responsibility in preparing for a disaster, evacuating, and seeking post-disaster care. Older adults who "aged in place" may find themselves with a weakened social network as older neighbors die or move away and new relationships with younger neighbors are not established. Informal caregivers, many of whom are family members, provide at least some support to 90% of in-home care for older adults with chronic health conditions (IOM, 2008b). Informal caregivers, such as family, neighbors, and friends, are often first on the scene after a disaster and are instrumental in arranging for shelter, medical care, food, and water and providing moral support. For older adults, informal social networks buffer or mitigate the negative effects of normal life stressors. During times of crisis, informal social support systems are integral to the well-being of older adults (see chap. 9 for an in-depth exploration of family caregiving of older adults).

Deterioration of the social support system is likely to result in adverse short- and long-term psychological consequences (Kaniasty and Norris, 1993). Although social support is often mobilized when older adults' life or health is threatened after a disaster, assistance is less available when property is damaged or destroyed, electricity or phone communication is lost, or daily routines are disrupted (Kaniasty and Norris, 1999). Because many members of an older adult's social support network will also be survivors of the same disaster, an adequate public health response is paramount in providing temporary support and assistance in rebuilding support systems (for additional information on social engagement and a healthy aging society, see chap. 10).

Preparation for a disaster may be hindered if help is not available to assist with securing home and personal property, and personal safety may be threatened if evacuation transportation is not made available. Significant barriers to using public sheltering include difficulty finding a pet-friendly shelter prior to an event and completing the necessary paperwork to receive special needs sheltering services. Special needs shelters provide accommodations and assistance with basic medical needs during and after a disaster for older adults who medically qualify for services. However, community emergency planning efforts, including access to appropriate transportation to evacuate disabled people and elders to public shelters, remain a challenge (Fugate, 2010).

Frail, homebound older adults are at significant risk during disasters. During a disaster, services provided through the aging services network by health aides or other providers, such as Meals on Wheels, may be interrupted. Family responsibilities, transportation problems, and personal health issues are a few of the reasons why formal support services may not be available in the event of a disaster. Without assistance, vulnerable homebound adults may not have the ability to use transportation, seek help from disaster assistance centers, or replenish basic supplies such as food and water. Public health workers will need to locate people who are homebound and may not have the physical ability to leave their homes and stand in line for assistance. Public health emergency response should work with aging network providers to receive lists of older adults who need services or who may need transportation to shelters.

During the recovery phase, older adults living in the community may elect to use recovery programs that are available to the general population or services that are developed and offered through local organizations that provide care and services only to older adults. Services might be available through existing local mental health clinics, state agencies, community centers, or, if specific to older adults, the aging network services such as AAA, ADRCs, or senior centers. Many communities have implemented phoning 2-1-1 to identify social services, housing, and counseling resources available in the local community (for further information on housing see chap. 3). Some barriers to care include limited public transportation, long-distance travel for older adults living in rural communities, and damaged roads and bridges.

Research suggests that the subsequent low-level but chronic stressors, also called daily hassles, may be more potent than past trauma exposure in predicting post-disaster distress and speed of recovery (Norris et al., 2002). Effective outreach is particularly important during the recovery phase, as many may feel overwhelmed by forms, information, insurance adjusters, FEMA representatives, and others selling services such as home repair to windows and roofs. Public health workers should be trained to recognize the signs of disaster-related distress, provide survivors with written information about disaster recovery services and crisis counseling programs, and be taught how to encourage acceptance of assistance, if needed.

Community Housing with Services

Community housing with services is a term that includes a range of housing options. Rarely licensed by the state or localities, these entities vary widely by size, services included, and price. Support services generally include access to housekeeping, meal preparation, laundry, transportation services, and help with administration of medication. As a person's requirements move from instrumental activities of daily living (IADL) services to ADL assistance, the living arrangements move along a continuum from completely independent, to independent with services, and then to assisted living (American Association of Homes and Services for the Aging, Assisted Living Federation of America, American Seniors Housing Association, National Center for Assisted Living, and the National Investment Center for the Seniors Housing & Care Industry, 2009). Some state regulation is more likely in assisted living facilities. If all three housing options are available on one campus, the community may be a continuing care retirement community and subject to some regulations regarding the contract for health and personal care, or the structure of the entrance fee or initial purchase of the residence. In community living with services, the individual may be expected to develop a personal emergency response plan, or if older adults are congregated in one geographic locality, the community may have plans to shelter residents or help them evacuate if needed. Families and consumers should be encouraged to ask questions about emergency plans during disasters and how the community will care for residents.

The inability of older adults living in community settings and people living with a disability to receive adequate services during disasters can have devastating consequences. After Hurricane Katrina, the Louisiana Department of Health estimated that 1,300 community-living older adults were permanently placed in nursing homes because their health and well-being were so compromised. Thus, the ability of public health officials to work with aging network providers who can identify and then provide help to frail older adults during disasters is critical. Because planning prior to an event is especially important for older adults, CDC's efforts to encourage individual and then provider-level disaster plans are important steps in ensuring adequate disaster readiness for vulnerable populations, including older adults.

Assisted Living

Nationwide, about 1 million adults reside in "assisted living" communities, and this housing option has grown dramatically over the past 10 years (National Center for Assisted Living [NCAL], 2010). Between 1990 and 2002, the capacity of assisted living doubled (Smith and Feng, 2010). Generally a state-licensed program, the regulation of this housing option varies by state as do the size, price, services offered, and emergency planning requirements. In addition to providing a private room or apartment, services usually include meals, laundry, housekeeping, medication reminders, and assistance with ADLs and IADLs. Initially, assisted living services were privately financed by residents, but an estimated 131,000 residents (13% of residents nationally) receive some assistance from state Medicaid programs (NCAL, 2010). Since 1981, when Medicaid established the home- and community-based waiver program under Section 1915c of the Social Security Act, states have encouraged persons who are eligible for nursing home care to live in lower-cost community-based alternatives, including assisted living facilities (Ng, Harrington, and Kitchner, 2010). Consequently, assisted living residents are increasingly likely to have higher levels of functional needs and cognitive disabilities over time (Smith and Feng, 2010). During a disaster, the staffs are likely to be challenged to manage this highly vulnerable population. It is therefore critical that assisted living facilities develop disaster preparedness plans and file these plans with local emergency management systems to avoid adverse outcomes. An established relationship with emergency operation managers prior to an event is likely to enhance access to needed resources during the event and increase the likelihood of restoring electricity and other services during the recovery phase of a disaster. Assisted living facilities, like nursing homes, need to be integrated into the emergency response network and be recognized as sheltering frail and vulnerable older adults during disasters (Hyer et al., 2010).

Nursing Homes

Nursing homes, unlike assisted living facilities, are mandated to provide residents a safe environment during all phases of a disaster. With approximately 1.5 million individuals, the nation's 16,000 nursing homes accepting Medicaid and Medicare payment for services are expected to have well-developed disaster plans, but state laws and regulations also drive disaster preparedness. In a study comparing emergency preparedness requirements among eight Gulf Coast and hurricane-prone states, Brown, Hyer, and Polivka-West (2007) reported widely varying state requirements for food supply, emergency power, and hazard analysis.

In an investigation of disaster preparedness after Hurricane Katrina, the U.S. Department of Health and Human Services Office of the Inspector General's (U.S. DHHS OIG, 2006) *Nursing Home Emergency Preparedness and Response during Recent Hurricanes* noted that nursing homes, unlike hospitals, were excluded from emergency response systems and did not have well-developed disaster plans. Focus groups of nursing home staff conducted by the Agency for Healthcare Research and Quality (2007) found that nursing homes were rarely involved in regional all-hazards planning and disaster preparedness. IOM's (2008a) *Research Priorities Report* also noted the need to improve preparedness and disaster response between providers of services and government entities.

To improve national disaster preparedness the Centers for Medicare and Medicaid (CMS) released emergency preparedness guidelines for all health care providers and urged development of all-hazards planning (CMS, 2009). Because these are guidelines rather than regulations, public health officials should work with local health departments and licensing agencies to encourage adoption of these guidelines. From a public health perspective, nursing homes need to be identified as health care facilities housing a vulnerable group of older adults and disabled residents. Nursing home administrators acknowledged the importance of emergency management offices during all phases of the 2004 hurricanes (Hyer et al., 2010). Depending on the advance warning of the event, the emergency management office may help by providing transportation to evacuate an entire building or particular populations, such as individuals who need dialysis. Access to transportation for evacuation is often unavailable because resources are oversubscribed during a disaster or the assets may be commandeered by local emergency management offices (Hyer, Polivka-West, and Brown, 2007; Hyer, Brown, Polivka-West, and Berman, 2010). Nursing homes' access to critical supplies and services such as food, fuel, water, and restoration of electrical power is essential to resident well-being to ensure that refrigerated medications don't spoil and air conditioning can be restored to avoid heat strokes (Hyer, Brown, Berman, and Polivka-West, 2006; Laditka et al., 2008). Nurses providing care in the aftermath of hurricanes describe the danger of distributing medications by flashlight and the difficulty of keeping incontinent residents comfortable without the use of washing machines to provide frequently needed clean linens (Hyer, Brown, Christensen, and Thomas, 2009). The likelihood of increased pressure sore development as a result of skin breakdown and inadequate continence care are additional public health consequences for this population if nursing homes do not receive adequate support during the recovery phase of the disaster.

Nursing home administrators in New Orleans interviewed after Hurricane Katrina reported feeling abandoned by public health and emergency management offices that did not provide assistance (Dosa, Grossman, Wetle, and Mor, 2007). In a study of mortality in Mississippi and Louisiana nursing homes compared with the same experience 2 years prior to Hurricane Katrina, Dosa et al. (2010) estimated an excess of 148 nursing home resident deaths 30 days after Katrina and a total of 230 excess deaths 90 days after Katrina. Hospitalization rates were also greater at 30 days (204 extra hospitalizations) for those same nursing homes compared with the prior 2 years and at 90 days (132 extra hospitalizations).

It is important to note that the increased mortality and hospitalization rates occurred in facilities that evacuated as well as facilities that did not evacuate. As the bus fire and death of 23 residents fleeing Hurricane Rita demonstrates, evacuation is fraught with difficulty (Dosa et al., 2008), and reimbursement to nursing homes may not be covered (Thomas, Hyer, Brown,

Polivka-West, and Branch, 2010). Evacuation, while appropriate in homes that may flood, is clearly not without risk. Finally, it is important to note that during the recovery phase of the disaster, nursing homes may need assistance with police security. The aforementioned report (U.S. DHHS OIG, 2006) also noted that some nursing homes evacuated after hurricanes because the nursing home was the only building that had medications, cash, food, electrical power, and supplies and attracted people from all over the community. Emergency management offices, recognizing the need to ensure adequate police protection for nursing homes after disasters, should work with local police to avoid an evacuation of frail residents under these conditions.

Since Hurricane Katrina, the disaster planning efforts for nursing home residents have greatly improved, as has the recognition of nursing homes as health care facilities by emergency management operations centers. Blanchard and Dosa (2009) reported that administrators evacuating for Hurricane Gustav in 2008 reported much better coordination of services as compared with Katrina.

Between FY 2002 and 2007, CDC allocated $4.9 billion in funding for its Public Health Emergency Preparedness Program to support state and local public health agencies' efforts to build a public health preparedness infrastructure (Association of State and Territorial Health Officials, the National Association of County and City Health Officials, the Association of Public Health Laboratories, and the Council of State and Territorial Epidemiologists, 2008). The Departments of Homeland Security and Health and Human Services have also allocated additional billions to improve preparedness. While many of the aforementioned programs supported disaster preparedness efforts of states and community-based preparedness, few efforts have concentrated specifically on older adults, and only one to our knowledge, the John A. Hartford Foundation (JAHF), focused specifically on improving nursing homes' disaster preparedness planning efforts. With a 3-year grant, *Hurricane and Disaster Preparedness for Long-Term Care Facilities*, LuMarie Polivka-West, the principal investigator and Senior Vice President of Policy at FHCA, worked in partnership with the authors to incorporate nursing home association representatives within ESF #8's public health support during emergencies. In addition, the grant provided money to create all-hazards planning materials, including software, to improve nursing home disaster preparedness planning, response, and recovery. The guide and software, available through FHCA (2008), have been used to help nursing homes create all-hazards disaster plans that are applicable for wildfires, tornados, floods, and other types of disasters.

PUBLIC HEALTH RESPONSE DURING DISASTERS:
NEEDS AND FUTURE DIRECTIONS

As this chapter demonstrates, during natural or human-made disasters, older adults are disproportionately affected. The sheer number of and the growing proportion of older adults in the U.S. population indicate the urgent need to encourage seniors to make personal and family plans for disasters. Public health workers should receive training on health care needs of older adults as part of CDC's public health preparedness centers. The aging of the population provides an opportunity to train public health professionals to recognize the physical, social, and mental health needs of older adults and why they are so susceptible to adverse outcomes following a disaster. However, given the pervasive negative attitudes about elders (Cuddy, Norton, and Fiske, 2005), public health training should also explore workers' potential ageist attitudes and assumptions about older adults, as well as develop skills in appropriate pre- and post-intervention disaster preparedness, response, and recovery.

To encourage better disaster preparedness, CDC and many states have developed campaigns to encourage all Americans to develop a personal disaster plan through its website, Emergency Preparedness and You (http://emergency .cdc.gov/preparedness/). Older adults can receive additional age-specific preparedness information under CDC's Health Aging Initiative (www2c.cdc .gov/podcasts/player.asp?f=10778). The U.S. AoA has developed emergency preparedness materials for aging service providers, plans for their own agencies to work with local emergency management offices, and has materials to encourage older adults to develop emergency personal plans, including plans for those caring for persons with dementia (www.aoa.gov/aoaroot/Preparedness/ Resources_Individuals/index.aspx). By developing plans and lists of clients, aging service providers can identify older adults at risk and work with local EOCs to provide services or support, if needed. For older adults receiving services from a licensed health care provider, CMS (2009) created emergency provider checklists for all licensed health care facilities, residents of nursing homes, and ombudsman programs. All these programs are geared to improve disaster preparedness and all-hazards planning for all Americans, but with a special emphasis on elders.

Many public health emergency preparedness services and supports for vulnerable elders have improved since Hurricane Katrina, but much work remains. The dramatic increase in home- and community-based care services raises concerns about the community supports and infrastructure to sustain frail elders at home during disasters. Public shelters are rarely suited to the needs of older adults with medical conditions or with cognitive impairment. The number of beds designated as special needs shelters are far fewer than the need given the growing numbers of disabled and older adults with serious chronic conditions. These shelters, while staffed by medical personnel, are also not always staffed by personnel trained to work with older adults.

However, new and evolving technologies such as geographic information systems (GIS) offer promise to improve identification and surveillance of vulnerable communities or populations to plan prevention programs and ways to minimize the impact of disasters on these populations (Holt et al., 2008). CDC has led efforts to profile vulnerable communities and to develop strategies to adapt the public health response system to accommodate the multiple vulnerable populations and scenarios of potential events. Emerging social networks such as Facebook, Twitter, and apps for mobile devices provide public health responders and risk communications experts new opportunities to disseminate educational programs and information to individuals as disasters unfold. It is anticipated that between 2008 and 2030, the over-65 population will double to approximately 72 million older adults and compose 20% of the total U.S. population. Given the frequency of disasters and the growing number of older people with cognitive impairment and disability, the public health system will continue to be challenged to promote public health preparedness in an aging society.

REFERENCES

Administration on Aging (AoA). 2006. *Administration on Aging: Emergency Assistance Guide*. Washington, DC: U.S. Department of Health and Human Services. Retrieved October 15, 2010, from www.aoa.gov/aoaroot/Preparedness/Resources_Network/pdf/Attachment_1357.pdf.

Agency for Healthcare Research and Quality (AHRQ). 2007. Research Findings #7: *Emergency Preparedness Atlas: U.S. Nursing Homes and Hospital Facilities*. Rockville, MD: AHRQ. Retrieved December 21, 2010, from www.ahrq.gov/prep/nursing homes/atlas.htm.

Aldrich, N., and W. F. Benson. 2008. Disaster preparedness and the chronic disease needs of vulnerable older adults. *Preventing Chronic Disease* 5(1):1–7.

American Association of Homes and Services for the Aging, Assisted Living Federation of America, American Seniors Housing Association, National Center for Assisted Living, and the National Investment Center for the Seniors Housing & Care Industry. 2009. *Overview of Assisted Living: 2009*. Washington DC: Authors.

Association of State and Territorial Health Officials, the National Association of County and City Health Officials, the Association of Public Health Laboratories, and the Council of State and Territorial Epidemiologists (2008). *Public Health*

Emergency Preparedness: Six Years of Achievements. Retrieved May 19, 2011, from www.aphl.org/aphlprograms/phpr/ahr/Documents/PHEP_Partners_Report.pdf.

Below, R., A. Wirtz, and D. Guha-Sapir. 2009. *Disaster Category Classification and Peril Terminology for Operational Purposes.* Brussels, Belgium: Louvain-la-Neuve.

Blanchard, G., and D. Dosa. 2009. A comparison of the nursing home evacuation experience between Hurricanes Katrina (2005) and Gustav (2008). *Journal of the American Medical Directors Association* 10:639–43.

Brown, L. M., M. L. Bruce, K. Hyer, W. L. Mills, E. Vongxaiburana, and L. Polivka-West. 2009. A pilot study evaluating the feasibility of psychological first aid for nursing home residents. *Clinical Gerontologist* 32:293–308.

Brown, L. M., D. Cohen, and J. Kohlmaier. 2007. Older adults and terrorism. In *Psychology and Terrorism,* ed. B. Bongar, L. M. Brown., L. Beutler, P. Zimbardo, and J. Breckenridge, pp. 288–310. New York: Oxford University Press.

Brown, L. M., K. Hyer, and L. Polivka-West. 2007. A comparative study of laws, rules, codes and other influences on nursing homes' disaster preparedness in the Gulf Coast states. *Behavioral Sciences and the Law* 25:655–75.

Brown, L. M., K. Hyer, J. A. Schinka, A. Mando, D. Frazier, and L. Polivka-West. 2010. Use of mental health services by nursing home residents after hurricanes. *Psychiatric Services* 61(1):74–77.

Brown, L. M., M. Rothman, and F. Norris. 2007. Issues in mental health care for older adults during disasters. *Generations* 31(4):25–30.

Centers for Medicare and Medicaid Services (CMS). 2009. *Survey and Certification. Emergency Preparedness Checklist: Recommended Tool for Effective Health Care Facility Planning.* Washington, DC: U.S. Department of Health and Human Services. Retrieved August 16, 2010, from www.cms.gov/SurveyCertEmergPrep/downloads/ S&C_EPChecklist_Provider.pdf.

Cuddy, A. J. C., M. I. Norton, and S. T. Fiske. 2005. This old stereotype: The pervasiveness and persistence of the elderly stereotype. *Journal of Social Issues* 61:267–85.

Dosa, D., Z. Feng, K. Hyer, L. M. Brown, K. Thomas, and V. Mor. 2010. Effects of Hurricane Katrina on nursing facility resident mortality, hospitalizations, and functional decline. *Disaster Medicine and Public Health Preparedness* 4:S28–32.

Dosa, D., N. Grossman, T. Wetle, and V. Mor. 2007. To evacuate or not to evacuate: Lessons learned from Louisiana nursing home administrators following Hurricanes Katrina and Rita. *Journal of the American Medical Directors Association* 8:142–49.

Dosa, D. M., K. Hyer, L. M. Brown, A. W. Artenstein, L. M. Polivka-West, and V. Mor. 2008. The controversy inherent in managing frail nursing home residents during complex hurricane emergencies. *Journal of the American Medical Directors Association* 9:599–604.

Federal Emergency Management Agency (FEMA). 2010. *Declared Disasters by Year or State.* Retrieved November 4, 2010, from www.fema.gov/news/disaster_totals_ annual.fema.

Federal Interagency Forum on Aging-Related Statistics. 2010. *Older Americans 2010: Key Indicators of Well-Being.* Washington, DC: U.S. Government Printing Office.

Florida Health Care Association (FHCA). 2008. *Emergency Management Guide for*

Nursing Homes. Tallahassee, FL: Author. Available from www.fhca.org/emerprep/guide.php.

Ford, E. S., A. H. Mokdad, M. W. Link, W. S. Garvin, L. C. McGuire, R. B. Jiles, and L. S. Balluz. 2006. Chronic disease in health emergencies: In the eye of the hurricane. *Preventing Chronic Disease* 3(2):A46 [serial online] 2006 Apr [October 15, 2010]. Retrieved October 15, 2010, from www.cdc.gov/pcd/issues/2006/apr/05_0235.htm.

Fugate, C. 2010. Are disabled still at risk in disasters? *CNN.com.* Atlanta: CNN; 2010 July 26. Retrieved August 21, 2010, from www.cnn.com/2010/OPINION/07/26/fugate.disabled.disasters/index.html.

Fullerton, C. S., R. J. Ursano, A. E. Norwood, and H. H. Holloway. 2003. Trauma, terrorism and disaster. In *Terrorism and Disaster Individual and Community Mental Health Interventions*, ed. R. J. Ursano, C. S. Fullerton, and A. E. Norwood, pp. 1–22. New York: Cambridge University Press.

Guha-Sapir, D. 2000. Disaster preparedness in schools of public health. In *Disaster Preparedness in Schools of Public Health: A Curriculum for the New Century*, ed. L. Y. Landesman, sect. 1.0, 1.1. Washington, DC: Association of Schools of Public Health.

Holt, J. B., A. H. Mokdad, E. S. Ford, E. J. Simoes, W. P. Bartoli, and G. A. Mensah. 2008. Use of BRFSS data and GIS technology for rapid public health response during natural disasters. *Preventing Chronic Disease* 5. Retrieved October 26, 2010, from www.cdc.gov/pcd/issues/2008/jul/07_0159.htm.

Huus, K. 2005. Lost in the shuffle: Katrina leaves elderly evacuees displaced, disconnected. *MSBNC.com.* Retrieved December 29, 2010, from www.msnbc.msn.com/id/10180296.

Hyer, K., L. M. Brown, A. Berman, and L. Polivka-West. 2006. Establishing and refining hurricane response systems for long-term care facilities. *Health Affairs* 25(5): w407–11. doi:10.1377/hlthaff.25.w407.

Hyer, K., L. M. Brown, J. J. Christensen, and K. S. Thomas. 2009. Weathering the storm: Challenges to nurses providing care to nursing home residents during hurricanes. *Applied Nursing Research* 22(4):e9–14.

Hyer, K., L. M. Brown, L. Polivka-West, and A. Berman. 2010. Helping nursing homes prepare for disasters. *Health Affairs* 29(10):1961–65.

Hyer, K., L. M. Brown, K. S. Thomas, D. Dosa, J. Bond, L. Polivka-West, and J. A. Schinka. 2010. Improving relations between emergency management offices and nursing homes during hurricane-related disasters. *Journal of Emergency Management* 8(1):57–66.

Hyer, K., L. Polivka-West, and L. M. Brown. 2007. Nursing homes and assisted living facilities: Planning and decision-making for sheltering in place or evacuation. *Generations* 31(4):29–33.

Inouye, S. K. 2006. Delirium in older persons. *New England Journal of Medicine* 354:1157–65.

Institute of Medicine (IOM). 2003. *Preparing for the Psychological Consequences of Terrorism: A Public Health Strategy*, ed. A. S. Butler, A. M. Panzer, and L R. Goldfrank. Washington, DC: National Academies Press.

Institute of Medicine (IOM). 2008a. *Research Priorities in Emergency Preparedness and Response for Public Health Systems: A Letter Report.* Washington, DC: National Academies Press.

Institute of Medicine (IOM). 2008b. *Retooling for an Aging America: Building the Health Care Workforce.* Washington, DC: National Academies Press.

Kaniasty, K., and F. H. Norris. 1993. A test of the social support deterioration model in the context of natural disaster. *Journal of Personality and Social Psychology* 64:395–408.

Kaniasty, K., and F. H. Norris. 1999. The experience of disaster: Individuals and communities sharing trauma. In *Responses to Disaster*, ed. R. Gist and B. Lubin, pp. 25–61. Ann Arbor, MI: Braun-Brumfield.

Karter, M. J. 2009. *Fire Loss in the United States 2008.* Quincy, MA: National Fire Protection Association Fire Analysis and Research Division.

Kessler, R., A. Sonnega, E. Bromet, M. Hughes, C. Nelson, and N. Breslau. 1999. Epidemiological risk factors for trauma and PTSD. In *Risk Factors for Posttraumatic Stress Disorders*, ed. R. Yehuda, pp. 23–60. Washington, DC: American Psychiatric Press.

Knight, B. G., M. Gatz, K. Heller, and V. L. Bengston. 2000. Age and emotional response to the Northridge Earthquake: A longitudinal analysis. *Psychology and Aging* 15:627–34.

Laditka, S. B., J. N. Laditka, S. Xirasagar, C. B. Cornman, C. B. Davis, and J. V. Richter. 2008. Providing shelter to nursing home evacuees in disasters: Lessons from Hurricane Katrina. *American Journal of Public Health* 98:1288–93.

Mensah, G.A., R. A. Goodman, S. Zaza, A. D. Moulton, P. L. Kocher, W. H. Dietz, T. F. Pechacek, and J. S. Marks. 2004. Law as a tool for preventing chronic diseases: Expanding the spectrum of effective public health strategies. *Preventing Chronic Disease* (January). Retrieved October 15, 2010, from www.cdc.gov/pcd/issues/2004/apr/04_0009.htm.

Mokdad, A. H., G. A. Mensah., S. F. Posner, E. Reed, E. J. Simoes, M. M. Engelgau, and the Chronic Diseases and Vulnerable Populations in Natural Disasters Working Group. 2005. When chronic conditions become acute: Prevention and control of chronic diseases and adverse health outcomes during natural disasters. *Preventing Chronic Disease* (Special Issue). Retrieved October 15, 2010, from www.cdc.gov/pcd/issues/2005/nov/05_0201.htm.

National Center for Assisted Living (NCAL). 2010. *Assisted Living State Regulatory Review 2010.* Washington, DC: Author.

Ng, T., C. Harrington, and M. Kitchner. 2010. Medicare and Medicaid in long-term care. *Health Affairs* 29(1):22–28. doi:10.1377/hlthaff.2009.0494.

Norris, F. H., M. J. Friedman, and P. J. Watson. 2002. 60,000 Disaster victims speak: Part II. Summary and implications of the disaster mental health research. *Psychiatry* 65(3):240–60.

Phifer, J. F., and F. H. Norris. 1989. Psychological symptoms in older adults following natural disaster: Nature, timing, duration, and course. *Journal of Gerontology* 44(6):S207–17.

Raphael, B. 2003. Early intervention and the debriefing debate. In *Terrorism and*

Disaster: Individual and Community Mental Health Interventions, ed. R. J. Ursano, C. S. Fullerton, and A. E. Norwood, pp. 146–61. London: Cambridge University Press.

Robert T. Stafford Disaster Relief and Emergency Assistance Act. 1988. Public Law 100–707, 100th Congress. Retrieved December 19, 2010, from www.fema.gov/pdf/about/stafford_act.pdf.

Rothman, M., and L. M. Brown. 2007. The vulnerable geriatric casualty: Medical needs of frail older adults during disasters. *Generations* 31(4):20–24.

Simerman, J., D. Ott, and T. Mellnik, T. 2005. Early data challenge assumptions about Katrina victims. *Austin American Statesman*, December 30.

Smith, D. B., and Z. Feng. 2010. The accumulated challenges of long-term care. *Health Affairs* 29(1):29–34.

Thomas, K. S., K. Hyer, L. M. Brown, L. Polivka-West, and L. G. Branch. 2010. Florida's model of nursing home Medicaid reimbursement for disaster-related expenses. *Gerontologist* 50:263–70.

U.S. Department of Health and Human Services Office of Inspector General (U.S. DHHS OIG). 2006. *Nursing Home Emergency Preparedness and Response during Recent Hurricanes.* Retrieved October 28, 2010, from http://oig.hhs.gov/oei/reports/oei-06–06–00020.pdf.

U.S. Department of Homeland Security (U.S. DHS). 2004. *National Response Plan December.* Retrieved May 19, 2011, from www.iir.com/Information_Sharing/global/resources/fusioncenter/NRPbaseplan.pdf. *Notice of Change to the National Response Plan*, Version 5.0. Retrieved May 19, 2011, from www.albany.edu/ncsp/docs/NRP/NRP%202006%206–30%20%20Revisions/NRP_Notice_of_Change_5–22–06.pdf.

U.S. Department of Homeland Security (U.S. DHS). 2008. *National Response Framework.* Washington, DC: Author. Retrieved October 28, 2010, from www.fema.gov/pdf/emergency/nrf/nrf-core.pdf.

PART V

Emerging Issues

CHAPTER 15

Planned and Built Environments
in Public Health

William A. Satariano, PhD, MPH
Marcia G. Ory, PhD, MPH
Chanam Lee, PhD, MLA

Patterns of health and well-being in populations are affected by a dynamic interplay of biological, behavioral, and environmental factors. Thus, ecological models, which incorporate this interplay, are especially well suited to plan, execute, and evaluate best practices and policies needed to promote and preserve health and well-being in a growing and increasingly diverse aging population (Smedley and Syme, 2001; Sallis et al., 2006; Satariano, 2006). Ecological public health models combined with gerontological theories underscore the systematic unfolding of interactive forces over the life course of individuals, families, and communities (Ory, Abeles, and Lipman, 1992; Smedley and Syme, 2001; Satariano, 2006). This perspective also recognizes that chronological age, along with gender, race, ethnicity, and socioeconomic differences, shapes the context in which individuals function and thereby directly and indirectly influences health risks and resources. In addition, the ecological model serves to identify multiple points of possible interventions, from the microbiological to the environmental levels; to postpone the risks of disease, disability, and death; and to enhance the chances for

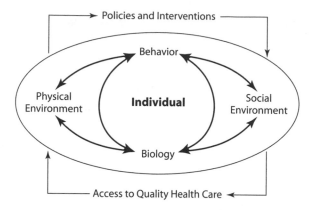

Fig. 15.1. Determinants of health. *Source*: Adapted from U.S. Department of Health and Human Services, 2000

health, mobility, and longevity (Smedley and Syme, 2001; Li et al., 2005). There are a number of different renderings of the ecological model. Figure 15.1 is an adaptation of a version included in *Healthy People 2010*, a government report that outlines the U.S. public health agenda for the first decade of the twentieth century (U.S. Department of Health and Human Services, 2000).

Although the ecological model by definition emphasizes the *interplay* of biological, behavioral, and environmental domains, there has always been something special about the *environment* itself in public health (Corburn, 2009). The environment, really "place" in all of its various forms, represents a spatial entrée for promoting and preserving health, mobility, and longevity in the *population* itself. The environment represents the context or setting of everyday life. Following Rose's (1985) insightful distinction between "sick individuals" and "sick populations," environmental interventions hold the promise of shifting the distribution of human behavior in a positive direction to improve health and well-being for the general population, not just the relatively small number of individuals at greatest risk for disease. Put differently, environmental interventions represent effective and efficient ways of "moving upstream" to promote health and well-being in populations (McKinlay, 1979). Along these lines, there is a growing recognition that elements of the "built environment," that is, human constructions such as buildings and streets and the relevant properties such as safety, land-use patterns, and infrastructure conditions, are associated with "healthy aging." This is reflected best in the definition of healthy aging offered by the Healthy Aging Network (HAN) of the Centers for Disease Control and Prevention (CDC) (https://depts.washington.edu/harn/): "Healthy aging is the development and maintenance of optimal physical, mental and social well-being and function in older adults. It is most likely to be achieved when physical environments and communities are safe, and support the adoption and maintenance by individuals of attitudes and behaviors known to promote health and well-being; and by the effective use of health services and community programs to prevent or minimize the impact of acute and chronic disease on function."

The built environment covers many domains and has special significance for the study and enhancement of health and well-being in aging populations. Our purpose here is to consider (a) the possible pathways by which the built environment can affect patterns of health behaviors and health outcomes among older populations; (b) the key research findings on the environment, walking, and physical activity; (c) methodological issues; (d) current applications of research to practice and policy; and (e) new directions for research, practice, and policy in this area. Our focus is on the interaction of age, environment, and health-related outcomes. Although critical for understanding environmental influences on aging and health, we will not focus on housing or transportation service. We recommend the following sources for comprehensive reviews of these topics: the U.S. Centers for Disease Control and Prevention and U.S. Department of Housing and Urban Development (2006); the U.S. Environmental Protection Agency (2009); and the U.S. Transportation Research Board, U.S. National Academies of Science (2004).

ENVIRONMENTAL PATHWAYS

There are three pathways that characterize the possible effects of the built environment on patterns of health behaviors and health outcomes (fig. 15.2). One pathway captures the *main effects* of the environment. In this case, the path reflects situations in which elements of the environment (e.g., presence and quality of sidewalks) directly account for differences in health behaviors/ outcomes (e.g., levels of walking among older people). A second pathway highlights elements of the built environment that are "on the causal pathway" to an outcome and thus serve to *mediate* the association between an independent and outcome variable. For example, elements of the environment (e.g., relative proximity of a grocery store to place of residence) may mediate or help to explain differences in walking or body mass (outcome variable) between African American and non-Hispanic white seniors (independent variable). A third possible pathway reflects situations in which elements of the environment *moderate* the relationship between an independent and outcome variable. Known as either statistical interaction or effect modifica-

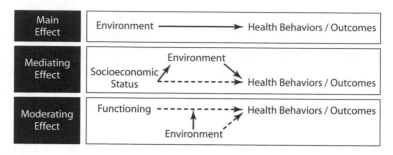

Fig. 15.2. Environment and health behaviors and outcomes: main, mediating, and moderating effects.

tion, it refers to situations in which the direction and strength of the relationships between two variables (e.g., lower-body function and walking) are affected by a third (moderating) variable (e.g., "neighborhood walkability"). For example, among older people with reduced lower-body function, those who live in more walkable neighborhoods are more likely to walk than those with the same level of reduced lower-body capacity who live in less walkable neighborhoods. The moderating effects of the environment come closest to the tenets of an "environmental theory of aging," first proposed by Powell Lawton and colleagues in the 1970s (Lawton and Nahemow, 1973; Lawton, 1986). This theory, also known as the "Press-Competence model," assumes that with age-related declines in individual competence or capacity, the effects of the environment on health and well-being become more salient for older adults, again, a moderating effect.

ENVIRONMENT, WALKING, AND PHYSICAL ACTIVITY

A growing number of research studies have examined the associations between the built environment and a variety of health behaviors and outcomes in older populations, including walking, physical activity, diet and nutrition, obesity, falls and injuries, depression, disability, and overall mortality (Dannenberg et al., 2003; Frank, Saelens, Powell, and Chapman, 2007). We focus here on walking and physical activity, the most common subject of study in this area (Cunningham and Michael, 2004; Saelens and Papadopoulos, 2008; Yen, Michael, and Perdue, 2009). No doubt, one reason that walking and physical activity have attracted so much attention is because they are associated with a variety of health conditions. Inactivity, for example, is associated with an elevated risk for leading health conditions, such as cardiovascular disease, breast and colorectal cancers, and diabetes (Prohaska et al., 2006; Lee and Buchner, 2008; Chodzko-Zajko et al., 2009). Walking is also associated with problems and disorders associated with movement and mobility, such as falls and injuries, obesity, and specific types of disability. Finally, walking is associated with social interactions such as contact with friends and relatives and access to goods and services, also related to positive health outcomes and quality of life.

We frame this presentation and characterize the state of the science in terms of the three environmental pathways described previously, i.e., main, mediating, and moderating effects. It is important to note that most research studies on the built environment, walking, and physical activity are based on cross-sectional designs (Cunningham and Michael, 2004; Saelens and Papadopoulos, 2008; Yen et al., 2009), which means that assessments of the environment and walking/physical activity are conducted at the same point in time and can only provide limited evidence for establishing main, mediating, and moderating effects. It may be, for example, that active older people elect to reside in more "walkable communities" so that they can more easily be active and have better access to goods and services. In this case, the environment itself is not affecting or causing their behavior. In contrast to cross-sectional projects, longitudinal studies, which include temporal assessment, are better able to assess to what extent and under what circumstances the built environment affects patterns of walking and physical activity over time (Frank et al., 2007), yet these are often difficult or expensive to implement, leaving much of our knowledge base dependent on cross-sectional studies.

Main Effects

Cross-sectional studies identify some consistent associations between elements of the built environment and walking/physical activity in older populations (Saelens and Papadopoulos, 2008; Yen et al., 2009). Walking for transportation (destination walking), compared with leisure walking, for example, is shown to be more strongly related to environmental conditions (Shigematsu et al., 2009). Specifically, land-use patterns are associated with walking for transportation in older populations. Older residents of mixed-use communities (e.g., residence in areas in proximity to goods and services) are more likely to walk than other people who live in residential-only communities commonly found in suburban areas (Gauvin et al., 2008; Nagel, Carlson, Bosworth, and Michael, 2008; Frank, Greenwald, Winkelman, Chapman, and Kavage, 2010; Satariano et al., 2010). Certain destinations are shown to encourage older adults' walking, including grocery stores, restaurants, convenience stores, parks, open spaces, trails, religious institutions, malls, and post offices (King et al., 2000; Wen, Kandula, and Lauderdate, 2004; Michael, Beard, Choi, Farguhar, and Carlson, 2006; Lee, 2007). In addition to mixed-use areas with more walkable destinations, older people who reside in more compact areas, generally characterized by higher densities and shorter block length or more street intersections (grid-like street pattern), are more likely to walk (Frank, Kerr, Sallis, Miles, and Chapman, 2008; Rodriguez, Evenson, Diez Roux, and Brines, 2009; Frank et al., 2010). With regard to leisure-time walking and other forms of physical activity, older adults who reside in areas in closer proximity to parks, recreational facilities, and walking trails are more likely to be physically active than older people who do not (Owen, Humpel, Leslie, Bauman, and Sallis, 2004). Older people who perceive their neighborhoods as safe are more likely to walk or engage in other outdoor activities than those who perceive their neighborhoods as unsafe (Li, Fisher, Brownson, and Bosworth, 2005; King, 2008; Mendes de Leon et al., 2009; Satariano et al., 2010). Finally, living in neighborhoods with higher levels of social cohesion and/or lower levels of socioeconomic deprivation also promotes physical activity among older adults (Fisher, Li, Michael, and Cleveland, 2004; King, 2008; Annear, Cushman, and Gidlow, 2009).

A limited number of longitudinal studies also identify prospective associations between elements of the built environment, most notably perceived safety and walking/physical activity in older populations (Balfour and Kaplan, 2002; Li, Fisher, and Brownson, 2005; Clark, Ailshire, and Lantz, 2009; Clark et al., 2009). Li, Fisher, and Brownson (2005) report that neighborhood walking declined over a 12-month period among a sample of older residents of Portland, Oregon. However, the decline in walking was less precipitous among older residents who perceived their neighborhoods as safe and with greater access to physical activity facilities. In a separate study, Clark et al. (2009) noted that older residents of New Haven, Connecticut, who reported more concerns about safety from crime in their neighborhoods were more likely to later report greater subsequent disability with regard to basic mobility, i.e., ability to climb stairs and walk a half mile, over an 8-year period than those who had earlier perceived their neighborhoods as safe with better access to physical activity facilities. It is important to note that Balfour and Kaplan (2002) also report a longitudinal association between reported neighborhood problems and overall and lower-body functional loss among older residents of Alameda County, California, over the course of 1 year. While the measures of general and lower-body function include reported difficulty in climbing stairs and walking a half mile, it is not possible to examine the independent effects on those two measures of mobility. Finally, Clarke and colleagues (2009) provide evidence from the Americans' Changing Lives Study that adults aged 75 and older who reside in areas with greater traffic volume report greater difficulty walking two or more city blocks for any given year over a 15–year period than adults of the same age who live in more pedestrian-friendly areas.

Mediating Effects

There is also evidence that elements of the built environment help to mediate the association that demographic (e.g., age, gender, and race/ethnicity) and socioeconomic factors have with walking and physical activity in older populations. Socioeconomic status is defined in terms of both individual- and neighborhood-level characteristics (Do et al., 2008). Although less attention has been given to the mediating effects than to the main effects of the environment, it is reported from cross-sectional studies in Australia and the Netherlands that older residents of lower socioeconomic status are less likely to walk as part of everyday activities or recreation, primarily because of issues of safety and aesthetics (Giles-Corti and Donovan, 2002; Kamphuis et al., 2009). It is interesting, however, that in a Pittsburgh study older women of lower socioeconomic status are more likely than those of higher socioeconomic status to engage in physical activity (King et al., 2005). King et al. (2005) hypothesize that the older, lower-income neighborhoods are more likely to have mixed land use, which tends to be associated with walking. In addition, with less ready access to other forms of transportation, older residents are more likely to walk to stores and services out of necessity (King et al., 2005). These cross-sectional studies indicate the complexity of this topic, especially when involving the "age" factor that appears to interact with socioeconomic, environmental, and other demographic variables. To our knowledge, there are no longitudinal studies addressing the extent to which elements of the built environment serve to mediate or explain the relationship between demographic/socioeconomic factors and health behaviors/outcomes for older adults.

Moderating Effects

There is evidence from cross-sectional studies that elements of the built environment may moderate the association between functional capacity and basic mobility disability. Among older Chicago residents with lower-extremity impairments, the odds of reporting severe mobility difficulty (i.e., not being able to walk two blocks or climb one flight of stairs) are over four times greater for those living in neighborhoods with streets in poor conditions (e.g., cracks, broken curbs, potholes) compared with those living in neighborhoods with streets in good condition (Clarke, Ailshire, Bader, Morenoff, and House, 2008). These results are consistent with an earlier study that demonstrated that environmental factors moderate the association between lower-extremity functional limitations and both ADL and IADL disability among a sample of older residents from North Carolina (Clarke and George, 2005). There is no significant association (main effect) between a measure of housing density and either activity of daily living (ADL) or instrumental activity of daily living (IADL) disability. However, older residents with functional limitations living in lower-density areas report more ADL disability than those in higher-density tracts. In addition, older residents with functional limitations living in lower-mixed-use areas report more difficulty with IADL than older people with the same level of functional limitations who reside in high-mixed-use areas. Shumway-Cook et al. (2002, 2003) also examine environmental demands associated with walking and mobility among disabled older people, compared with those without disabilities. Compared with disabled seniors, those without disabilities travel greater distances, complete more errands, and, most importantly, are better able to circumvent environmental barriers, such as poor street conditions. Finally, from cross-sectional interviews with older people from four locations across the United States, perceived crime is associated with less walking, but only among those with poor lower-body functioning (Satariano et al., 2010). However, when median block length is included, the statistical interaction between lower-body functioning and walking by level of perceived safety is no longer significant. Further examination reveals that older residents of compact areas, associated here with walking, are most likely to view their neighborhoods as unsafe, shown here to be associated with less walking. Short block length and perception of neighborhood danger are associated, but each neighborhood factor is associated in opposing directions with walking (Satariano et al., 2010). These results demonstrate the complexity of this issue. Additional longitudinal studies are needed to clarify some of these ambiguities.

Summary

Given the relative consistency of the cross-sectional findings and the few longitudinal studies conducted, there is evidence that elements of the built environment, especially perceived safety, independently affect patterns of walking and physical activity (i.e., a main effect). The evidence is not as strong, however, for possible mediating and moderating effects. Although the cross-sectional studies suggest mediating and moderating effects of perceived and objective measures of the built environment, the more definitive evidence from longitudinal studies is not currently available.

METHODOLOGICAL ISSUES: CONCEPTUALIZATION AND MEASUREMENT

In addition to elements of research design (e.g., cross-sectional vs. longitudinal studies noted previously), there are a number of underlying methodological issues that should be addressed to provide a more complete understanding of the relationships between aging, health, and environmental factors. In this section we address conceptualization and measurement issues associated with walking, physical activity, and the built environment. This discussion highlights the strengths and limitations of various measurement strategies.

Walking and Physical Activity

As the most common form of physical activity among older adults, walking is the most researched health behavior examined in the context of the environment. Walking is assessed with surveys, interviews, and travel diaries as self-reports (frequency, duration, location/destination, and purpose) and with pedometers (step counts) as objective measures. Pedometers are reasonably inexpensive for large epidemiological studies. However, the fact that subjects can easily see the number of steps traveled has raised concerns among researchers that this assessment strategy may actually have an intervention effect. For measuring overall physical activities, most commonly used tools are surveys and accelerometers (the average amplitude of body accelerometers during a defined period) (Tudor-Locke, Ainsworth, and Thompson, 2002).

Most surveys, as well as pedometers and accelerometers, do not record the location of the activity. Travel/walking diaries or activity logs are the self-report instruments designed to collect information about location. These require the subjects to record the origin and destination locations, departure and arrival items, and the travel mode and purpose of each trip. The recording of this information, while critical for studies of place and walking, may be perceived by older adults as burdensome. The popularization of newer technologies may reduce some of these concerns. For example, Global Positioning System (GPS) technology has now advanced to the point that devices can be easily worn on a belt or wrists, and such GPS units are reasonably inexpensive for field studies (Wieters, Kim, and Lee, 2008). A small number of recent studies have shown the potential of wearable GPS units as useful research tools (Rodriguez, Brown, and Troped, 2005; Troped et al., 2008). However, more evidence is needed to confirm its utility for studying older people.

The Built Environment

Built environmental measures assess a range of settings, including the home, the household site, the immediate surroundings, and the neighborhood. The measures also include geographic areas visited and routes taken outside the immediate neighborhood as part of everyday activities (Moudon and Lee, 2003). The built environment can be measured subjectively with self-reports (e.g., surveys and interviews) and objectively with environmental audits and geographic information systems (GIS). Most existing assessment tools, which are used in studies of place and outdoor walking, focus on the neighborhood environment. However, conceptualizing and defining the neighborhood and its spatial boundaries still remains a subject of debate. We highlight the advantages and disadvantages of some of the most common assessment technologies.

Surveys

Questionnaires and interviews are especially well suited to older residents' perceptions of the neighborhoods. The Neighborhood Environment Walkability Survey (NEWS), developed by Saelens, Sallis, Black, and Chen (2003), includes a standard set of questions divided into subscales: perceived residential density, land-use mix diversity, land-use mix access, street connectivity, walking/cycling facilities, aesthetics, pedestrian/automobile traffic safety, and crime safety. Additional questionnaires include the Environmental Supports for Physical Activity Questionnaire by Ainsworth, Wilcox, Thompson, Richeter, and Henderson (2003) and the St. Louis Environment and Physical Activity Instrument by Brownson, Chang, and Eyler (2006). The reliability of these three questionnaires has been judged as acceptable from a comparative reliability study by Brownson, Chang, et al. (2004).

Geographic Information Systems

GIS refers to the systematic ascertainment and collection of archival and computerized sources of spatially referenced data for specific geographic areas. GIS provides multilevel data for specific geographic areas that are structured based on points, lines, and polygons. The U.S. Census is an excellent source for GIS analyses because of its extensive coverage of the entire nation (while most other existing GIS data sets are available for specific local areas) and the possibility of linking with many other data elements compiled utilizing the census units. There are also limitations. Data on the built environment can only be spatially aggregated to one of the census units (blocks, block groups, and tracts), thus limiting the specificity of analyses in this area.

GIS is also used for more fine-grained and disaggregated measures, for example, neighborhood characteristics around individual residences utilizing various buffer and proximity functions. Lee and Moudon (2006), for example, identify 3Ds + R (density, destination, distance, and route) to be key components of the neighborhood environment important for walking, which can be measured in GIS. Examples of common buffer-based measures are the number/density of land uses (e.g., restaurants, grocery stores, parks, or pharmacies) within a prespecified distance from home. Examples of proximity measures are the distance from home to those land uses. Route variables that can be captured in GIS, upon data availability, include presence/completeness of sidewalks, street block size, traffic conditions, and route directness to a destination (Moudon et al., 2006). An important prerequisite for valid buffer-based measures is the selection of buffer distances appropriate for the study population and target outcome variables. For older people, especially for studies on walking, 400 meters (approximately one-quarter of a mile) is generally recommended.

The strengths of GIS are clear. It provides a multilevel and quantitative view of the spatial elements and their approximate patterns/distributions within a specific geographic area. Potential problems include the relative timeliness of the data, incompleteness and errors in the data, insufficient levels of specificity, lack of data comparability between different geographic units/jurisdictions, and labor-intensive data processing and analysis for large geographic areas and/or involving a large number of data layers.

Environmental Audits

Environmental audits represent a systematic procedure for characterizing street-level elements. Audit instruments are designed to characterize the factual and perceptual characteristics of the built environment. The factual items include land uses, street designs, pedestrian facilities, bicycle facilities, amenities, barriers, and hazards. The perceptual items often include safety, maintenance, cleanliness, and aesthetics. Several instruments have been developed, tested for validity and/or reliability, and used in empirical studies on walking and physical activity (e.g., Brownson, Hoehner, et al., 2004). Other instruments, such as the HAN Environment Audit, were developed to ensure coverage of elements important for older populations, for example, street benches and public restrooms (Kealey et al., 2005). The HAN instrument also includes an assessment of intersections and items relevant to rural areas, for example, the inclusion of paths and other walkways in addition to sidewalks. Other targeted instruments include the Senior Walking Environment Assessment Tool by Cunningham, Michael, Farquhar, and Lapidues (2005) and the Rural Active Living Assessment by Yousefian et al. (2010).

Most environmental audits are designed to assess the street environments, but several instruments are also available for assessing other settings, such as trails and parks (Bedimo-Rung, Gustat, Tompkins, Rice, and Thomson, 2006; Troped et al., 2006). Environmental audits are often necessary to capture street-level environmental data that are not available from GIS. Because the collection of these data is typically labor-intensive, some studies have utilized systematic and/or random-type sampling strategies to select a feasible number of streets that can reasonably represent larger areas, for example, 25% of streets within 400 meters of a residence (e.g., Kelly, Schootman, Baker, Barnidge, and Lemes, 2007; Zhu and Lee, 2008; McMillan, Cubbin, Parmenter, and Lee, 2010).

Several studies have utilized more qualitative methods to elicit additional in-depth information specific to particular groups of people. For example, a Canadian study, utilizing photovoice and focus groups, reported that connected and barrier-free walking routes and amenities along the routes (e.g., benches and washrooms) are important for older adults' walking (Lockett, Willis, and Edwards, 2005). Another focus group study involving older African American and white women in South Carolina found convenient and inexpensive facilities/programs and churches to be important incentives for exercise (Wilcox, Oberrechit, Bopp, Kammermann, and McElmurray, 2005). Other examples of more qualitative environmental assessments involve the use of videotape to capture the manner in which older adults interact with the environment (e.g., streets taken and barriers avoided) as they travel from one destination to another (Shumway-Cook et al., 2002, 2003).

This brief overview highlights the pros and cons of different approaches. Thus, it is important not only to match a particular assessment approach to the underlying question being addressed but also to consider factors such as populations, settings, and available resources for both data collection and analysis in choosing a particular assessment methodology. Finally, another popular strategy is to triangulate findings with various assessment tools (e.g., combine different approaches to obtain a richer picture of different environmental aspects).

CURRENT APPLICATIONS OF RESEARCH TO
PRACTICE AND POLICY

Place matters. There is a growing body of research indicating that the built environment is associated with—and, in some instances, directly affects— patterns of walking and physical activity in older populations. Brownson, Hoehner, Day, Forsyth, and Sallis (2009) characterize this work as representing the first generation of studies. The state of the science in this area is compelling but not definitive, especially with regard to the possible main, mediating, and moderating effects of specific elements of the built environment. For example, based on reports prior to 2006, the Guide to Community Preventive Services identified a limited number of studies that examined the association between the built environment and physical activity in general adult populations (Heath et al., 2006), not focusing specifically on older adults. These studies, in most cases with a cross-sectional design, demonstrated activity differences across environments. The Task Force recommends relatively minor environmental changes such as construction and access to walking trails, improvement in street lighting, and installation and repair of sidewalks as reasonable environmental modification that should improve walking and physical activity (Heath et al., 2006). Since the Task Force recommendations, the strongest evidence for an environmental effect on patterns of walking and physical activity in older adults comes from the few longitudinal studies, noted previously, that demonstrate independent, main effects of perceived levels of neighborhood safety. Brownson et al. (2009) argue that the next generation of studies will be based increasingly on longitudinal studies in diverse populations, which presumably include more studies of older adults. While the second-generation studies, no doubt, will improve the state of the science and provide a stronger evidence base for future interventions, environmentally based practices and policies are already being proposed and introduced today. A number of reports and publications, issued by organizations such as the World Health Organization, CDC, and Environmental Protection Agency, have recommended environmental policies and programs to enhance health and mobility in older populations (table 15.1).

The state of the art in this field depends on several factors. First, as noted previously, there is a substantial body of cross-sectional studies that consis-

TABLE 15.1

Selected publications recommending environmental policies and programs to enhance health and mobility in older populations

Title	Publisher/author	Year	Website
Global Age-Friendly Cities: A Guide	World Health Organization	2007	www.who.int/ageing/publications
Why Place Matters: Building a Movement for Healthy Communities	California Endowment and PolicyLink	2007	www.policylink.org
Where We Live Matters for Our Health: The Links between Housing and Health *Where We Live Matters for Our Health: Neighborhoods and Health*	Commission to Build a Healthier America and Robert Wood Johnson Foundation	2008	www.commissiononhealth.org
Growing Smarter, Living Healthier: A Guide to Smart Growth and Active Aging	Environmental Protection Agency	2009	www.epa.gov/aging/bhc/guide
Promoting Physical Activity: Environmental and Policy Approaches (Guide to Community Preventive Services)	The Task Force on Community Preventive Services and Centers for Disease Control and Prevention	Online (updated 2010)	www.thecommunityguide.org/pa/environmental-policy
Building Healthy Communities for Active Aging National Recognition Program	Environmental Protection Agency	Online (updated 2010)	www.epa.gov/aging
Environmental Policy Change: Building Communities to Support Healthy Aging	Centers for Disease Control and Prevention, Healthy Aging Network	2010	www.prc-han.org

tently indicate an association between elements of the built environment (based on both self-report and objective measures) and patterns of walking and physical activity. Second, recommendations for improving the quality of life in neighborhoods by enhancing their aesthetic and utilitarian characteristics make sense ("face validity") and do no apparent harm. Finally, environmental practices and policies designed to improve walkability among older adults appear to positively affect the community at large. Perhaps for all of these reasons, there are a number of stakeholders recommending "walkable neighborhoods." With these points in mind, it is still necessary to establish a stronger evidence base to improve the design of environmentally based programs and policies. With a better research base, one that takes into account main, mediating, and moderating environmental effects, the interventions and policies to improve walking in older populations could be made more efficient and effective. Environmental programs and policies can take at least three forms.

Environmental Modification

Most environmental policies proposed by governmental bodies and private foundations recommend neighborhood modifications. These recommendations have included the construction of "aging-friendly" communities, infill developments, and "complete streets" to benefit pedestrians, bicyclists, and motorists. Although these recommendations, in keeping with the principles of "universal design," are designed to benefit people in all age groups, there are also specific environmental modifications, however modest, that would benefit older people in particular. These environmental elements include an increase in the presence of shaded park benches and access to clean restrooms (Kealey et al., 2005). Many research publications on the built environment and walking and physical activity conclude by outlining the implications of the findings for practice and policy. These sections often include general recommendations for modifications to the neighborhood, typically in the form of changes to city and county zoning requirements (e.g., encouragement of mixed land-use development). As noted previously, these changes may be recommended for a variety of reasons, but, as with many public health interventions, it is important to acknowledge the level of evidence for recommending large-scale changes to the environment as a vehicle of improving walking and physical activity in older populations (Heath et al., 2006). The research-to-practice base can be strengthened by the inclusion of more definitive evidence generated from longitudinal observational studies and, what would be even more compelling and far more difficult, randomized community trials (Heath et al., 2006; Brownson et al., 2009; Frank and Savage, 2009; Yen et al., 2009).

Environmental Adaptation

This type of program or policy is designed to promote adaptation to the environment by locating or linking residents to the best features of their neighborhood or community. It does not entail constructing new facilities or making major modifications to existing facilities. It may include, for example, the extension of timed signals for pedestrian crossing to take better account of the slower walking speed of the majority of older adults. It also may include the provision of neighborhood walking maps to encourage walking in "safe" areas or reasonable routes to access services, such as full-service grocery stores. There is at least one report from a pilot study indicating the feasibility of developing and implementing these environmental adaptations, such as the provision of walking maps among older residents (Rosenberg et al., 2009). Because this type of program or policy does not involve environmental change or modification, it can be implemented more quickly at less cost. It also may be possible to develop community-based trials in which the intervention (e.g., walking maps) could be randomized to different groups or neighborhoods. This, in turn, may lead to the establishment of a stronger evidence base to guide the refinement of such programs in the future.

Individual-Environmental Intervention

This type of program is designed to provide a multilevel intervention to affect change at both the individual and environmental levels. It follows directly from the tenets of the ecological model (Satariano and McAuley, 2003). To our knowledge, this type of intervention has only been used to reduce the risk of indoor falls and injuries in older people by addressing concurrently individual factors (e.g., improvement in lower-body strength, balance, and vision) and environmental factors (e.g., removal of tripping hazards in the home) (McClure et al., 2005; Sleet, Moffet, and Stevens, 2008). Following from the description of environmental adaptation, it may be possible to design a community-based randomized study to assess whether the provision of neighborhood walking maps, in conjunction with an individually based program, enhances walking in older populations beyond what could be realized with only an individually based walking program.

NEW DIRECTIONS FOR ENVIRONMENTAL RESEARCH,
PRACTICE, AND POLICY

The development of evidence-based environmental programs and policies is a key objective for public health and aging. The research to date is promising. The question is, where do we go from here? What is the next generation of research in this area? How does the need for evidence-based programs and policies guide this research and, in turn, benefit from it? In this section, we offer five recommendations to that end.

1. *Develop an integrated conceptual model of the built environment, mobility, and activities of everyday life.* It is important to develop a more comprehensive and integrated view that better captures everyday life. Currently, there is a distinction between research on housing and the neighborhood, in contrast to how most people live their lives. A more comprehensive conceptual model will be more effective in understanding and enhancing the environmental effects of mobility and activities of everyday life. Consider falls and injuries as "mobility disorders" that represent one of the leading causes of accidental death in older populations. Even though outdoor falls are slightly more common than indoor falls (approximately 60% vs. 40% across studies), less research has been conducted on the epidemiology of outdoor falls (Lai, Low, Wong, Wong, and Chan, 2009). Of the relatively few studies in this area, there is evidence suggesting the importance of environmental factors. Outdoor falls are most likely to occur during walking and most likely to take place on sidewalks, curbs, and streets, as well as gardens, patios, yards, decks or porches, parks and recreational areas, parking garages, and parking lots (Li et al., 2006; Lai et al., 2009). Uneven surfaces and abrupt changes in walking surfaces (e.g., an unexpected step) are especially problematic. In addition to these design elements, situational factors (e.g., wet or slippery surfaces) also contribute to the likelihood of an outdoor fall (Li et al., 2006; Lai et al., 2009). It is also reported that frail seniors are more likely to fall indoors, whereas seniors who are more fit with better lower-body capacity are more likely to fall outdoors.

This is an interesting issue with important policy implications. It may be that while seniors at risk for an outdoor fall are generally fit and sufficiently mobile to venture from their homes, they may have other individual characteristics, such as poor vision or depressive symptoms, that elevate their risk for an outdoor fall (Bergland, Jarnio, and Laake, 2003). In fact, it may be the combination of these individual factors in conjunction with outdoor environmental hazards that increases the likelihood of an injurious fall.

Beyond research on place and falls, it is also necessary to have a more comprehensive view of the environment and mobility. It is clear that walking and physical activity improve the health and well-being of older people, but what are the potential risks relative to the known benefits? To what extent and under what circumstances does encouraging older people to leave their homes and take part in walking programs elevate the risk of an outdoor fall? What are the relative risks involved, and what can be done at both the individual and environmental levels to reduce those risks?

2. *Develop strategies to conduct better longitudinal studies.* Longitudinal observational studies will make possible a better understanding of the main, mediating, and moderating effects of the built environment on the temporal patterns of mobility and activities of everyday life. In keeping with the tenets of the ecological model, the elements of the built environment itself, as well as the characteristics of individuals and populations, should be assessed over time. A more comprehensive understanding of temporal patterns should also consider "memory of place." It may be, for example, that the reason older people elect to walk in one area as opposed to another is their memory of those places rather than how they look today (King, Satariano, Marti, and Zhu, 2008). In addition, given the time and expense of longitudinal studies, we should consider the utility of computerized simulations of the effect of specific built and planned environments on walking and physical activity in older populations.

3. *Expand the study of diverse aging populations.* Most studies have focused on older populations in specific regions. It is necessary to examine urban, suburban, and rural populations of older residents in different locations around the country. In the 1980s, the National Institute on Aging (NIA) sponsored the Established Populations for Epidemiologic Studies of the Elderly (EPESE). This collaboration, involving population-based studies in New Haven, Connecticut, and East Boston, Massachusetts, as well as selected counties in Iowa and North Carolina, served as the basis for a rich set of studies that advanced our understanding of the epidemiology of aging. It may be that a new national collaborative study, patterned after the NIA EPESE, could advance our understanding of the effects of the built and planned environments on health and well-being. This should enhance our understanding of racial, ethnic, socioeconomic, and regional differences in health and well-being and the extent to which differences in the built environment contribute to that diversity. The protocol for this type of project should include a full range of environmental measures, including GIS, environmental audits, and questionnaires to capture objective and perceived as-

sessments of the environment at the community, neighborhood, housing sites, and housing levels. This protocol may lead to the establishment of a more standardized approach for the conduct of research in this area.

4. *Explore the biological and behavioral mechanisms to explain the effects of the built environment on health and well-being in older populations.* The ecological model, described previously, assumes that patterns of health and well-being are due to a dynamic interplay of biological, behavioral, and environmental factors. For a more comprehensive understanding of the effects of the built environment, it is necessary to determine how biological and behavioral factors help to understand the effects of the built environment on health and well-being. There is a growing body of research to understand the physiological mechanisms associated with social and behavioral factors and population health. There is evidence, for example, that prolonged and persistent exposure to stressors, often associated with residence in particular communities, reduces host immunity, enhances susceptibility to disease, and leads to "weathering" and premature aging (Taylor, Repetti, and Seeman, 1997). It is also necessary to consider whether some older adults have enhanced biological susceptibility to particular environmental characteristics and thus enhanced behavioral reactions to the environment for good or ill (Hertzman and Boyce, 2010; Uchino, Birmingham, and Berg, 2010). Finally, it is necessary to consider whether residence and exposure to particular types of environments over the life course from childhood to the present affect patterns of health and well-being in older populations (Hertzman and Boyce, 2010).

5. *Develop strategies to develop a new generation of evidence-based environmental programs and policies to enhance health and well-being in aging populations.* To develop new strategies, it is important to be alert to the dangers of environmental ageism. Following from Butler (2002) and others (Palmore, Branch, and Harris, 2005), we see ageism in environmental programs and policies that reinforce the stereotypical position that aging and age-related limitations reflect reduced competence and societal worth, deserving, then, of less attention, compensation, and respect. Environmental ageism can be manifested in calls to ensure that environments are not made to be too accommodating for older adults, for fear of reducing the overall efficiency, effectiveness, and well-being of the larger community. On the other hand, environmental ageism can also be reflected in calls to ensure that older adults be protected from environments perceived to be too challenging, somewhat akin to Binstock's (1983) notion of "compassionate ageism." While the two forms of ageism may appear to be quite different, in both cases the assumption is that older adults, because of age-related limitations, cannot participate

fully in everyday life, preventing them from making useful contributions to the larger society. With the specter of environmental ageism present, the overall objective of programs and policies should be, to quote again from the CDC definition of healthy aging, "the development and maintenance of optimal physical, mental and social well-being in older adults." And, most important for our purposes here, "it is most likely to be achieved when physical environments and communities are safe, and support the adoption and maintenance by individuals of attitudes and behaviors known to promote health and well-being; and by the effective use of health services and community programs to prevent or minimize the impact of acute and chronic disease on function."

CONCLUSION

One of the important objectives in public health is to understand and promote health and well-being in a diverse aging population. The expanding body of research on the built environment holds the promise for the development, evaluation, and dissemination of a new generation of programs and policies to promote "healthy aging." The fulfillment of that promise will necessitate new ideas and resources to advance a new multidisciplinary research agenda involving researchers in public health, gerontology, architecture, landscape architecture, urban planning, transportation, and parks and recreation. More important, it will involve new collaborations among researchers, practitioners, policy makers, and older people themselves to advance and enhance healthy aging. We have indicated first- and second-generation research activities—the third stage is interdisciplinary research that bridges research and practice and better informs the development of environments that are better suited for the promotion of healthy aging.

REFERENCES

Ainsworth, B. E., S. Wilcox, W. W. Thompson, D. L. Richeter, and K. A. Henderson. 2003. Personal, social, and physical environmental correlates of physical activity in African American women in South Carolina. *American Journal of Preventive Medicine* 25:23–29.

Annear, M. J., G. Cushman, and B. Gidlow. 2009. Leisure time physical activity difference among older adults from diverse socioeconomic neighborhoods. *Health and Place* 15:482–90.

Balfour, J. L., and G. A. Kaplan. 2002. Neighborhood environment and loss of physical function in older adults: Evidence from the Alameda County Study. *American Journal of Epidemiology* 155:507–15.

Bedimo-Rung, A. L., J. Gustat, B. J. Tompkins, J. Rice, and J. Thomson. 2006. Development of a direct observation instrument to measure environmental characteristics of parks for physical activity. *Journal of Physical Activity and Health* 3:S176–89.

Bergland, A., G. B. Jarnio, and K. Laake. 2003. Predictors of falls in the elderly by location. *Aging Clinical and Experimental Research* 15:43–50.

Binstock, R. H. 1983. The aged as scapegoat. *Gerontologist* 23:136–43.

Brownson, R. C., J. J. Chang, and A. Eyler. 2006. The St. Louis Environment and Physical Activity Instrument measures perceived environmental influences on physical activity. Retrieved October 29, 2010, from www.activelivingresearch.org/node/10644.

Brownson, R. C., J. J. Chang, A. A. Eyler, B. E. Ainsworth, K. A. Kirtland, B. E. Saelens, and J. F. Sallis. 2004. Measuring the environment for friendliness toward physical activity: A comparison of the reliability of 3 questionnaires. *American Journal of Public Health* 94:473–83.

Brownson, R. C., C. M. Hoehner, L. K. Brennan, R. A. Cook, M. B. Elliott, and K. M. McMullen. 2004. Reliability of two instruments for auditing the environment for physical activity. *Journal of Physical Activity and Health* 1:189–207.

Brownson, R. C., C. M. Hoehner, K. Day, A. Forsyth, and J. F. Sallis. 2009. Measuring the built environment for physical activity: State of the science. *American Journal of Preventive Medicine* 36(Suppl. 4):S99–123.

Butler, R. N. 2002. *Why Survive? Being Old in America*. Baltimore: Johns Hopkins University Press.

Chodzko-Zajko, W. J., D. N. Proctor, S. Fiatarone, C. T. Minson, C. R. Nigg, G. J. Salem, and J. S. Skinner. 2009. American College of Sports Medicine position stand: Exercise and physical activity for older adults. *Medicine & Science in Sports & Exercise* 41:1510–30.

Clark, C. R., I. Kawachi, L. Ryan, K. Ertel, M. E. Fay, and L. F. Berkman. 2009. Perceived neighborhood safety and incident mobility disability among elders: The hazards of poverty. *BMC Public Health* 9:162–77.

Clarke, P., J. A. Ailshire, M. Bader, J. D. Morenoff, and J. S. House. 2008. Mobility disability and the urban built environment. *American Journal of Epidemiology* 168:506–13.

Clarke, P., J. A. Ailshire, and P. Lantz. 2009. Urban built environments and trajectories of mobility disability: Findings from a national sample of community-dwelling American adults (1986–2001). *Social Science & Medicine* 69:964–70.

Clarke, P., and L. K. George. 2005. The role of the built environment in the disablement process. *American Journal of Public Health* 95:1933–39.

Corburn, J. 2009. *Toward the Healthy City*. Cambridge, MA: MIT Press.

Cunningham, G. O., and Y. L. Michael. 2004. Concepts guiding the study of the impact of the built environment on physical activity for older adults: A review of the literature. *American Journal of Health Promotion* 18:435–43.

Cunningham, G. O., Y. L. Michael, S. A. Farquhar, and J. Lapidues. 2005. Developing a reliable senior walking environmental assessment tool. *American Journal of Preventive Medicine* 29:215–17.

Dannenberg, A. L., R. J. Jackson, H. Frumkin, R. A. Schieber, M. Pratt, C. Kochtiz-

ky, and H. H. Tilson. 2003. The impact of community design and land-use choices on public health: A scientific research agenda. *American Journal of Public
Health* 93:1500–1508.

Do, D. P., B. K. Finch, R. Basurto-Davila, C. Bird, J. Escarce, and N. Lurie. 2008.
Does place explain racial health disparities? Quantifying the contribution of resi-
dential context to the black/white health gap in the United States. *Social Science
& Medicine* 67:1258–68.

Fisher, K. J., F. Li, Y. Michael, and M. Cleveland. 2004. Neighborhood-level influences on physical activity among older adults. *Journal of Aging and Physical Activity* 11:45–63.

Frank, L., and S. Savage. 2009. A national plan for physical activity: The enabling
role of the built environment. *Journal of Physical Activity and Health* 6:S186–95.

Frank, L. D., M. J. Greenwald, S. Winkelman, J. Chapman, and S. Kavage. 2010.
Carbonless footprints: Promoting health and climate stabilization through active
transportation. *Preventive Medicine* 50:S99–105.

Frank, L. D., J. Kerr, J. F. Sallis, R. Miles, and J. Chapman. 2008. A hierarchy of sociodemographic and environmental correlates of walking and obesity. *Preventive
Medicine* 47:172–78.

Frank, L. D., B. E. Saelens, K. E. Powell, and J. E. Chapman. 2007. Stepping towards
causation: Do built environments or neighborhood and travel preferences explain
physical activity, driving, and obesity? *Social Science & Medicine* 65:1898–914.

Gauvin, L., M. Riva, T. Barnett, C. L. Craig, M. Spivock, S. Laforest, S. Laberge,
M.-C. Fournel, H. Gagon, and S. Gagne. 2008. Association between neighborhood active living potential and walking. *American Journal of Epidemiology* 167:
944–53.

Giles-Corti, B., and R. J. Donovan. 2002. Relative influences of individual, social
environmental, and physical environmental correlates of walking. *American Journal of Public Health* 93:1583–89.

Heath, G., R. C. Brownson, J. Kruger, R. Miles, K. E. Powell, L. T. Ramsey, and the
Task Force on Community Preventive Services. 2006. The effectiveness of urban
design and land use and transport policies and practices to increase physical activity:
A systematic review. *Journal of Physical Activity and Health* 3 (Suppl. 1):S55–76.

Hertzman, C., and T. Boyce. 2010. How experience gets under the skin to create
gradients in developmental health. *Annual Review of Public Health* 31:329–47.

Kamphuis, C. B. M., F. J. van Lenthe, K. Giskes, M. Huisman, J. Brug, and
J. P. Mackenbach. 2009. Socioeconomic differences in lack of recreational walking among older adults: The role of neighbourhood and individual factors. *International Journal of Behavioral Nutrition and Physical Activity* 6:1–11.

Kealey, M., J. Kruger, R. Hunter, S. Ivey, W. Satariano, C. Bayles, B. Ramirez,
L. Bryant, C. Johnson, C. Lee, D. Levinger, K. McTigue, G. Moni, A. V. Moudon,
D. Pluto, T. Prohaska, C. Sible, S. Tindal, S. Wilcox, K. Winters, and K. Williams. 2005. Engaging older adults to be more active where they live: Audit tool
development. *Preventing Chronic Disease* [serial online]. Available from www.cdc
.gov/pcd/issues/2005/apr/pdf/04_0142q.pdf.

Kelly, C. M., M. Schootman, E. A. Baker, E. K. Barnidge, and A. Lemes. 2007. The association of sidewalk walkability and physical disorder with area-level race and poverty. *Journal of Epidemiology and Community Health* 29:978–83.

King, A. C., C. Castro, S. Wilcox, A. A. Eyler, J. F. Sallis, and R. C. Brownson. 2000. Personal and environmental factors associated with physical inactivity among different racial-ethnic groups of U.S. middle-aged and older-aged women. *Health Psychology* 19:354–64.

King, A. C., W. A. Satariano, J. Marti, and W. Zhu. 2008. Multilevel modeling of walking behavior: Advances in understanding the interactions of people, place, and time. *Medicine & Science in Sports & Exercise* 40:S584–93.

King, D. 2008. Neighborhood and individual factors in activity in older adults: Results from the Neighborhood and Senior Health Survey. *Journal of Aging and Physical Activity* 16:144–70.

King, W., S. H. Belle, J. S. Brach, L. R. Simkin-Silverman, T. Soska, and A. M. Kriska. 2005. Objective measures of neighborhood environment and physical activity in older women. *American Journal of Preventive Medicine* 28:461–69.

Lai, P. C., C. T. Low, M. Wong, W. C. Wong, and M. H. Chan. 2009. Spatial analysis of falls in an urban community of Hong Kong. *International Journal of Health Geographics* 8:14–28.

Lawton, M. P. 1986. *Environment and Aging*. Albany, NY: Center for the Study of Aging.

Lawton, M. P., and L. Nahemow. 1973. Ecology and the aging process. In *The Psychology of Adult Development and Aging*, ed. C. Eisdorfer and M. P. Lawong, pp. 619–74. Washington, DC: American Psychological Association.

Lee, C. 2007. Environment and active living: The roles of health risk and economic factors. *American Journal of Health Promotion* 21:S293–304.

Lee, C., and A. V. Moudon. 2006. The 3Ds + R: Quantifying land use and urban form correlates of walking. *Transportation Research Part D* 11:204–12.

Lee, I.-M., and D. M. Buchner. 2008. The importance of walking to public health. *Medicine & Science in Sports & Exercise* 40:S512–18.

Li, F., K. J. Fisher, A. Bauman, M. G. Ory, W. Chodzko-Zajko, P. Harmer, M. Bosworth, and M. Cleveland. 2005. Neighborhood influences on physical activity in middle-aged and older adults: A multilevel perspective. *Journal of Aging and Physical Activity* 13:87–114.

Li, F., K. J. Fisher, and R. C. Brownson. 2005. A multilevel analysis of change in neighborhood walking activity in older adults. *Journal of Aging and Physical Activity* 13:145–59.

Li, F., K. J. Fisher, R. C. Brownson, and M. Bosworth. 2005. Multilevel modeling of built environment characteristics related to neighbourhood walking activity in older adults. *Journal of Epidemiology and Community Health* 59:558–64.

Li, W., T. H. Keegan, B. Sternfeld, S. Sidney, C. P. Quesenberry, and J. L. Kelsey. 2006. Outdoor falls among middle-aged and older adults: A neglected public health problem. *American Journal of Public Health* 96:1192–200.

Lockett, D., A. Willis, and N. Edwards. 2005. Exploratory qualitative study to identify environmental barriers to and facilitators of walking. *Canadian Journal of Nursing Research* 37:48–65.

McClure, R. J., C. Turner, N. Peel, A. Spinks, E. Eakin, and K. Hughes. 2005.

Population-based interventions for the prevention of fall-related injuries in older people. *Cochrane Database of Systematic Reviews* 2005, Issue 1. Art. No.: CD004441. doi:10.1002/14651858.CD004441.pub 2.

McKinlay, J. (1979). A case for refocusing upstream: The political economy of illness. In *Patients, Physicians, and Illness: A Sourcebook in Behavioral Science and Health*, ed. J. Gartley, pp. 9–25. New York: Free Press.

McMillan, C., B. Cubbin, A. V. M. Parmenter, and R. E. Lee. 2010. Neighborhood sampling: How many streets must an auditor walk? *International Journal of Behavioral Nutrition and Physical Activity* 7:20.

Mendes de Leon, C. F., K. A. Cagney, J. L. Bienias, L. L. Barnes, K. A. Skarupski, P. A. Scherr, and D. A. Evans. 2009. Neighborhood social cohesion and disorder in relation to walking in community-dwelling older adults: A multilevel analysis. *Journal of Aging and Health* 21:155–71.

Michael, Y. L., T. Beard, D. Choi, S. Farguhar, and N. Carlson. 2006. Measuring the influence of built neighborhood environments on walking in older adults. *Journal of Aging and Physical Activity* 14:302–12.

Moudon, A. V., and C. Lee. 2003. Walking and biking: An evaluation of environmental audit instruments. *American Journal of Health Promotion* 18:21–37.

Moudon, A. V., C. Lee, A. D. Cheadle, C. Garvin, D. Johnson, T. L. Schmid, R. D. Weathers, and L. Lin. 2006. Operational definitions of walkable neighborhood: Theoretical and empirical insights. *Journal of Physical Activity and Health* 3(Suppl. 1):S99–117.

Nagel, C. L., N. E. Carlson, M. Bosworth, and Y. L. Michael. 2008. The relation between neighborhood built environment and walking activity among older adults. *American Journal of Epidemiology* 168:461–68.

Ory, M. G., R. Abeles, and P. D. Lipman, eds. 1992. *Aging, Health, and Behavior.* Newberry, CA: Sage.

Owen, N., N. Humpel, K. Leslie, A. Bauman, and J. F. Sallis. 2004. Understanding environmental influences on walking: Review and research agenda. *American Journal of Preventive Medicine* 27:67–76.

Palmore, E. B., L. Branch, and D. K. Harris, eds. 2005. *Encyclopedia of Ageism.* New York: Haworth Press.

Prohaska, T., E. Belansky, B. Belza, D. Buchner, V. Marshall, K. McTigue, W. Satariano, and S. Wilcox. 2006. Physical activity, public health, and aging: Critical issues and research priorities. *Journals of Gerontology Series B: Psychological Sciences and Social Sciences* 61B:S267–73.

Rodriguez, D. A., A. L. Brown, and P. J. Troped. 2005. Portable global positioning units to complement accelerometry-based physical activity monitors. *Medicine & Science in Sports & Exercise* 37(Suppl. 11):S572–81.

Rodriquez, D. A., K. R. Evenson, A. V. Diez Roux, and S. J. Brines. 2009. Land use, residential density, and walking. The multi-ethnic study of atherosclerosis. *American Journal of Preventive Medicine* 37:397–404.

Rose, G. 1985. Sick individuals and sick populations. *International Journal of Epidemiology* 14:32–38.

Rosenberg, D., J. Kerr, J. F. Sallis, K. Patrick, D. J. Moore, and A. King. 2009. Feasibility and outcomes of a multilevel place-based walking intervention for seniors: A pilot study. *Health and Place* 15:173–79.

Saelens, B. E., and C. Papadopoulos. 2008. The importance of the built environment in older adults' physical activity: A review of the literature. *Washington State Journal of Public Health Practice* 1:13–21.

Saelens, B. E., J. F. Sallis, J. B. Black, and D. Chen. 2003. Neighborhood-based differences in physical activity: An environment scale evaluation. *American Journal of Public Health* 93:1552–58.

Sallis, J. F., R. Cervero, W. W. Ascher, K. Henderson, M. K. Kraft, and J. Kerr. 2006. An ecological approach to creating active living communities. *Annual Review of Public Health* 27:297–322.

Satariano, W. A. 2006. *Epidemiology of Aging: An Ecological Approach.* Sudbury, MA: Jones and Bartlett.

Satariano, W. A., S. L. Ivey, E. Kurtovich, M. Kealey, A. E. Hubbard, C. M. Bayles, L. L. Bryant, R. H. Hunter, and T. R. Prohaska. 2010. Lower-body function, neighborhoods, and walking in an older population. *American Journal of Preventive Medicine* 38:419–28.

Satariano, W. A., and E. McAuley. 2003 Promoting physical activity among older adults: From ecology to the individual. *American Journal of Preventive Medicine* 25:184–92.

Shigematsu, R., J. F. Sallis, T. L. Conway, B. E. Saelens, L. D. Frank, K. L. Cain, J. E. Chapman, and A. C. King. 2009. Age differences in the relation of perceived neighborhood environments to walking. *Medicine & Science in Sports & Exercise* 41:314–21.

Shumway-Cook, A., A. Patla, A. Stewart, L. Ferrucci, M. A. Ciol, and J. M. Guralnik. 2002. Environmental demands associated with community mobility in older adults with and without mobility disabilities. *Physical Therapy* 82:670–81.

Shumway-Cook, A., A. Patla, A. Stewart, L. Ferrucci, M. A. Ciol, and J. M. Guralnik. 2003. Environmental components of mobility disability in community-living persons. *Journal of the American Geriatrics Society* 51:393–98.

Sleet, D. A., D. B. Moffett, and J. Stevens. 2008. CDC's research portfolio in older adult fall prevention: A review of progress, 1985–2005, and future research directions. *Journal of Safety Research* 39:259–67.

Smedley, B. D., and S. L. Syme, eds. 2001. *Promoting Health: Intervention Strategies for Social and Behavioral Research.* Washington, DC: National Academies Press.

Taylor, S. E., R. L. Repetti, and T. E. Seeman. 1997. Health psychology: What is an unhealthy environment and how does it get under the skin? *Annual Review of Psychology* 48:411–47.

Troped, P. J., K. K. Cromley, M. S. Fragala, S. J. Melly, H. H. Hasbrouch, S. L. Gortmaker, and R. C. Brownson. 2006. Development and reliability and validity testing of any audit tool for trail/path characteristics: The Path Environment Audit Tools (PEAT). *Journal of Physical Activity and Health* 3(Suppl. 1):S158–75.

Troped, P. J., M. S. Oliveria, C. E. Mathews, K. K. Cromley, S. J. Melly, and B. A. Craig. 2008. Prediction of activity mode with global positioning system and accelerometer data. *Medicine & Science in Sports & Exercise* 40:958–78.

Tudor-Locke, C., R. Ainsworth, and R. Thompson. 2002. Comparison of pedometer and accelerometer measures of free living physical activity. *Medicine & Science in Sports & Exercise* 34:2045–51.

Uchino, B. N., W. Birmingham, and C. A. Berg. 2010. Are older adults less or more physiologically reactive? A meta-analysis of age-related differences in cardiovascular reactivity to laboratory tasks. *Journals of Gerontology Series B: Psychological Sciences and Social Sciences* 65B:154–62.

U.S. Centers for Disease Control and Prevention and U.S. Department of Housing and Urban Development. 2006. *Healthy Housing Reference Manual.* Washington, DC. www.cdc.gov/nceh/publications/books/housing/2006_HHM_FINAL_front_matter.pdf.

U.S. Department of Health and Human Services. 2000. *Healthy People 2020. Understanding and Improving Health.* Washington, DC: Author.

U.S. Environmental Protection Agency. 2009. *Growing Smarter, Living Healthier: A Guide to Smart Growth and Active Aging.* Washington, DC. www.epa.gov/aging/bhc/guide/2009_Aging.pdf.

U.S. Transportation Research Board, U.S. National Academies of Science. 2004. *Transportation in an Aging Society: A Decade of Experience.* Conference Proceedings 27. Technical Papers and Reports from Conference, November 7–9, 1999, Bethesda, MD. http://onlinepubs.trb.org/onlinepubs/conf/reports/cp_27.pdf.

Wen, M., N. R. Kandula, and D. S. Lauderdate. 2004. Walking for transportation or leisure: What difference does the neighborhood make? *Journal of General Internal Medicine* 22:1674–80.

Wieters, M., J. Kim, and C. Lee. 2008. Assessments of available research instruments for measuring physical activity. Chicago: Association of Collegiate Schools of Planning.

Wilcox, S., L. Oberrechit, M. Bopp, S. K. Kammermann, and C. T. McElmurray. 2005. A qualitative study of exercise in older African American and white women in rural South Carolina: Perceptions, barriers, and motivations. *Journal of Women & Aging* 17:37–53.

Yen, I. H., Y. L. Michael, and L. Perdue. 2009. Neighborhood environments in studies of health of older adults: A systematic review. *American Journal of Preventive Medicine* 37:455–63.

Yousefian, A., E. Hennessy, M. R. Umstattd, C. D. Economos, J. S. Hallam, R. R. Hyatt, and D. Hartley. 2010. Development of the rural active living assessment tools: Measuring rural environments. *Preventive Medicine* 50(Suppl. 1):S86–92.

Zhu, X., and C. Lee. 2008. Walkability and safety around elementary schools: Economic and ethnic disparities. *American Journal of Preventive Medicine* 34:282–90.

CHAPTER 16

Genomics and Aging

Steven M. Albert, PhD, MSPH, MA
M. Michael Barmada, PhD

Public health genomics is a new field that began only in the mid- to late 1990s. The field focuses on the use of genetic information to improve population health, but it bears no relation to the crude eugenics programs of the earlier part of the century. Its focus is the entirety of genetic information—the genome—and the ways genes and gene-environment interactions contribute to mechanisms of disease. Thus, the U.S. Office of Public Health Genomics (OPHG), established in 1997, "promotes the integration of genomics into public health research, policy, and practice to prevent disease and improve the health of all people" (www.cdc.gov/genomics/). The journal *Public Health Genomics*, which first appeared in 1998, similarly aims to apply genome-based knowledge to disease prevention and promote gains in population health.

The field of genomics and aging is even more recent. It is similar to the broader field of public health genomics in that it also seeks to discover mechanisms of chronic disease and use genomic knowledge to help target therapies to groups at high risk for such diseases. The genomic approach to aging is similar as well in its focus on behavioral risk factors and environment as these interact with gene expression. But it differs in one important way. While most genome-based aging research seeks to identify mechanisms involved in the chronic diseases of later life, genomic approaches have also been used to understand mechanisms of longevity and the basis of optimal aging itself.

BACKGROUND

The *genome* is the full DNA sequence of an organism, the whole of an organism's hereditary information. When the genome of an organism is sequenced, we obtain the complete ordering of base pairs (or nucleotides) along every chromosome. Variations in nucleotide order and content are seen when sequencing many individuals and occur on many different levels (e.g., variations at single nucleotides, rearrangements of segments of DNA from one position to another, repetitions or deletions of segments of DNA). The most common form of variation in the human genome is the *single nucleotide polymorphism* (SNP), which is variation in a nucleotide (substitution in a single chemical base pair of DNA, for example, AACGCTA to AACGTTA). SNPs can be used in genetic association or linkage studies to identify genetic variation and pinpoint genes involved in disease, development, or potentially aging and senescence.

The combination of alleles at any particular SNP is called a *genotype*, and the sequence of consecutive alleles on a chromosome is termed a *haplotype*. The International HapMap Project succeeded in mapping several million well-defined SNPs (SNPs where each allele occurs in at least 1% of the population), genotyping those SNPs in a sample of individuals from various ethnic populations, identifying the common haplotypes and associations between them in different ethnic populations, and making these results available to researchers worldwide. Completed in 2006, the HapMap has allowed researchers to compare human samples with and without a phenotype of interest (for example, Alzheimer's disease or reaching age 90) and identify relevant genes responsible for such variation.

In *genome-wide association studies* (GWAS), the genomes of samples differing in such phenotypes are compared by automated microarray genotyping of genome-wide SNPs predicted by HapMap data to have the highest likelihood of capturing variation in the region (i.e., in linkage disequilibrium with a large number of SNPs in the immediate vicinity), or of SNPs with known or predicted functional consequences (e.g., changing the amino acid coding of a protein-coding region). If the frequency of SNP alleles differs in the two samples, the phenotype is likely to be associated with haplotypes defined by SNPs at these particular locations on chromosomes.

This approach may lead to the identification of genetic variation influencing the phenotype but is limited by the frequency of the SNP alleles assayed. Under the assumptions of the Common Disease–Common Variant (CDCV) hypothesis (Chakravarti, 1999; Reich and Lander, 2001), phenotypes that are "common" in the population (with prevalence >1%) are likely to be influenced by genetic variants (e.g., SNPs) with a similarly common frequency (>5%). Thus, though the human genome contains approximately 20,000–25,000 genes and perhaps 3 billion base pairs, SNPs and the HapMap make it unnecessary to sequence the whole genome to identify genes associated with a disease. Rather, fine gene mapping can be reserved for regions pinpointed by GWAS. While there have certainly been notable successes of this approach (Crohn's disease being an often-mentioned example), the majority of GWAS to date have produced associations that do not appear to be highly predictive and do not (as of yet) yield insights into disease mechanisms. Newer genome-wide SNP arrays are now being constructed using SNP variants with much lower allele frequencies (<1%).

If the genome is the full set of an organism's genes, *genomics* is the study of the full DNA sequence of an organism, which is sometimes extended beyond genes and DNA (genome) to mRNA (the transcriptome) and to proteins produced by genes (the proteome). *Functional genomics* seeks to describe gene function from the perspective of the genome, examining the effect of multiple genes on protein function and protein-protein interaction. Major collaborative efforts in this area include ENCODE (Encyclopedia of DNA Elements), which seeks to identify all functional elements of human genomic DNA, in both coding and noncoding regions (i.e., regions clearly associated with genes that code for proteins as well as regions without obvious function) (ENCODE, www.genome.gov/10005107). In research on the genomics of aging, important online databases and search tools have been collected in the Human Ageing Genomic Resources project. This includes GenAge, a database of genes potentially associated with aging and longevity, and AnAge, a database on aging for over 4,000 species.

These efforts should be seen as part of the larger goals of the National Human Genome Research Institute at the National Institutes of Health (NIH) (Collins, Green, Guttmacher, and Guyer, 2003) and the Office of Population Genomics (Manolio et al., in press). Thus, we can add *population genomics* to this growing and fast-moving field, which continues to evolve with progress in microarray technologies, high-throughput computing, and bioinformatics.

The central question in genomics and aging is how to find the genes that really count, that is, genes that distinguish long-lived from short-lived species and also regulate aging, disease, and longevity within a species (Miller, 1999). This effort has been frustrated so far by the inability of conventional genetic approaches (candidate gene studies) to uncover genes with large effects in these areas, at least in human studies. The genomic approach holds the promise of studying the function of large networks of genes, which may change our understanding of longevity assurance genes and emphasize instead the ways these networks maintain biological systems over time (Vigh and Suh, 2003, 2005).

The rise of genomics has important implications for public health and aging. These include the following, which we discuss below:

—*Greater focus on the aging phenome, or the complete phenotypic representation of the aging process, rather than on particular aspects of aging.* The many genes involved in regulation of aging (such as genes governing insulin signaling, cellular defense, and stress response, which may act in combination) likely affect multiple domains of aging.

—*Greater focus on a multifactorial etiology for the aging phenome.* Aspects of aging are likely to be determined by many genetic influences interacting with a host of social and environmental factors. Moreover, the specific gene variants involved in disease, as well as the influence of genetic and environmental factors, may vary even among people with the same disease or similar experience of aging (Burke, Khoury, Stewart, and Zimmern, 2006). This complexity should not be neglected when we think of genomics as paving the way for a truly personalized medicine.

—*Greater focus on the public health value of disease-associated genotypes.* Knowing that a person has the APOE-ε4 genotype, and hence greater risk for Alzheimer's disease, adds only marginal accuracy to the diagnosis. It does not offer guidance on treatment and is equivocal for predicting disease progression. For these reasons, relying on genetic information may lead to suboptimal decision making by patients and families. (Mayeux and Schupf, 1995). Without a specific therapy to reduce the risk of disease (as in the case of BRCA1 for risk of breast cancer), the public health value of disease-associated genotypes is limited.

—*Recognition of the potential for genetic information to change health risk behaviors.* In prior studies, knowing that one has a genetic risk for lung cancer did not change smoking behavior, but knowledge of colorectal cancer risk increased the likelihood of screening colonoscopy (McBride et al., 2002). How knowledge of genetic risk affects health behaviors is still emerging, but it is clear that people are likely to misinterpret probabilistic risk information without adequate education. Apart from this challenge, the public health establishment has had little experience in directing interventions to subpopulations based on genetic risk (McBride et al., 2008).

WHAT IS THE MOST APPROPRIATE PHENOTYPE FOR GENOMIC STUDIES OF AGING?

Healthy or optimal aging is a complex trait in both phenotype and underlying genetic influence (Manolio, 2007). So far research has not identified an underlying pacemaker or clock for the rate of human aging, so we are forced to use surrogate phenotypes of aging. Phenotypes of optimal aging usually include late age at death or extreme longevity (reaching age 90 and greater); disease-free survival; high physical, cognitive, or social function late in life; and slow rate of change in physiologic parameters. Yet it is also possible that these are not good indicators of optimal aging because they reflect strong environmental as well as genetic effects. It is difficult, for example, to monitor assessment of environmental exposures over a lifetime. Nevertheless, since reaching very old age is clearly heritable, is relatively easy to assess, and presumes long periods of the life span free of disease and with high functional status, it has so far been the phenotype of choice.

While a number of candidate genes have been associated with longevity in GWAS, these associations have been quite modest and hard to replicate. A recent meta-analysis of GWAS findings for longevity in four large community-based cohort studies also failed to find strong associations between SNPs and survival to age 90+ (Newman et al., 2010). While 273 SNPs were associated with the longevity phenotype, none reached prespecified genome-wide levels of significance. A strength of this study was to compare people reaching age 90+ with people who died before age 80 in the same community cohorts. The 22 SNPs that had the largest association with longevity were assessed in two different replication cohorts. Only 1 of 16 SNPs successfully genotyped for the replication analysis gained in its association with longevity. Thus, a powerful genomic analysis of longevity using excellent samples and state-of-the-art analysis was unable to unequivocally identify genes for this healthy aging phenotype.

Why did this GWAS fail to find associations with longevity? The authors suggest that heterogeneity in environmental exposures and gene-environment interactions may have obscured true genome-phenome associations. In this case, genomic analyses will falter until we find better ways to measure environmental exposures across the life span, or until we can define populations with greater homogeneity in environmental exposures. Alternatively, the authors suggest that still larger samples may be required to uncover associations that meet the very stringent levels of significance appropriate for GWAS. Finally, the authors raise questions about this phenotype of optimal aging. They suggest the use of more extreme survival phenotypes (survival to centenarian status) or evaluation of more specific phenotypes, such as disease-free survival. At this point the jury is out on the most appropriate phenotype for genomic studies of aging.

ANALYTIC CHALLENGES IN GENOMIC STUDIES OF AGING

Genome-wide research depends on three key developments. First, as mentioned earlier, the International HapMap Project created a public, genome-wide database of genotype and haplotype frequencies in different ethnic populations. This map allows researchers with DNA samples to scan hundreds of thousands of chromosomal SNPs to determine their association with clinical conditions and other traits of interest (Manolio and Collins, 2009). Second, advances in high-throughput array-based genotyping allow increasingly inexpensive and efficient genome-wide assessment of associations between SNPs and phenotypes of interest. Finally, refinements in statistical methodology have been critical for adequately assessing the thousands of potentially significant associations that invariably emerge in such studies.

Progress in the field is dizzying. In the pre-genomics era, research mostly focused on associations between clinical conditions and a small number of mutations in single genes. Most studies were negative, and positive associations proved difficult to replicate. Today, studies examine potentially millions of variations in DNA across the entire genome. A comparison between the field in 2002, when genome-wide studies were just beginning, and the field in 2010 is instructive. In 2002, examining a representative number of base-pair variations in a sample required months of laboratory work and hundreds of electrophoresis gels at a cost of over $500,000. In 2010, a single silicon chip can detect well over 1 million different base-pair variations in a person's genome in a few hours for a few hundred dollars (Feero, Guttmacher, and Collins, 2010). The result has been an increase in GWAS studies from a trickle to a flood (Visscher and Montgomery, 2009). In 2009, over 200 GWAS publications appeared (in a field that began in 2005, with the first such publication). Likewise, reports of genomic associations have correspondingly increased. GWAS studies went from reporting hardly any significant associations between SNPs and disease phenotypes (with genome-wide significance defined as $p < 10^{-7}$) to a mean of about 250 such associations per publication (Visscher and Montgomery, 2009). A total of about 1,000 genetic variants have been associated with human disease through GWAS.

Making sense of these associations is a central challenge. GWAS reveal significant SNP variants for virtually any disease investigated. But these SNPs are often in regions of the genome without known genes or instead are in genes without any obvious relationship to the biology of the disease or trait at issue. Moreover, effect sizes for SNPs are small; odds ratios associated with putative risk variants are typically less than 1.5 (median, 1.28) (Witte, 2010). Finally, SNPs identified in GWAS account for only a small part of the heritability, or genetic variation, in a condition (Maher, 2008). For example, the heritability of autism or schizophrenia, identified in twin studies, is estimated to be as high as 80%–90%. Yet the genes identified in GWAS together account for only a small proportion of this variance, leading to concern about missing heritability.

These limitations have dampened enthusiasm for the current approach to GWAS. Frustration with inconsistent findings has led some investigators to dismiss GWAS and seek instead sequencing of whole genomes rather than genotyping of SNPs. This is the goal of the 1000 Genomes Project of the National Human Genome Research Institute (NHGRI). By full sequencing of more than 1,000 unrelated individuals across the globe, the project will extend the HapMap to cover virtually all genetic variants, allowing more extensive genotyping studies (www.genome.gov). Other investigators have turned instead to assessment of copy-number variations (CNVs), or other differences in genetic architecture that do not alter SNP sequences (and hence do not appear in the HapMap) and yet be may be important for gene function. CNVs are stretches of DNA that are deleted or duplicated across individuals. These may be one source of the missing heritability evident in current GWAS, although the observation that more than 80% of common CNVs are well assayed by current SNP genotyping tools suggests otherwise (Barnes et al., 2008).

The absence of large genetic effects in GWAS may also genuinely reflect the polygenic nature of healthy aging and other complex phenotypes. Hundreds or perhaps thousands of rarer genetic variants may contribute to the risk of disease or presence of a trait. This scenario would imply a greater role for epigenetics (effect of gene environment on gene function) and likely lead to the reclassification of many diagnostic entities based on genetics, since multiple overlapping sets of genes likely underlie diseases or phenotypes we consider homogeneous.

KEY EFFORTS IN THE GENOMICS OF AGING

Aging has not been a predominant focus of GWAS. Apart from the study of longevity to age 90+, described above, we concentrate on a few key findings from collaborative efforts examining SNP-trait associations in aging. Some of the major efforts to date include STAMPEED: SNP Typing for Association with Multiple Phenotypes from Existing Epidemiologic Data (http://public .nhlbi.nih.gov/GeneticsGenomics/home/stampeed.aspx). This collaborative GWAS effort has identified genetic variants associated with blood pressure and hypertension, stroke, waist circumference, cardiac structure and function, glucose metabolism and diabetes, and heart failure. STAMPEED collects genomic information from participants in the CHARGE consortium, which includes four community-based prospective cohorts: the Atherosclerosis Risk in Communities Study, the Cardiovascular Health Study, the Framingham Heart Study, and the Rotterdam Study.

Another important effort is the Cancer Genetic Markers of Susceptibility (CGEMS). This initiative seeks to identify common, inherited gene mutations that increase the risks for breast and prostate cancer (http://cgems.cancer .gov). The CGEMS study uses cases and controls from a series of large epidemiological studies and clinical trials, including the Prostate, Lung, Colorectal, and Ovary (PLCO) study and NCI Breast and Prostate Cancer Cohort Consortium. This effort has resulted in identifying a number of associations between SNPs and risk of prostate, gastrointestinal, and breast cancer, as well as a study of genomic predictors of smoking (Caporaso et al., 2009).

The Genes, Environment, and Health Initiative (GEI) (http://gei.nih.gov/) involves both genomic analysis and exposure biology. The latter seeks to develop new tools for measuring environmental exposures. GEI was developed to examine the role of changes in environments, diets, and activity levels and the extent to which these may produce disease in genetically predisposed persons. It is thus a very good example of public health genomics applied to risk factors that may affect health across the life span.

Other efforts include the Genetic Association Information Network (GAIN; www.genome.gov/19518664), which has reported GWAS results for a variety of aging-related phenotypes, including psoriasis, depressive disorders, and diabetic nephropathy. The Welcome Trust Case Control Consortium (WTCCC, 2007) has conducted GWAS of seven major diseases: bipolar disorder, coronary artery disease, Crohn's disease, hypertension, rheumatoid arthritis, and diabetes (types 1 and 2). Affected individuals (totaling 14,000) were compared with controls drawn from the 1958 British Birth Cohort and UK National Blood Service. The deCODE/Icelandic Studies (Gulcher and Stefansson, 1998) group has collected phenotypic and genotypic information on over 40,000 residents of Iceland. One advantage of deCODE is access to national health system records of participants for diagnostic and treatment information. The cohort has been extremely useful for GWAS in establishing genomic associations for bone mineral density and age at menarche, among many other efforts. The Long-Life Family Study (https://dsgweb.wustl.edu/llfs/) has collected extensive aging-related phenotype data from over 5,000 members of more than 1,000 U.S. and Danish families with extreme longevity, in the hopes of using family-based SNP analyses to examine multiple aging phenotypes and to better define the components of aging under genetic control. The New England Centenarians Study (www.bumc.bu.edu/centenarian/), originally begun as an Alzheimer's study in 1994, is now collecting genetic data on individuals older than 100 years of age and their families (Sebastiani et al., 2010).

STUDY DESIGN CONSIDERATIONS FOR GENOMIC STUDIES OF AGING

As mentioned previously, the first challenge in identifying genotype-phenotype associations in aging is to establish a well-defined phenotype. The healthy or optimal aging phenotype would ideally involve more than simple longevity, allow standardization across studies, and be easily measurable. It should also have high heritability and a close relationship to gene products or known genetic pathways. At this point, GWAS have supplanted family-based linkage and candidate gene association studies, and soon GWAS will likely be supplanted by whole-genome sequencing and fine mapping.

Population-based (case-control) genome-wide studies offer many advantages over family-based studies. Once an association has been found, the segment of genomic DNA that needs to be investigated is much smaller in the case of unrelated individuals than in related family members (Manolio, 2007). Case-control genomic studies are also much easier to conduct, since registries of affected individuals and population-based controls are available, with banked blood. Finding families and constructing pedigrees is much more laborious. Nonetheless, family-based studies also offer several advantages over population-based studies, particularly when trying to identify appropriate phenotypes for study. Because families allow measurement of similar phenotypes in multiple generations, along with measurement of the segregation of those traits through generations, family-based studies facilitate identification of phenotypes that are most likely to be under genetic control. However, for aging studies the problem becomes that younger generations have not yet aged sufficiently to exhibit exceptional aging (i.e., they are not yet old enough to determine if they will exceed the average life expectancy of their age-cohort), so to properly study aging in a family-based design would require many years of follow-up.

GWAS usually rely on a multiple-stage approach. In a recent GWAS, genetic loci associated with Alzheimer's disease were identified in three stages and replicated in a fourth (Seshadri et al., 2010). By combining cohorts and multiple pooled data sources, researchers were able to identify four SNPs that were significantly associated with Alzheimer's disease. All cohorts used in the analysis relied on the same definition of dementia, and all cases met standard criteria used to define Alzheimer's. While this study design is somewhat unusual (taking advantage of the large number of studies that formed this mega-consortium), the use of the different cohorts helped to eliminate variance associated with differences in population structure and genotyping methodology. More commonly, only two stages are undertaken, a discovery stage (identifying SNPs associated with the phenotype) and a replication stage (in which significant SNPs from the discovery stage are examined in an independent cohort with a different genotyping platform).

Results from GWAS efforts are shown in a regional association plot, the so-called Manhattan plot, in which the significance level of different SNPs is plotted against their chromosomal position. Results are replicated with an independent cohort to determine whether effect sizes for significant SNPs are similar (for the Alzheimer's study mentioned above, the intent was to examine whether identified SNPs near the APOE locus were independently associated with Alzheimer's) and whether previously associated SNPs were confirmed. Finally, the investigators assessed the extent to which identified genes from the analysis improved prediction of Alzheimer's disease in incident cases beyond age, sex, and APOE status. Addition of these genetic markers increased prediction (as measured in receiver operator characteristic curves), but only marginally.

Here too an exemplary study using GWAS and state-of-the-art efforts to ensure quality and replication failed to produce clinically significant results. Why? The authors point to limited statistical power, phenotypic heterogeneity, and misclassification in controls (Seshadri et al., 2010). It is also possible that the genetic basis of Alzheimer's may depend on many rare genetic variants not easily identified by analysis of common SNPs (Maniolo, 2007). Finally, it is also possible that environmental factors may contribute to the absence of strong effects. Gene-environment interactions may obscure the detection of genetic associations. An important example of such an environmental effect is evident in the case of the hepatic lipase gene (LIPC) polymorphism and the effects of diet on plasma high-density lipoprotein cholesterol (HDL-C). The association between LIPC and HDL-C depends heavily on both LIPC genotype (TT, CT, CC) and the proportion of animal fat in daily diets (Ordovas et al., 2002). Without attention to the effect of diet, it is hard to see genotype-phenotype associations clearly. Many of the small and contradictory effects established in GWAS may require similar attention to environmental effects to establish accurate and reproducible genetic associations.

BEHAVIORAL AND ETHICAL QUESTIONS IN GENOMIC STUDIES OF AGING

Personal genomic tests provide comprehensive genetic risk information directly to consumers. Test results may include profiles for many diseases or other genetic information, such as ancestry. Major providers of personalized genomics testing include 23andMe, which provides individual genomic analysis of 156 disease and trait risks, as well as ancestry information, at a cost of $500; Navigenics, which provides testing for a similar number of disease and trait risks, but only provides information on confirmed associations (and also provides customers with access to genetic counselors), all for a slightly higher premium (approximately $800); and deCODEme, which provides a product similar to that of 23andMe at a similar cost. These personal genomic testing services process an individual's saliva, which is mailed to the company, and provide results on a secure website.

The main difference between the testing services lies primarily in how the genetic information (genotypes, ancestry information) is converted into risk profiles for the individual. These differences in fact lead to variation in estimated risks and have led some to question the accuracy of the information being provided (Ng, Murray, Levy, and Venter, 2009). 23andMe advertises its services this way: "With the advent of chip-based genome-wide association studies, the era of personalized genomics is finally here. It is now possible for individuals to obtain their own genotypes with the same technologies as those used in large association studies, then compare their genotypes to those discussed in the scientific literature" (www.23andme.com/for/scientists/). They also state that providing personalized genetic information may result in people taking more responsibility for their health and well-being and help educate the public about genetics.

A recent workshop sponsored by several NIH institutes along with the Centers for Disease Control and Prevention (CDC) examined the scientific basis for personal genomics testing (Khoury et al., 2009). The workshop sought to assess what genetic information from personal genomics testing adds to risk algorithms currently available for guiding patient decision making. It also addressed the potential for personal genomics testing to improve patient outcomes. Workshop participants noted that individual genomics testing could become part of the disease prevention–health promotion armamentarium in a variety of ways.

For *primary prevention*, testing for susceptibility to cancer or diabetes, for example, could be used to reduce disease risk by targeting interventions (such as lifestyle changes, e.g., cholesterol reduction or weight loss) long in advance of typical ages at onset. As *secondary prevention*, personal genomics testing could be used for earlier disease detection through targeted screening. Individuals with high susceptibility to prostate or colorectal cancer based on genetic risk factors, for example, could be targeted for earlier and more frequent testing. *Tertiary prevention* would involve personalized treatments based on genomic profiles. This form of prevention would likely be most valuable in light of pharmacogenomic findings. For example, GWAS have shown genetic differences in responsiveness to warfarin and SSRIs, and personal genomics testing may allow more rational use of therapies. Finally, *quaternary prevention* would allow use of genetic information to plan for care in the case of diseases without treatments, such as Alzheimer's disease. One could imagine families planning for disease management (by arranging long-term care or advanced directives, for example) based on results of personalized genomics information that would convey information about progression. This testing might also raise the index of suspicion for unclear symptoms, leading to earlier planning and adoption of caregiver roles in families.

These applications depend on reasonable clinical validity and utility for personalized testing. However, the NIH-CDC Workshop raised doubts about the clinical value of these tests. *Clinical validity* is defined by the strength of the association between the genetic variant and phenotype and the predictive value of this association, that is, what proportion of disease or health outcome can be attributed to the variant. The jury is still out on the credibility of genetic associations. One study found that only half the associations reported in personal genomic tests had been subjected to appropriate meta-analytic tests (Janssens et al., 2008). Workshop participants concluded that access to credible and rapidly updated genomic information is urgently needed (Khoury et al., 2009).

The HuGE Navigator (http://hugenavigator.net/) is a constantly updated database for citations on human genomics studies and will help in this regard (Yu, Gwinn, Clyne, Yesupria, and Khoury, 2008). Some of the initiatives included in the HuGE Navigator include (i) the Genotype Prevalence Catalog, which provides U.S. population prevalence for selected genetic variants genotyped in the National Health and Nutrition Examination Survey (NHANES); (ii) Genopedia and Phenopedia applications, which allow users to look up genetic associations and human genome epidemiology summaries by disease; and (iii) the GWAS Integrator, which allows data mining of all published GWAS.

Even if an association is supported in the literature, does this association separate people who are at risk from those who are not, and would knowledge of this association lead one to reclassify risk status? The small effect sizes identified in GWAS mean that identified genetic associations will contribute only marginally to prediction beyond other risk factors, such as family history. Also, to date reclassification of risk status based on genetic associations has proven difficult. One variant on chromosome 9p21.3 has been reliably associated with increased risk of cardiovascular disease (Paynter et al., 2009), but the effect of this variant is small and hence such information would lead to reclassification of a person's risk status only in the presence of other acknowledged risk factors. Only a small proportion of people may fall into this group.

Clinical utility is the net health benefit of a personal genomics test. Ideally, harms resulting from testing (such as psychological burden, loss of insurance) should be outweighed by the benefits of testing (such as targeting of treatment and reduction in risk of disease). Little research is available on whether personalized testing actually improves health outcomes. At this point, research suggests that such testing at least does not in itself do harm. In the Risk Evaluation and Education for Alzheimer's disease study, families opting for APOE testing on the whole did not report adverse psychological effects from testing (Green et al., 2009). However, results were communicated as part of a genetic counseling protocol, which is not the case for Web-based personalized genomic testing. Also, it is possible that people likely to have the most negative reactions self-select not to be screened.

Will knowledge of genetic risk profiles influence health practices among individuals and families? This is the subtitle of an important review of behavioral responses to personalized genetic information (McBride, Koehly, Sanderson, and Kaphingst, 2010). Personalized genetic information may have particularly potent health behavior effects. It is in some sense an undeniable risk factor, unlike many other risk indicators (such as family history). It also affects whole families, encouraging collective behavioral responses. People must understand the nature of these risks, which, as mentioned earlier, are not obvious. Evidence is mounting that genetic information may motivate behavior change. Also noted earlier, BRCA1/2 carriers are more likely to receive mammography than noncarriers 1 year post-testing (Watson, Foster, Eeles, Eccles, and Ashley, 2004), while results are equivocal for smoking and communication of genetic information involving susceptibility to lung cancer (Sanderson et al., 2008). Communication of APOE status led ε4 carriers to adopt diet, exercise, or nutritional supplements more frequently than people with standard risk factors (e.g., family history) (Chao et al., 2008).

To explore who is receptive to genetic assessment and what people do with such information, the NHGRI and National Cancer Institute teamed up with Group Health Cooperative in Seattle and Henry Ford Health System in Detroit to develop the Multiplex Initiative (www.multiplex.nih.gov/) (McBride et al., 2008). This study examined whether healthy, young adults would consent to genetic testing of 15 different genes for eight common conditions (type 2 diabetes, coronary heart disease, high blood cholesterol, high blood pressure, osteoporosis, lung cancer, colorectal cancer, and malignant melanoma). Results suggest that a key factor in determining whether people choose genetic assessment is the perception of the relative role of behavior and genes in disease risk. Those who think behavior is central to risk of disease appear to be more likely to have genetic tests. This suggests that health activism, which motivates people to practice healthy behaviors, apparently extends to genetic testing as well.

CONCLUSION: THE GENOMICS OF AGING AND INSIGHTS ON AGING

This brief review suggests that exemplary application of genomic methods has explained only a small fraction of the genetics of aging and has not shed as much light as hoped for in understanding mechanisms associated with optimal aging. Reasons for this low yield are unclear. It may be that rare variants or structural variation (such as copy-number repeats), not captured in current SNP genotyping technologies, are responsible for variation in the aging phenome. Or it may be that genetic associations will not become clear until we understand epigenetic or environmental factors better. Here genomic investigations and public health efforts clearly overlap. Better understanding of the presence and timing of behavioral exposures over the life span (including agent interactions with the physical, social, and built environment) may help clarify genetic influences on health in later life. Or it may be that the diseases of interest for aging are polygenic and we will need to identify many genes, each with small effect. Population genomics is still evolving and will no doubt evolve more sophisticated technologies and analytics.

In the meantime, genomic approaches have already changed the landscape of health decision making. People have begun to request personal genomic information, and a number of commercial providers have emerged to sell it. How such knowledge will change behavior or affect health outcomes remains unclear. We can expect new ethical and policy challenges with continuing evolution of genomic science.

REFERENCES

Barnes, C., V. Plagnol, T. Fitzgerald, R. Redon, J. Marchini, D. Clayton, and M. E. Hurles. 2008. A robust statistical method for case-control association testing with copy number variation. *Nature Genetics* 40:1245–52.

Burke, W., M. Khoury, A. Stewart, and R. Zimmern. 2006. The path from genome-based research to population health: Development of an international collaborative public health genetics initiative. *Genetics in Medicine* 8:451–58.

Caporaso, B., F. Gu., N. Chatterjee, J. Sheng-Chih, K. Yu., M. Yeager, C. Chen, K. Jacobs, W. Wheeler, M. Landi, R. Ziegler, D. Hunter, S. Chanock, S. Hankinson, P. Kraft, and A. Bergen. 2009. Genome-wide and candidate gene association study of cigarette smoking behaviors. *PLoS ONE* 4:e4653.

Chakravarti, A. 1999. Population genetics—making sense out of sequence. *Nature Genetics* 21:56–60.

Chao, S., J. S. Roberts, T. M. Marteau, R. Silliman, L. A. Cupples, and R. C. Green. 2008. Health behavior changes after genetic assessment for Alzheimer's disease: The REVEAL study. *Alzheimer Disease and Associated Disorders* 22:94–97.

Collins, F. S., E. D. Green, A. E. Guttmacher, and M. S. Guyer. 2003. A vision for the future of genomics research. *Nature* 422:835–47.

Feero, W. G., A. E. Guttmacher, and F. S. Collins. 2010. Genomic medicine—an updated primer. *New England Journal of Medicine* 362:2001–11.

Green, R. C., J. S. Roberts, L. A. Cupples, N. R. Relkin, P. J. Whitehouse, T. Brown, S. LaRusse-Eckert, M. Butson, A. D. Sandounick, K. Quaid, C. Chen, R. Cook-

Deegan, and L. A. Farrer. 2009. Disclosure of APOE genotype for risk of Alzheimer's disease. *New England Journal of Medicine* 361:245–54.

Gulcher, J., and K. Stefansson. 1998. Population genomics: Laying the groundwork for genetic disease modeling and targeting. *Clinical Chemistry and Laboratory Medicine* 36:523–27.

Janssens, A. C., M. Gwinn, L. A. Bradley, B. A. Oostra, C. M. Van Dujin, and M. J. Khoury. 2008. A critical appraisal of the scientific basis of commercial genomic profiles used to assess health risks and personalize health interventions. *American Journal of Human Genetics* 82:593–95.

Khoury, M. J., C. M. McBride, S. D. Schully, J. Ioannidis, W. G. Feero, C. Janssens, M. Gwinn, D. G. Simons-Morton, J. M. Bernhardt, M. Cargil, S. J. Chanock, G. M. Church, R. J. Coates, F. S. Collins, R. T. Croyle, B. R. Davis, G. J. Downing, A. Duross, S. Friedman, M. H. Gail, G. S. Ginsburg, R. C. Green, M. H. Greene, P. Greenland, J. R. Gulcher, A. Hsu, K. L. Hudson, S. L. Kardia, P. L. Kimmel, M. S. Lauer, A. M. Miller, K. Offit, D. F. Ransohoff, J. S. Roberts, R. S. Rasooly, K. Stefansson, S. F. Terry, S. M. Teutsch, A. Trepanier, K. L. Wanke, J. S. Witte, and J. Xu. 2009. Centers for Disease Control and Prevention. The scientific foundation for personal genomics: Recommendations from a National Institutes of Health-Centers for Disease Control and Prevention multidisciplinary workshop. *Genetics in Medicine* 11:559–67.

Maher, B. 2008. Personal genomes: The case of missing heritability. *Nature* 456:18–21.

Manolio, T. A. 2007. Study designs to enhance identification of genetic factors in healthy aging. *Nutrition Reviews* 65:S228–33.

Manolio, T. A., G. L. Burke, J. C. Murray, L. R. Cardon, S. J. Chanock, and R. L. Chisholm. In press. Research frontiers in population genomics.

Manolio, T. A., and F. S. Collins. 2009. The HapMap and genome-wide association studies in diagnosis and therapy. *Annual Review of Medicine* 60:443–56.

Mayeux, R., and N. Schupf. 1995. Apolipoprotein E and Alzheimer's disease: The implications of progress in molecular medicine. *American Journal of Public Health* 85:1280–84.

McBride, C. M., S. H. Alford, R. J. Reid, E. B. Larson, A. D. Baxevanis, and L. C. Brody. 2008. Putting science over supposition in the arena of personalized genomics. *Nature Genetics* 40:939–42.

McBride, C. M., G. Bepler, I. M. Lipkus, P. Lyna, G. Samsa, J. Albright, S. Datta, and B. K. Rimer. 2002. Incorporating genetic susceptibility feedback into a smoking cessation program for African-American smokers with low income. *Cancer Epidemiology, Biomarkers, and Prevention* 11:521–28.

McBride, C. M., L. M. Koehly, S. C. Sanderson, and K. A. Kaphingst. 2010. The behavioral response to personalized genetic information: Will genetic risk profiles motivate individuals and families to choose more healthful behaviors? *Annual Review of Public Health* 31:89–103.

Miller, R. A. 1999. Kleemeier Award lecture: Are there genes for aging? *Journal of Gerontology: Biological Sciences* 54A:B297–307.

Newman, A. B., S. Walter, K. L. Lunetta, M. E. Garcia, P. E. Slagboom, K. Christensen, A. M. Arnold, T. Aspelund, Y. S. Aulchenko, E. J. Benjamin, L. Christiansen, R. B. D'Agostino, Sr., A. L. Fitzpatrick, N. Franceschini, N. L. Glazer, B. Gudnason, A. Hofman, R. Kaplan, D. Karasik, M. Kelly-Hayes, D. P. Kiel, L. J. Launer, K. D. Marciante, J. M. Massaro, I. Miljkovic, M. A. Nalls, D. Hernandez, B. M. Psaty, F. Rivadeneira, J. Rotter, S. Seshadri, A. V. Smith, K. D. Taylor, H. Tiemeier., H-W. Uh, A. G. Uitterlinden, J. W. Vaupel, J. Walston, R. G. J. Westendorp, T. B. Harris, T. Lumley, C. M. van Duijn, and J. M. Murabito. 2010. A meta-analysis of four genome-wide association studies of survival to age 90 years or older: The Cohorts for Heart and Aging Research in Genomic Epidemiology Consortium. *Journal of Gerontology: Medical Sciences* 65A:478–87.

Ng, P. C., S. S. Murray, S. Levy, and J. C. Venter. 2009. An agenda for personalized medicine. *Nature* 461:724–26.

Ordovas, J. M., D. Corella, S. Demissie, L. A. Cupples, P. P. Couture, O. Coltell, P. W. Wilson, E. J. Schaefer, and K. L. Tucker. 2002. Dietary fat intake determines the effect of a common polymorphism in the hepatic lipase gene promoter on high-density lipoprotein metabolism: Evidence of a strong dose effect in this gene-nutrient interaction in the Framingham Study. *Circulation* 29:2315–21.

Paynter, N. P., D. I. Chasman, J. E. Buring, D. Shiffman, N. R. Cook, and P. M. Ridker. 2009. Cardiovascular disease risk prediction with and without knowledge of genetic variation at chromosome 9p21.3. *Annals of Internal Medicine* 150:65–72.

Reich, D. E., and E. S. Lander. 2001. On the allelic spectrum of human disease. *Trends in Genetics* 17:502–10.

Sanderson, S. C., S. F. Humphries, C. Hubbart, E. Hughes, M. J. Jarvis, and L. Wardle. 2008. Psychological and behavioral impact of genetic testing smokers for lung cancer: A phase II exploratory trial. *Journal of Health Psychology* 13:481–94.

Sebastiani, P., N. Solovieff, A. Puca, S. W. Hartley, E. Melista, S. Andersen, D. A. Dworkis, J. B. Wilk, R. H. Myers, M. H. Steinberg, M. Montano, C. T. Baldwin, and T. T. Perls. 2010. Genetic signatures of exceptional longevity in humans. *Science*, ePub ahead of print.

Seshadri, S., A. L. Fitzpatrick, M. A. Ikram, A. L. DeStefano, V. Gudnason, M. Boada, J. C. Bis, A. V. Smith, M. M. Carassquillo, J. C. Lambert, D. Harold, E. M. Schrijvers, R. Ramirez-Lorca, S. Debette., W. T. Longstreth, Jr., A. C. Janssens, V. S. Pankratz, J. F. Dartigues, P. Hollingworth, T. Aspelund, I. Hernandez, A. Beiser, L. H. Kuller, P. J. Koudstaal, D. W. Dickson, C. Tzourio, R. Abraham, C. Antunez, Y. Du, J. I. Rotter, Y. S. Aulchenko, T. B. Harris, R. C. Petersen, C. Berr, M. J. Owen, J. Lopez-Arrieta, B. N. Varadarajan, J. T. Becker, F. Rivadeneira, M. A. Nalls, N. R. Graff-Radford, D. Campion, S. Auerbach, K. Rice, A. Hofman, P. V. Jonsson, H. Schmidt, M. Lathrop, T. H. Mosley, R. Au, B. M. Psaty, A. G. Uitterlinden, L. A. Farrer, T. Lumley, A. Ruiz, J. Williams, P. Amouyel, S. G. Younkin, P. A. Wolf, L. J. Launer, O. L. Lopez, C. M. van Duijn, M. M. Breteler, CHARGE Consortium; GERAD1 Consortium; and EADI1 Consortium. 2010. Genome-wide analysis of genetic loci associated with Alzheimer's disease. *Journal of the American Medical Association* 303:1832–40.

Vigh, J., and Y. Suh. 2003. Functional genomics of ageing. *Mechanisms of Ageing and Development* 124:3–8.

Vigh, J., and Y. Suh. 2005. Genetics of longevity and aging. *Annual Review of Medicine* 56:193–212.

Visscher, P. M., and G. W. Montgomery 2009. Genome-wide association studies and human disease: From trickle to flood. *Journal of the American Medical Association* 302:2028–29.

Watson, M., C. Foster, R. Eeles, D. Eccles, and S. Ashley. 2004. Psychosocial impact of breast/ovarian (BRCA1/2) cancer-predictive genetic testing in a UK multicenter clinical cohort. *British Journal of Cancer* 91:1787–94.

Welcome Trust Case Control Consort (WTCCC). 2007. Genome-wide association study of 14000 cases of seven common diseases and 3000 shared controls. *Nature* 447:661–78.

Witte, J. S. 2010. Genome-wide association studies and beyond. *Annual Review of Public Health* 31:9–20.

Yu, W., M. Gwinn, M. Clyne, A. Yesupria, and M. J. Khoury. 2008. A navigator for human genome epidemiology. *Nature Genetics* 40:124–25.

CHAPTER 17

Global Perspectives on Public Health and Aging

Laurence G. Branch, PhD
Hongdao Meng, PhD

> Population aging may be seen as a human success story—
> the triumph of public health, medical advancements, and
> economic development over diseases and injuries that had
> limited human life expectancy for millennia.
>
> —*Kinsella and Phillips, 2005*

CONTEXT

Population aging is indeed a global phenomenon, as evidenced by the staggering growth in both the size of the world population as a whole and the share of older adults. During the twentieth century, the world population nearly quadrupled, growing from 1.65 billion to 6.12 billion (United Nations, 2009). Today, 10 years into the new millennium, the world is entering a period of rapid population aging. In more developed countries, the population aged 60 and over is increasing at an annual rate of 1.9%. As a result, the older adult population in developed countries is projected to increase by more than 50% from 264 million to 416 million between 2009 and 2050 (United Nations, 2009). In contrast, the trend in population aging among the developing countries is expected to exhibit an even sharper increase at an annual rate of 3%, with a growth of the older adult population from 475 million to 1.6 billion, or more than triple the current level (United Nations, 2009). This unbalanced trend in the global population aging is expected to present substantial challenges to medical, social, economic, and ethical aspects of improving population health across countries (McMorrow and Roeger, 2004).

Figure 17.1 presents the world population growth and projected growth to the year 2050, while table 17.1 provides populations of older adults (60 and older and 80 and older) for major areas and regions in the world. As can be seen in the figure, population increments have tapered since 1980–90, while the world population continues to increase through 2050. Table 17.1 shows that 1 in 10 (10.8%) of the world population was aged 60 and older in 2009, of whom over 100 million were age 80 or older. There is also a linear decline in the percent of the older population to total population as the regions/countries move from more developed to least developed.

Building upon the economic growth and major advancement in science and technology during the past century, the trend in global aging is driven by two related factors: declining fertility (defined as the birth rate of women of childbearing age [aged 15–44 years] and calculated by dividing the total number of births in a given year by the number of women aged 15–44 and multiplying by 1,000) and longer average life expectancies (defined as the mean number of additional years a person of a given age [typically at birth, but which can be calculated at any age] can expect to live) (United Nations, 2009). Ironically, both factors are directly or indirectly the result of unprecedented achievements in public health, medicine, and economic development (Kinsella, 2005). For example, life expectancy at birth in the United States has increased from 68.2 (65.6 years for males, 71.1 for females) in 1950 to 76.6 (73.9 for males, 79.5 for females) in 2000—a laudable accomplishment to add approximately 8 years to life expectancy over a 50–year span. In comparison, according to United Nations World Population Prospects 2008 Revision (United Nations, 2009), the average life expectancy at birth for the world as a whole is 67.2 years (65.0 years for males and 69.5 years for females). Therefore, in terms of life expectancy at birth, the world on average in 2010 is not that different from the United States in 1950. While the trend toward increasing life expectancy among more developed countries is likely to slow down, owing in part to the diminishing returns of spending in health care according to the U.S. National Institute on Aging (NIA, 2006), developing countries will face major challenges as their population aging coincides with early stages of economic growth. Lack of preparation, inadequate public health and public policy development, and understaffed and undertrained

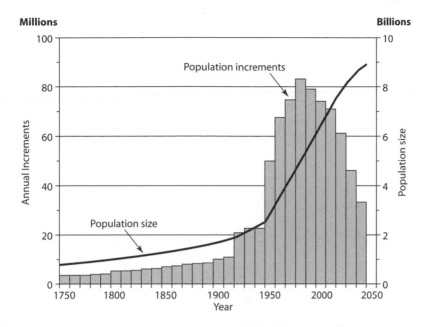

Fig. 17.1. Long-term world population growth, 1750-2050. *Source*: United Nations Population Division

medical care providers can have detrimental consequences in population health, as limited health care resources can easily be overwhelmed by the sustained increase in demand because more people are living longer with more chronic conditions.

Is it reasonable to anticipate that life expectancies around the world will follow a similar trajectory as experienced in the United States during the second half of the twentieth century? We will argue that there is no need for worldwide trajectories to be limited by the advances seen in the United States during the past 50 years. In our judgment, the potential exists for much more rapid gains in life expectancy around the world because of the increasing rate of diffusion in knowledge and technologies associated with information technology and globalization. However, the accelerating changes in life expectancy will likely require that countries with lower life expectancies understand and learn the lessons that other countries learned somewhat slowly and in some cases somewhat painfully in the second half of the twentieth century.

VARIATION AROUND THE WORLD

According to the most recent United Nations data (United Nations, 2009), Japan has the longest life expectancy at birth for females at 86.1 years, while

TABLE 17.1
Population (in thousands) aged 60 or over and 80 or over and percentages, 2009

Major areas and regions	60 or over					
	Total	%	Male	%	Female	%
World	737,275	10.8	335,464	9.7	401,811	11.9
More developed regions	263,905	21.4	112,205	18.7	151,700	23.9
Less developed regions	473,370	8.5	223,259	7.9	250,111	9.1
Least developed countries	42,922	5.1	19,769	4.7	23,153	5.5
Africa	53,770	5.3	24,639	4.9	29,131	5.8
Asia	399,881	9.7	189,301	9.0	210,580	10.5
Europe	158,503	21.6	65,372	18.5	93,131	24.5
Latin America and the Caribbean	57,039	9.8	25,737	8.9	31,301	10.6
North America	62,744	18.0	27,915	16.2	34,828	19.7
Oceania	5,338	15.1	2,499	14.1	2,839	16.0

Source: United Nations, 2009

Iceland has the longest life expectancy for men at 80.2 years (table 17.2). There are 15 countries in the world with overall life expectancy at birth of over 80 years. Notably absent among the 15 is the United States. From the Western Hemisphere, there are only two (Iceland and Canada); there are none from Central or South America, four from Asia, six from Europe, two from Oceania (Australia and New Zealand), one from the Middle East (Israel), and none from Africa. In total, 41 countries have life expectancies over 80 years for females; only one (Iceland), as noted earlier, has life expectancy over 80 years for males. There are 126 countries with overall life expectances above the world average; there are 68 countries below the world average. Countries with overall life expectancy below the world average include India, with its nearly 1.2 billion people, the second most populous country in the world; Haiti, with the lowest overall life expectancy in the Western Hemisphere; and Bolivia and Guyana in South America. At the same time, there are 44 countries with overall life expectancies of 60.0 years or less, and all but three (Afghanistan, Iraq, and Cambodia) are from Africa.

In summary, despite much progress in higher global life expectancy, disparities continue to exist across continents and between more developed and less developed countries. For example, the single most influential factor contributing to the low life expectancy in Africa is HIV/AIDS (Weinberger, 2007). In addition, general economic development and the specific diffusion of population health and medical care technologies among less developed

Major areas and regions	80 or over					
	Total	%	Male	%	Female	%
World	101,873	1.5	37,768	1.1	64,105	1.9
More developed regions	51,827	4.2	17,110	2.9	34,717	5.5
Less developed regions	50,046	0.9	20,658	0.7	29,388	1.1
Least developed countries	3,282	0.4	1,396	0.3	1,887	0.5
Africa	4,136	0.4	1,680	0.3	2,456	0.5
Asia	45,235	1.1	18,251	0.9	26,983	1.3
Europe	29,994	4.1	9,419	2.7	20,575	5.4
Latin America and the Caribbean	8,331	1.4	3,277	1.1	5,054	1.7
North America	13,179	3.8	4,758	2.8	8,420	4.8
Oceania	998	2.8	382	2.2	616	3.5

countries remain major challenges facing public health professionals around the world.

LIFE SPAN PUBLIC HEALTH PERSPECTIVE TO LIFE EXPECTANCY

If the United Nations considered a policy to increase life expectancy world-wide by 1% every 5 years, is this a feasible goal? Let's address the issue by applying a public health approach to the task of increasing life expectancy. The primary factor driving life expectancy, of course, is death. As noted earlier, the causes of death and age at death vary considerably by region and country. A public health perspective to improving life expectancy globally would not only take into account age and major causes of death but also address the conditions and factors contributing to mortality. From a practical perspective, the death of a 5–year-old will reduce the total number of person-years lived by the cohort more than the death of a 50–year-old would, while the death of a 75–year-old would add less to the total mean number of person-years lived by the cohort than the death of a 90–year-old. However, the causes of death and the contributing factors resulting in the cause of death would likely be significantly different among those aged 5, 50, 75, and 90 years and would present different public health strategies to increase life expectancy.

In the classic article by McKinlay and McKinlay (1959/2009), the authors

TABLE 17.2

The ten countries or areas with the highest and the lowest life expectancy at birth, 2005–10

Rank	Country or area	Life expectancy at birth (years)
Highest life expectancy at birth		
1	Japan	82.7
2	China, Hong Kong SAR	82.2
3	Switzerland	81.8
4	Iceland	81.8
5	Australia	81.5
6	France	81.2
7	Italy	81.2
8	Sweden	80.9
9	Spain	80.9
10	Israel	80.7
Lowest life expectancy at birth		
1	Afghanistan	43.8
2	Zimbabwe	44.1
3	Zambia	45.2
4	Lesotho	45.3
5	Swaziland	45.8
6	Angola	46.8
7	Central African Republic	46.9
8	Sierra Leone	47.4
9	Democratic Republic of the Congo	47.5
10	Guinea-Bissau	47.6

state that "the introduction of specific medical measures and/or the expansion of medical services are generally not responsible for most of the modern decline in mortality." They note a role for medical advancements and services but also pointed out that improved nutrition, air quality, better hygiene, and rise in real income are among the major contributors to the increased life expectancy in the past century. The public health perspective would focus on the predominant risk factors to poor health for acute and chronic conditions across the life span of the population and, working with the resources and limitations of the setting, provide strategies to minimize or eliminate these risk factors.

An important consideration in global aging is the change in the average life expectancy among older adults and the factors contributing to these increases. While it was noted that the average life expectancy increased considerably over the past 100 years, much of this increase among the industrialized countries in the earlier part of the century was driven by improvements in infant mortality and advances in maternal and child health. However, more recently, average life expectancy has improved among those aged 60 years and older. Public health and aging focuses on improvements in mortality (and morbidity) across the life span and the (mutable and non-mutable) risk factors contributing to them.

The public health perspective takes into account premature or preventable mortality. As an illustration, in the United States at the turn of the twentieth century, slightly more than 30% of mortality was attributable to a group of infectious diseases like pneumonias, influenza, tuberculosis, and diarrhea, but by the middle of the century those causes of mortality dropped to less than 6%. Logically the mortality attributable to those diseases at the beginning of the twentieth century was imminently preventable; they might not have been at that time, but they are preventable and therefore were causes of premature mortality. If one were to die before age 40 of one of those infectious diseases, that person did not become a candidate for mortality due to cardiovascular diseases and cancers, which typically occur in people aged 50 and over. But once those causes of infectious disease mortality were eradicated, the population became eligible for cardiovascular and cancer mortality, which reached a peak at about 60% of the mortality in 1980 in the United States. But the majority of cardiovascular and cancer mortality is also preventable, and its percentage of mortality in the United States is decreasing, so that by the end of the twentieth century they accounted for slightly more than half of the mortality (Mokdad, Marks, Stroup, and Gerberding, 2004). McLeroy and Crump (1994) provide a cogent discussion of these *epidemiologic transitions*, that is, the shifts accompanied by the decline in the birth rate and subsequent aging of the population. They discuss the transition from the first stage, which they call the "age of pestilence and famine," to the "age of declining pandemics," in which the major causes of death are due primarily to endemic infectious diseases (e.g., tuberculosis and pneumonia/influenza). They describe the third stage of the epidemiologic transition as the "age of degenerative and man-made diseases," which is characterized by a shift from infectious to chronic diseases as the primary influences on life expectancy. The major point is that public health and clinical medicine unite to reverse causes of preventable mortality, resulting in increasing life expectancies and changes in the mortality patterns (Crimmins, 2004; Parker and Thorslund, 2007).

When cardiovascular diseases were the single largest cause of death in the United States in the mid- to late 1970s, one of us (LGB) recalls that conventional clinical wisdom at the time was that systolic pressure should be 100 plus one's age. Clearly the conventional clinical wisdom was incorrect, and it was around that time that clinical norms began to change based on better understanding of optimal cardiovascular functioning. What occurred was both a change in clinical medical practice and a textbook example of mistaking normal aging for optimal aging. It was indeed true that systolic blood pressure for most people increased slowly but surely with advancing age during that era, but that process actually represented unrecognized hypertension, not optimal aging. A better understanding of optimal cardiovascular function led to more appropriate clinical guidelines, which in turn led to declines in cardiovascular mortality.

OPTIONS FOR GLOBAL AGING

Given a basic understanding of the calculation of life expectancy, and given the knowledge of how to prevent premature mortality from certain infectious diseases, from most forms of cardiovascular disease, and from most cancers, the options available to the nonindustrialized countries of the world are much clearer at the start of the twenty-first century than they were for the nations embarking on industrialization at the start of the twentieth century. Many would agree that the most significant activity a nonindustrialized country could do to increase its overall life expectancy would be to minimize its infant and child mortality rates. The mortality rates during the first year of life (usually called "infant mortality" and presented as the number of deaths per 1,000 live births) and mortality rates among those under 5 years of age (also presented as the number of deaths per 1,000 live births) among those countries with the lowest overall rates could be assumed to be an appropriate target for the nonindustrialized countries. The five countries with the lowest infant mortality have rates between 2.9 and 3.3; the five countries with the lowest child mortality rates have rates between 3.9 and 4.4 (United Nations, 2010). Over 40% of the countries in the world have infant mortality rates more than 10 times higher than the rate of the country with the lowest rate (more than 29.0 per 1,000 compared with 2.9 per 1,000). Similarly, there was a nearly identical pattern for child mortality: over 40% of the countries have child mortality rates more than 10 times the country with the lowest rate (more than 39.0 per 1,000 compared with 3.9 per 1,000). The most common causes of infant mortality are pneumonia and dehydration typically secondary to diarrhea. If improvement on overall life expectancy is a goal in countries with low life expectancy, they should focus on causes of infant and child mortality rather than older populations. Depending on the health risks (e.g., infectious diseases), individuals of all ages would benefit from public health interventions.

The next area of focus for nonindustrialized countries would be to prevent the premature mortality that strikes so many in their fifties to eighties in the form of cardiovascular diseases and cancers. Again, McLeroy and Crump (1994) would label this the age of degenerative and man-made diseases. The diets and physical activities that many people describe as normal in some nonindustrialized countries are considered by some to be superior from the perspective of health promotion and disease prevention to the diets and exercise regimens one finds in many industrialized countries. Walking is an example of this. While destination walking is part of normal daily activities for many people in nonindustrialized countries, the transition to automobiles and mass transit in industrialized countries minimizes destination walking. For example, while walking for exercise is the most common form of physical activity among older adults in the United States (Rafferty, Reeves, McGee, and Pivarnik, 2002), less than 25% of those who walk for leisure activity meet current recommended levels of activity (Eyler, Brownson, Bacak, and Housemann, 2003). While acknowledging that malnutrition and protein deficiencies can be serious problems in many nonindustrialized countries, remediating that dietary problem does not have to include the overconsumption of fats that characterize too much of the diet in some industrialized countries. Unfortunately, as industrialization increases the standard of living in the developing countries, some societies appear to suffer from the same pattern of overconsumption of food and reduced energy expenditures that the United States experienced. In the United States from 1991 to 2000, the prevalence of overweight and obesity has increased from 9.6% and 0.6%, respectively, to 20% and 3.0% (Wildman et al., 2008). The increase was evident across regions, in both urban and rural settings, and for all age groups. Therefore, public health and public policy interventions are urgently needed to reverse the tremendous disease burden associated with overweight and obesity across all age groups of the population. Choices can be made based on public health evidence. Sedentary lifestyles and high-fat diets are not necessary consequences of rising standards of living. For the most part, the countries that succeeded in industrialization in the twentieth century did not have the health information that countries embarking on industrialization in the twenty-first century have. Appropriate public health education should enable countries entering industrialization during the twenty-first century to avoid some of the health consequences that accompanied industrialization in the twentieth century.

WORLD HEALTH ORGANIZATION INITIATIVES IN GLOBAL AGING

The international community has recognized the importance of a collaborative approach in addressing these challenges of global aging in the twenty-first century. International organizations have spearheaded efforts to build consensus and develop practical actionable plans for adoption by its members. For example, the Second World Assembly on Ageing adopted the Madrid Political Declaration and International Plan of Action on Ageing in Madrid, Spain, in 2002 (United Nations, 2002).

The World Health Organization (WHO) has contributed to the Plan of Action by developing a policy framework, which defines active aging as "the process of optimizing opportunities for health, participation and security in order to enhance quality of life as people age" (WHO, 2002, p. 12). The policy framework reviewed evidence regarding the determinants of health (personal, social, economic, and environmental factors) throughout the life course and has helped to shape aging research and policies at national, regional, and community levels.

RETIREMENT AGE

An issue likely to receive renewed discussion around the world is the age at which a person is eligible for lifelong pension and how global aging will influence labor and create economic challenges (Börsch-Supan, 2004). German chancellor Otto von Bismarck, who presided over the world's first successful implementation of industrialization, faced the dilemma of how to bring younger workers into the labor force (Hufner, 2003). His planners proposed to furlough older workers to allow younger workers to have their places in the labor market. Chancellor von Bismarck implemented the idea and thereby introduced Germany's first social security system in 1889—and the world's first old-age social security program. Historians report that the retirement age was initially set at 70 in Germany, when the average life expectancy at birth was only 35.6 years for males and 38.4 for females (it was not until 1916 that the retirement age was reduced to 65). Clearly, under the first implementation of a social security program in Germany, pensioners were not expected to be collecting their pensions for 15 (male) to 20 (female) years, as they do in 2005.

The United States enacted its Social Security system in 1935, selecting 65 as the retirement age. At that time those aged 65 could expect to live another 13 to 15 years. However, only about 1 in 2 (54%) males and 3 of 5 females

(61%) survived from age 21 to age 65 at that time (Social Security Online, 2010). One implication is that nearly twice as many workers were expected to begin paying into the U.S. Social Security system than were expected to receive pensions from it. But over time the mortality patterns in the United States—as well as mortality patterns around the world—have changed. Now 3 out of 4 male workers and 4 out of 5 female workers who begin to pay into the U.S. Social Security system at age 21 will survive to collect benefits, and their additional life expectancies will be approximately 16 and 20 years, respectively. In addition, when a country's social security system is a "pay-as-you-go" program, which means that today's workers are paying for the benefits of today's beneficiaries, the ratio of the total number of workers paying into the social security system to the total number of retirees receiving benefits is also a critical component to the viability of the system. In the United States, for example, there were 42 workers per retiree in 1940. In 1950, the ratio was 16 to 1. Currently there are slightly more than three workers per retiree, and within 40 years there may be just two workers per retiree. As the population ages and life expectancies continue to rise, many social security systems will not be able to sustain themselves without major reform. Suffice it to say that the declining fertility rates in the last half of the twentieth century in many of the industrialized countries create an additional challenge.

At the same time that these mortality patterns were changing to produce more pensioners surviving to claim their pensions, and surviving for more years once starting their pensions, the social security systems around most of the world lowered the age of eligibility for pensions. Whereas von Bismarck began with age 70 and the United States started with age 65, most of the industrialized world, including most of Europe and most of South and Central America, now use age 60 as the retirement age for pension purposes. Even Germany uses age 60. Since 2003, the United States has embarked on a plan to raise the retirement age from 65 to 67 years, but most of the industrialized world has not followed suit. But the public policy question and the economic policy questions continue—can the current industrialized countries continue to afford their retirement and public pension systems that begin at age 60, when additional life expectancy can approach 20 to 25 years? As this book is going to press, France has raised its minimum retirement age from 60 to 62 years and its full pension benefit age from 65 to 67 years in an attempt to address erosion of the pension fund as a result of population aging (Associated Press in Paris, 2010). There have been demonstrations in France over this action, and there are discussions of similar actions in other European countries.

ACTIVE LIFE EXPECTANCY

Rather than focusing simply on the remaining years of life, we should redirect our metrics to estimating the years of independence and vigor, the years of active life expectancy (Katz et al., 1983) or disability-free life expectancy (REVES, 2010). The goal is not to extend the number of years an older person is frail and dependent on others for basic activities of daily living, but rather to extend the number of years that an older person is robust and independent. Although there is no consensus, most researchers agree that mortality continues to decline in the United States, and some indicators of active life expectancy show trends of improvement (Crimmins, 2004), while some other trends suggest increases in chronic disease and functional impairments (Parker and Thorslund, 2007).

Some countries around the world are working on this goal of increasing active life expectancy already. Globalization implies learning from one another. Some countries will find innovative approaches that expand active life expectancies that other countries can emulate; other countries will try programs to expand active life expectancy that will not be successful and can offer a lesson in mistakes to be avoided—just as the sedentary lifestyle, high-fat diets, smoking, and alcohol misuse were correlates of rising standards of living that also should be avoided.

Both industrialized and industrializing countries need to invest in public health statistical infrastructures that can reliably and validly monitor rates such as those of active life expectancy, various types of disabilities, and specific mortalities. They must also be capable of addressing the plethora of population statistical data that monitor population health, population health care costs, and population health care utilization. Without accurate health statistics, there is no ability to diagnose current problems, no ability to assess the success or failure of interventions, and no foundation for effective public health policies.

The impending global aging phenomenon is likely to have major implications for public health worldwide in areas such as disability, nutrition, physical activity, health education, and health promotion. First, more investment should be allocated to developing and promoting policy interventions aimed at curbing the epidemic of chronic diseases. In addition, continued development and promotion of age-friendly environments are essential to enable the maintenance of active aging around the world (WHO, 2006).

Finally, the complexity of chronic disease etiology and its interaction with social and cultural factors suggest that any public health solution needs to be multifaceted. For example, the WHO defines community health promotion as the process of enabling people to increase control over, and to improve, their health (WHO, 2009). Health promotion and prevention interventions can be implemented at various stages in the life course. Previous research reported that 80% of coronary heart disease, 90% of type 2 diabetes, and 33% of cancers can be avoided through behavioral changes such as healthy eating, exercise, and weight control throughout life (Darnton-Hill, Nishida, and James, 2004). Therefore, the extent to which developing countries can learn from the mistakes of the developed countries in preventing risk behavior–induced chronic diseases (e.g., heart disease, diabetes, and obesity) would have major implications for reducing the growth in total health care expenditures, population health, and demand for long-term care. In light of the importance of a systematic approach in designing public policy interventions to address the challenges posed by global aging, synthesizing evidence in disease prevention and health promotion from a life course perspective has the potential to contribute to a better understanding of the intersection between global aging and epidemiologic transitions (Binstock and George, 2011).

GLOBAL AGING INITIATIVE: A CASE STUDY

The following case study outlines a community-based framework for public health and aging in the Caribbean region and exemplifies strategies to address global aging from a public health perspective. Entitled *Pillars for the Care of Older Persons in the Caribbean: A Comprehensive Community-Based Framework*, it represents a joint effort among community organizations, academia, and professional organizations. It illustrates a state-of-the-art conceptual and development framework for dealing with global aging in a public health context (Partnership, 2010). It uses an evidence-based approach aimed at assisting the public and private sectors in determining polices and strategies necessary to address the rapid growth in the older adult population. The following four pillars represent a collection of potential programs and services delivered primarily in community settings that address the needs of older persons and their families across a continuum of care. The underlying premise of these four pillars is that current health care systems around the world are largely geared toward acute care and have become ineffective in promoting healthy living in the context of the chronic disease epidemic and population aging. The rapid growth in the number of elderly requiring primary care services has exacerbated the limitations of the current focus on diagnosis and treatment of acute symptoms and conditions instead of prevention and early detections. Some countries have realized that health care needs to try something other than the current expensive and clinically based treatment-centered practice, and a more prevention-focused framework with an emphasis on primary care to provide more cost-effective care with practice-based incentives and priorities is the option of choice. The hope is that through a shift to community-oriented services, health care systems can more effectively prevent and delay disability and illness.

Four Pillars Proposed by the Caribbean Community Partnership

Primary Care with Case Management

All persons should be assigned a primary care provider (primary care physician, nurse practitioner, clinics, etc.) so that their primary care (including preventive care) needs can be met, their specialty care needs can be coordinated, and their access to relevant information can be facilitated. The emerging Patient-Centered Medical Home (PCMH) model in the United States is such an example (Rittenhouse and Shortell, 2009).

Integrated Services Coordination

As a result of the increasing heterogeneity of health status and health care needs in older age, a wide range of medical and social services are needed to support community living for older adults. Service coordination and integration is a critically important approach to address the fragmentation of service provisions. Therefore, new systems of service delivery based on evidence-based practices should be developed and tested so that access to less restrictive settings (home- and community-based care) can be improved.

Population-Based Health Promotion

Health promotion is one area of public health and aging that has extensive research supporting the lifestyle risk factors influencing the health of older adults as well as behavioral interventions to improve their health. Lifestyle behavioral risk factors such as proper diet and nutrition and regular physical activity are desirable outcomes but are seldom achieved. Population-based health promotion should be integrated into day-to-day operations of the society across all settings (school, work, and faith).

Planning and Accountability

A moral, ethical, and legal commitment must be made to create an environment in which older adults can engage as members of the society. It is arguably the most important yet most understudied area. Fundamentally, the active process of community engagement, surveillance, monitoring, remediation, and policy development relies on accountability. Should the individuals, their families, health care providers, employers, and urban planners be held responsible for the health of the members of the society?

Community Partnership Consensus Recommendations for Policy Development
More Government Involvement

In order to ensure successful planning and accountability activities, the public sector (various levels of government) must be involved from the beginning of the process. For example, an indoor tobacco smoking ban was instituted in many U.S. states and cities by state and local governments and has been associated with reduced consumption and improved health outcomes (Darnton-Hill et al., 2004). This positive development in tobacco control should be adapted for obesity prevention policy. For example, the New York City Board of Health voted in 2006 to adopt the first major municipal ban in the United States of the use of all but tiny amounts of artificial trans fats in restaurant cooking (Lueck and Severson, 2006). By banning or increasing taxes on unhealthy foods, governments might positively influence obesity rates (Angell et al., 2009). Furthermore, local governments might improve the population health through the creation and maintenance of healthy living environments, such as parks and playgrounds, to promote physical activity and exercise, and they can ensure that their communities are safe and accessible.

More Team-Based Primary Care

The goal of a care management approach is to optimize self-care; decrease system and service fragmentation through improved continuity; improve costs, quality of life, and satisfaction; and decrease hospital care and negative health outcomes. A team approach to geriatric primary care with case management often starts with geriatric evaluations that can reduce hospital admission rates and improve functional abilities and survival. Teams typically consist of nurses, primary care physicians, social workers, therapists, and other important medical professionals. Teams can provide continuous and anticipatory care to ensure comprehensive treatment and access to a wide range of services to meet diverse needs.

Care managers serve an important role in many health care provider teams. Care managers can act as a liaison to link patients and health professionals with various services and areas of health care; provide patient education, screening, and needs assessment; and monitor health and outcomes. A community-based geriatric team approach (consisting of a general practitioner, geriatrician, social workers, nurses, and case managers) in the United Kingdom showed less decline in mental health and better cost outcomes compared with controls (Bernabei et al., 1998). Nurses are well suited to the role of care manager because they have proficient clinical backgrounds and education in health care and knowledge of a spectrum of services to link patients with various services. Geriatric nurse specialists work with geriatric physicians and social workers to cover a broad range of needs and services. However, the number of geriatric nurses does not meet the growing need in most geographic areas, and therefore perhaps adult and family practice nurse practitioners can receive additional training for work with older patients.

One model of integrated service coordination that has achieved some success in the United States is the Chronic Care Model (CCM), an integrated and multifaceted approach to the treatment of older adults, many of whom have at least one chronic condition, through which educated patients are empowered to control their health and a multidisciplinary team of health workers and professionals provides continuous, high-quality health care (Barr et al., 2003). The CCM shifts medical care away from acute illness treatment to prevention-based care. The role of nonphysician staff is to allow physicians to see and treat more patients while providing integrated quality care. The roles and tasks of team members are defined, and cultural sensitivity and patient-centered care are important to quality outcomes. Successful chronic disease management programs often focus on increasing patient knowledge, skills, and confidence in maintaining their conditions. The case for population-based health promotion stems from the recognition that a person's health is affected by the cumulative influences of one's behavioral choices, surrounding environment, and genetic factors. These factors can cause molecular, cellular, and organ damage throughout the life course, which disrupts the body's ability to regulate and function and causes physical decline and illness. Lifestyle choices made throughout life usually do not impact a person's well-being or significantly influence their health until later in life. In the country of Barbados, a recent study indicated that poor social conditions, a lack of education in childhood, and low-income levels were correlated with lower self-reported health throughout life (Cloos et al., 2010). Importantly, declining health status is generally reversible at any age, with the most benefits seen through adopting positive health behaviors earlier in life (Stanner, 2009). Some research suggests that access to health care throughout a person's life positively affects health and mortality, while a lack of health care can negatively impact a person's psychological and functional abilities in adulthood (Gu, Zhang, and Zeng, 2009). It is therefore important for people of all ages to have adequate access to health care services throughout their life span to ensure optimal health and aging.

More Emphasis on Disease Prevention and Health Promotion

The Declaration of Port of Spain noted the importance of disease prevention and health promotion throughout the life course through specific health care interventions targeting behaviors such as smoking, healthy eating, and exercise (Samuels, 2010). This declaration initiated one of the few community health promotion strategies targeting people throughout the life span in the Caribbean. Subsequent initiatives focused on preventing and delaying onset of disease, particularly chronic non-communicable diseases (CNCDs) in the elderly. The Healthy Caribbean Coalition, which supported the efforts of the Port of Spain Non Communicable Disease Summit Declaration, has documented such recent interventions. Several Caribbean countries, namely, Guyana, Suriname, Jamaica, Dominica, Saint Kitts/Nevis, Trinidad and Tobago, and SVG, have established taxes on tobacco products, but fewer countries, including Suriname, the Dominican Republic, and Trinidad, have formal policies regarding tobacco consumption (Haniff, 2009; Samuels, 2010). Ministers of health are advocating for legislation to reduce smoking and thereby prevent smoking-related diseases among people of all ages in the Caribbean (Haniff, 2009). Additionally, the Healthy Caribbean Coalition outlines goals for physical activity and healthy eating to reduce diseases, particularly CNCDs, and improve health in Caribbean elderly (Samuels, 2010). Population-based health promotion has achieved successes in increasing physical activities among older adults, changing dietary patterns to improve bone health and reduce the risk of diabetes, increasing compliance with vaccination programs to reduce annual infectious diseases among older people, and a variety of other applications.

More Emphasis on Public Health Statistics

If any country is to know if the health status of its aging population is improving or deteriorating, it must have reliable and valid indications of health status, health care utilization, and health care costs at both the population and individual levels. Establishing goals requires the ability to measure progress toward them. WHO provides excellent support to developing countries in how to establish appropriate population health status measurement systems.

CONCLUSION

The first half of the twenty-first century will be an interesting time. Countries that rapidly increase their economic growth and development during that time frame will have the opportunity to reflect on the public health correlates and consequences of the countries that underwent economic growth and development before them. Some of the circumstances that most of the first-generation developed countries experienced were a sedentary lifestyle, obesity, diabetes, and physical disability. These circumstances are avoidable. Creative alternatives to minimize these circumstances have been proposed and are being tested. The future is malleable.

REFERENCES

Angell, S. Y., L. Silver, G. Goldstein, C. Johnson, D. Deitcher, T. Frieden, and M. Bassett. 2009. Cholesterol control beyond the clinic: New York City's trans fat restriction. *Annals of Internal Medicine* 151:129–34.

Associated Press in Paris. 2010. French retirement age change to 62 becomes law. Retrieved December 23, 2010, from www.guardian.co.uk/world/2010/nov/10/french-retirement-age-reform-62.

Barr, V. J., S. Robinson, B. Marin-Link, L. Underhill, A. Dotts, D. Ravensdale, and S. Salivaras. 2003. The expanded Chronic Care Model: An integration of concepts and strategies from population health promotion and the Chronic Care Model. *Hospital Quarterly* 7:73–82.

Bernabei, R., F. Landi, G. Gambassi, A. Sgadari, G. Zuccala, V. Mor, L. Z. Rubenstein, and P. Carbonin. 1998. Randomised trial of impact of model of integrated care and case management for older people living in the community. *British Medical Journal* 316:1348–51.

Binstock, R. H., and L. K. George, eds. 2011. *Handbook of Aging and the Social Sciences*, 7th ed. San Diego: Academic Press.

Börsch-Supan, A. 2004. *Global Aging: Issue, Answers, More Questions*. Ann Arbor: University of Michigan, Retirement Research Center.

Cloos, P., C. F. Allen, B. E. Alvarados, M. V. Zunzunegui, D. T. Simeon, and D. Eldemire-Shearer. 2010. "Active ageing": A qualitative study in six Caribbean countries. *Ageing & Society* 30:79–101.

Crimmins, E. 2004.Trends in the health of the elderly. *Annual Review of Public Health* 25:78–98.

Darnton-Hill, I., C. Nishida, and W. P. James. 2004. A life course approach to diet, nutrition and the prevention of chronic diseases. *Public Health Nutrition* 7:101–21.

Eyler, A., R. Brownson, S. Bacak, and R. A. Housemann. 2003. The epidemiology of walking for physical activity in the United States. *Medicine and Science in Sports and Exercise* 35:1529–36.

Gu, D., Z. Zhang, and Y. Zeng. 2009. Access to healthcare services makes a difference in healthy longevity among older Chinese adults. *Social Science & Medicine* 68:210–19.

Haniff, F. 2009. Dr. Ramsammy aspires to introduce tobacco legislation. *Kaiteur News Online.* Retrieved October 28, 2010, from www.kaieteurnewsonline. com/2009/12/06/dr-ramsammy-aspires-to-introduce-tobacco-legislation.

Hufner, M. 2003. What would Bismarck have done? *Globalist,* December 2. Retrieved October 25, 2010, from www.theglobalist.com/StoryId.aspx?StoryId=3615.

Katz, S., L. G. Branch, M. H. Branson, J. A. Papsidero, J. C. Beck, and D. S. Greer. 1983. Active life expectancy. *New England Journal of Medicine* 309:1218–24.

Kinsella, K. G. 2005. Future longevity—demographic concerns and consequences. *Journal of the American Geriatrics Society* 53:S299–303.

Kinsella, K. G., and D. R. Phillips. 2005. Global aging: The challenge of success. *Population Reference Bureau* 60:1–42.

Lueck, T. J., and K. Severson. 2006. New York bans most trans fats in restaurants. Retrieved December 23, 2010, from www.nytimes.com/2006/12/06/nyregion/06fat .html?_r=1.

McKinlay, J., and S. McKinlay. 2009. Medical measures and the decline of mortality. In *The Sociology of Health and Illness: Critical Perspectives,* 8th ed., ed. P. Conrad, pp. 7–19. New York: Worth. (Original work published 1959)

McLeroy, K., and C. Crump. 1994. Health promotion and disease prevention: A historical perspective. *Generations* 18:9–17.

McMorrow, K., and W. Roeger. 2004. *The Economic and Financial Market Consequences of Global Ageing.* New York: Springer.

Mokdad, A., J. Marks, D. Stroup, and J. Gerberding. 2004. Actual causes of death in the United States, 2000. *Journal of the American Medical Association* 291:1238–45.

National Institute on Aging (NIA). 2006. The future of human life expectancy: Have we reached the ceiling or is the sky the limit? *Research Highlights in the Demography and Economics of Aging* 8:1–4.

Parker, M., and M. Thorslund. 2007. Health trends in the elderly population: Getting better or getting worse? *Gerontologist* 47:150–58.

Partnership of the Duke University School of Nursing Office of Global and Community Health Initiatives, the Pan American Health Organization Office of Caribbean Program Coordination, the Regional Nursing Body of CARICOM, and the University of the West Indies. 2010. *Pillars for the Care of Older Persons in the Caribbean: A Comprehensive Community-Based Framework.* Retrieved December 29, 2010, from www.google.com/search?ie=UTF-8&oe=UTF-8&sourceid=navcli ent&gfns=1&q=Pillars+for+the+Care+of+Older+Persons+in+the+Caribbean% 3A+A+Comprehensive+Community-Based+Framework.

Rafferty, A., M. Reeves, H. McGee, and J. Pivarnik. 2002. Physical activity patterns among walkers and compliance with public health recommendations. *Medicine and Science in Sports and Exercise* 334:1255–61.

REVES. 2010. Retrieved October 28, 2010, from http://reves.site.ined.fr.

Rittenhouse, D. R., and S. M. Shortell. 2009. The patient-centered medical home: Will it stand the test of health reform? *Journal of the American Medical Association* 301:2038–40.

Samuels, A. 2010. Chronic Diseases and Non Communicable Diseases in the Caribbean Community (CARICOM), at the Chronic Disease Research Centers Meeting, Barbados. 2010, University of the West Indies, Cave Hill.

Social Security Online. 2010. *Historical Background and Development of Social Security*. Retrieved August 30, 2010, from www.socialsecurity.gov/history/briefhistory3 .html/.

Stanner, S. 2009. Diet and lifestyle measures to protect the ageing heart. *British Journal of Community Nursing* 14(5):210–12.

United Nations. 2002. *Report of the Second World Assembly on Ageing*. Working Paper No. E.02.IV.4. New York: Author.

United Nations, Department of Economic and Social Affairs, Population Division. 2009. *World Population Prospects: The 2008 Revision, Highlights*. Working Paper No. ESA/P/WP.210. New York: Author.

United Nations. 2010. Population and Vital Statistics Report. *Statistical Papers*, ser. A, vol. 62, no. 2, New York. Retrieved December 29, 2010, from http://unstats .un.org/unsd/demographic/products/vitstats/Sets/SeriesA_July2010_complete.pdf.

Weinberger, M. B. 2007. Population aging: A global overview. In *Global Health & Global Aging*, ed. M. Robinson, W. Novelli, C. Pearson, and L. Norris, pp. 15–30. San Francisco: Jossey-Bass.

Wildman, R. P., P. Muntner, L. Reynolds, A. P. McGinn, S. Rajpathak, J. Wylie-Rosett, J., and M. R. Sowers. 2008. The obese without cardiometabolic risk factor clustering and the normal weight with cardiometabolic risk factor clustering: Prevalence and correlates of 2 phenotypes among the US population (NHANES 1999–2004). *Archives of Internal Medicine* 168:1617–24.

World Health Organization (WHO). 2002. *Active Ageing: A Policy Framework*, WHO/ NMH/NPH/02.8. Geneva, Switzerland: Author.

World Health Organization (WHO). 2006. *The World Health Report 2006—Working Together for Health*. Geneva, Switzerland: World Health Organization.

World Health Organization (WHO). 2009. *Milestones in Health Promotion: Statements from Global Conferences*. Geneva, Switzerland: World Health Organization.

CHAPTER 18

Resource Allocation in an Aging U.S. Society

Robert H. Binstock, PhD

The previous chapters in this book delineate a great many public health challenges posed by the aging of U.S. society. Prominent among them, explicitly and implicitly, is the need to increase financial resources for efforts to improve the health of the older population. Although chapter 3 makes clear that public resources devoted to the health and health care of older Americans are very substantial—including Medicare's national health insurance for most persons aged 65 and older—those resources still don't meet important contemporary health-related needs of older people. And chapter 2, emphasizing the rapid pace at which the United States will be transformed into an aging society in the years ahead, delineates a broad range of additional life course public health interventions needed for the health and health care of people aged 65 and older.

This chapter focuses on whether the public resources to effectively improve the quantity and quality of health-related ameliorative interventions for the older population will be sufficient in the near to longer term. It begins by providing a brief historical context of how the United States constructed an old-age welfare state despite a predominant ideology that emphasizes individualism over collectivism. Next, it delineates several contemporary pressures for cutting back on resources for old-age benefit programs. Then it presents an account of rhetoric calling for cutbacks in health care resources for older people and the emergence of public and private sector measures to do so. Finally, it examines how both the politics of aging and the politics of framing issues might maintain and possibly enhance resources needed for a healthy older population, despite the pressures to reduce those resources.

AMERICAN POLITICAL IDEOLOGY AND THE RISE OF THE OLD-AGE WELFARE STATE
Classical Liberalism

In sorting out different ideological approaches to issues of social risk—such as illness, unemployment, and poverty—Danish sociologist Gøsta Esping-Andersen has singled out the United States as the closest nation-state embodiment of *Homo liberalismus*, whose ideal is to pursue his personal welfare: "The well-being of others is their affair, not his. . . . His ethics tell him that a free lunch is amoral, that collectivism jeopardizes freedom, that individual liberty is a fragile good, easily sabotaged by sinister socialists or paternalistic institutions. Homo liberalismus prefers a welfare regime where those who can play the market do so, whereas those who cannot must merit charity" (Esping-Andersen, 1999, p. 171).

Most students of American political life would agree with Esping-Andersen's characterization of the predominant political ideology in the United States. Indeed, in his classic and influential treatise *The Liberal Tradition in America*, political theorist Louis Hartz (1955) argued that historically U.S. political ideas, institutions, and behavior have uniquely reflected a virtually unanimous acceptance of the tenets of the English political philosopher John Locke, whose ideas were in harmony with the laissez-faire economics subsequently propounded by Scotsman Adam Smith (1776/2003). In Lockean liberalism the individual is much more important than the collective, and one of the few important functions of a limited state is to ensure that the wealth that individuals accumulate through the market is protected (Locke, 1690/1924).

This ideological context helps explain why the United States did not establish a social security program until the mid-1930s, decades after such programs had become commonplace as a public policy in most Western European nations.

The Rise of Collective Concern: Compassionate Ageism

The dire collective and individual effects of the Great Depression, especially the manifest failures of the free market, made possible the acceptance (though hardly universal) of Franklin Roosevelt's New Deal programs to deal with market failures (Schlesinger, 1958). The classical liberal ideology that had characterized the American polity was temporarily submerged as a norm of activist government evolved from the New Deal, through World War II, and beyond. Both Republican and Democratic presidents maintained this norm through five decades (Altman, 2005).

The ideological bulwark of individual responsibility was overcome with Social Security's establishment in 1935—a policy that singled out older Americans as a special group that needed to be, and was worthy of being, collectively insured against the risks associated with old age. This new norm regarding older people, embodied in Social Security, was amplified in the years that followed. From the mid-1930s through the late 1970s the construction of an old-age welfare state was facilitated by a *compassionate ageism* (Binstock, 1983)—the attribution of the same characteristics, status, and just deserts to a heterogeneous group of "the aged" that tended to be stereotyped as poor, frail, dependent, objects of discrimination, and above all "deserving." American society accepted the oversimplified notion that all older persons are essentially the same, and all worthy of governmental assistance, even though many of them did not fit these stereotypes (see Neugarten, 1982).

The stereotypes expressed through this ageism, unlike those of racism or sexism, were far from prejudicial to the well-being of older people. During the 1960s and 1970s, the American polity implemented the construct of compassionate ageism by creating many old-age government benefit programs, as well as by enacting laws against age discrimination on the basis of old age. In those decades, just about every issue or problem affecting some older individuals that could be identified by advocates for older persons became identified as a governmental responsibility to some extent.

Medicare and Medicaid, enacted in 1965, have together provided almost all older Americans with government-financed health insurance. The Older Americans Act was legislated the same year and grew to support a nationwide network of nutritional, legal, transportation, and myriad other services and programs for seniors. The Age Discrimination in Employment Act of 1967 provided protection for older workers with respect to many dimensions of employment and, as subsequently amended in 1978 and 1986, has outlawed mandatory retirement at any age (except for workers with certain public safety responsibilities and high-level corporate executives). The Employee Retirement Income Security Act of 1974 vastly extended the nearly nonexistent regulation of old-age pension funds. It also created the Pension Benefit Guaranty Corporation, which provides pension benefits to retired workers if their employer pension plans fail to provide benefits. Also in 1974, culminating a 6–year lobbying effort by the Gerontological Society of America (see Lockett, 1983), the Research on Aging Act established a National Institute on Aging to fund and conduct research to improve the health of older people.

In addition to such major legislative landmarks, during these years older persons were identified as explicit beneficiaries of myriad programs and regulations focused on broader constituencies in areas such as housing, home repair, low-income energy assistance, and mental health. For instance, The Age Discrimination Act of 1975, which applied to all ages, prohibited discrimination on the basis of age in any programs and activities receiving federal assistance.

PRESSURES FOR RETRENCHING PUBLIC OLD-AGE EXPENDITURES

Since the late 1970s, however, various pressures for retrenching the American old-age welfare state have emerged and been continuous. They are stronger than ever in the second decade of the twenty-first century.

Neoliberalism and the Emergence of "Greedy Geezers"

By the late 1970s, after decades in which Social Security, Medicare, Medicaid, and the other old-age policies had become politically accepted as staples, the ideological pendulum swung back, away from collective concerns. Classical liberal ideology reemerged and flourished. This neoliberalism (popularly labeled as *conservatism*) once again emphasized the virtues of atomistic individualism and free-market capitalism, while also stressing the evils of "big government," including government regulation and welfare programs. The resurgence of classical liberalism was spearheaded by the presidency of Ronald Reagan and continued unabated through the presidency of George W. Bush. This ideological context is important for understanding public political discourse and proposals for changing old-age policies since the late 1970s.

As (the conservative) neoliberalism was reemerging, the compassionate stereotypes that had facilitated the building of an old-age welfare state did not disappear. But unflattering stereotypes emerged as competing themes of social construction in the U.S. media and in some policy circles, if not in the views of the American public. Older people came to be portrayed as one of the more flourishing and powerful groups in American society and, yet, attacked as a burdensome responsibility because of the growing costs of old-age benefit programs. Throughout the 1980s and into the 1990s the new stereotypes, readily observed in popular culture, depicted aged persons as prosperous, hedonistic, politically powerful, and selfish. For example, "Grays on the Go," a cover story in *Time*, portrayed older people as America's new elite — healthy, wealthy, powerful, and "staging history's biggest retirement party" (Gibbs, 1980). A dominant theme in such accounts of older Americans was that their selfishness was ruining the nation. A *New York Times* Op-Ed was headlined "Elderly, Affluent — and Selfish" (Longman, 1989). The *New Republic* (1988) highlighted this motif with a cover that displayed an unflattering caricature of aged persons, accompanied by the caption "greedy geezers." This theme soon was echoed widely, and "greedy geezers" became a familiar epithet in ongoing accounts of federal budget politics (e.g., Salholz, 1990) and remains so today. In the early 1990s, an article in *Fortune* magazine titled "The Tyranny of America's Old" asserted that the political and economic power of greedy older people was one of the most crucial issues facing U.S. society (Smith, 1992).

Why the New Stereotypes?

The immediate precipitating factor for these new stereotypes may have been the serious cash flow problem in the Social Security system that emerged within the larger context of a depressed economy during President Carter's administration (see Estes, 1983; Light, 1985). A high rate of unemployment substantially reduced the payroll tax base for Social Security revenue, while a simultaneous very high rate of inflation produced corresponding sharp increases in benefits through the program's annual cost-of-living adjustments. In order to deal with a projected cash flow problem in benefit payments for Old Age and Survivors Insurance (OASI) recipients, Congress authorized the Social Security Administration to borrow from the system's Disability Insurance and Hospital Insurance trust funds in order to help pay OASI benefits.

Two additional elements contributed importantly to the greedy-geezer image of older persons. One was the "graying of the budget," identified by political scientist Robert Hudson (1978). He highlighted a tremendous long-term growth in the amount and proportion of federal dollars expended on benefits to aging citizens, which at that time had come to be 25% of the budget and comparable to expenditures on national defense. Journalists quickly began to spread the word about this fact, asking, who will shoulder the "growing burden" of elderly Americans (e.g., Samuelson, 1978)?

Another element in the reversal of the stereotypes of old age was dramatic improvements in the aggregate status of older Americans, in large measure due to the impact of federal benefit programs. Social Security, for example, had helped to reduce the poverty rate of persons aged 65 and older from 30% in 1967 to 12% in 1984—a percentage that compared very favorably with a 21% rate for children that same year (U.S. Census Bureau, 2009).

"Intergenerational Equity" and Intergenerational Conflict

In this unsympathetic climate of opinion the aged emerged as a scapegoat for an impressive list of American problems, and the concept of "intergenerational equity"—but really intergenerational *inequity*—began to receive some prominence in public dialogue. Demographers and advocates for children blamed the political power of elderly Americans for the plight of youngsters experiencing inadequate nutrition, health care, and education and insufficiently supportive family environments. In an influential article, the president of the Population Association of America erroneously argued that rising poverty among children was the direct result of rising benefits to older people (Preston, 1984). One children's advocate even proposed that parents receive an "extra vote" for each of their children, in order to combat older voters in an intergenerational conflict (Carballo, 1981). The argument that old-age benefits are a major detriment to the health of the economy and younger generations has been persistently disseminated by Wall Street banker and former secretary of commerce Peter Peterson during the past three decades. In the mid-1980s, for instance, he suggested that a prerequisite for the United States to regain its stature as a first-class power in the world economy was a sharp reduction in programs benefiting older Americans (Peterson, 1987).

The themes of intergenerational inequity and conflict were adopted by the media and academics as routine perspectives for describing many social policy issues. They also gained currency in elite sectors of American society and among the Washington policy cognoscenti. For instance, the president of the prestigious American Association of Universities asserted at the Gerontological Society of America's 1990 annual meeting that "the shape of the domestic federal budget inescapably pits programs for the retired against every other social purpose dependent on federal funds" (Rosenzweig, 1990). This theme of zero-sum trade-offs between children and elders remains prominent in policy discussions today, especially among economists (e.g., Sawhill and Monea, 2008).

The Pressure of Population Aging

The issue of how to distribute public resources among older persons and other constituents and causes has been an issue in developed nations throughout the world as they experience population aging. In the United States, for example, 76 million individuals born between 1946 and 1964, described as the *baby boom*, are now beginning to enter the ranks of old age. The number of Americans aged 65 and older will increase from 40 million in 2010 to 72 million in 2030. At that point nearly 20% of the U.S. population will be aged 65 and older (Federal Interagency Forum on Aging-Related Statistics, 2010). This phenomenon will sharply escalate the aggregate demand for public health measures directed toward the U.S. older population (see chap. 2), including a retooling of the health care workforce (Institute of Medicine, 2008; also see chap. 13).

In European and some Asian nations *low fertility rates* are the major factor in population aging. Instead of baby booms, they have been experiencing "*baby busts.*" The consequences for the age structure of populations have already been felt substantially in these nations. About one in five Germans and Italians are currently aged 65 and older, and the proportion is slightly higher in Japan. The boomers will not have a comparable impact on the U.S. population structure until 2030. By then, however, if their low fertility rates continue, more than one in four Germans and Italians will be aged 65 and older, and more than 3 out of 10 Japanese will be in that age range (Vienna Institute of Demography, 2010).

For some years now, European nations have been responding to population aging by reforming their old-age welfare states to reduce their costs (Kohli and Arza, 2011). Now, as the leading edge of the baby boom cohort is becoming eligible for old-age benefit programs in the United States, serious attention is being paid to the fiscal implications of the fact that the number of old-age beneficiaries of these programs will more than double over the next 20 years and remain high for decades to come. These fiscal concerns regarding old-age policies are particularly acute with respect to the major sources of financing for health care and long-term care of older persons—the Medicare and Medicaid programs (see Gist, 2011). The growth in Medicare costs has been substantial to date and is projected to be explosive in the years ahead. Medicare was only 3.5% of the federal budget in the early 1970s but increased to nearly 16% in 2009 (Congressional Budget Office, 2009). The trustees of Medicare report that the program accounted for 3.5% of gross domestic product (GDP) in 2009 (Board of Trustees, 2010). It is projected to triple to about

8% of GDP by 2036 (Medicare Payment Advisory Commission, 2006), one-twelfth of the nation's wealth.

The Pressure of Fiscal "Crises" and "Deficit Reduction Mania"

A third pressure on the old-age welfare state has been fiscal problems experienced by a number of developed countries since 2008. The responses to these measures in a number of European nations were what Nobel laureate economist Paul Krugman (2010) characterized as a harmful fad—austere measures to reduce government deficits (see, e.g., Quinn, 2010).

In the United States a mania for reducing the federal deficit suddenly developed in 2010 (an election year) after 9 years of deficit spending on foreign wars, 9 years of substantial cuts in tax rates, and 2 years of expensive spending for economic stimulus, unemployment insurance, and government bailouts of private sector companies—such as large banks and financial firms, insurance companies, and the Ford and Chrysler automobile companies—in the context of the Great Recession. In February 2010, President Obama used an executive order to create a National Commission on Fiscal Responsibility and Reform (which became popularly known as the Deficit Reduction Commission). He charged the commission to recommend by early December measures "to improve the U.S. fiscal situation in the medium term and to achieve fiscal sustainability over the long term" (White House, 2010). At the same time, some members of Congress, the media, and various respected public policy and scientific sources turned a great deal of attention to the general issue of reducing the long-run cumulative deficit of the federal government (which had already reached over $12 trillion and was projected to keep growing). For instance, the National Research Council and the National Academy of Public Administration jointly issued a report titled *Choosing the Nation's Fiscal Future* (Committee on the Fiscal Future of the United States, 2010), in which it singled out the Social Security, Medicare, and Medicaid entitlement programs as essential major targets for deficit reduction reforms, including restraints on their growth and greater taxes to support them. Ben Bernanke, chairman of the Federal Reserve, persistently expressed this view throughout the year in speeches (e.g., Chan and Hernandez, 2010) and congressional testimony (Chan, 2010).

When the President's Commission released its report in December 2010, it included proposed cuts in Medicare and Medicaid, despite (or perhaps because of) the prospective entrance of tens of millions of baby boomers in these programs (National Commission on Fiscal Responsibility and Reform,

2010). Similarly, a few weeks earlier, a private commission of the Bipartisan Policy Center, co-chaired by a former Republican Senate Budget Committee chair and a former director of both the Congressional Budget Office and the Office of Management and Budget, released a report for dealing with the deficit. It called for including substantial increases in cost sharing and premiums to be paid by Medicare recipients and a cap on the growth of federal Medicaid expenditures (Horney, Van de Water, and Greenstein, 2010). Whether either of these sets of proposals (or others like them) for reducing financing of health care for older Americans would be enacted by Congress was unclear. But, as is discussed in the next section of this chapter, it was clear that pressures for limiting government financing for the health care and long-term care of older people would continue to mount.

LIMITING HEALTH RESOURCES FOR OLDER PEOPLE

The U.S. government has made health care far more readily available and affordable for older Americans than most other population groups. The 1965 enactment of Medicare and Medicaid singled out the older population as a group especially worthy of governmental support for receiving health care for two major reasons. One reason was that as older persons retired and were no longer part of an employer-based insured group, insurers were reluctant to insure them as individuals because of their comparatively high likelihood of requiring costly treatment. Consequently, health care insurers tended to deny them coverage, or to charge steep prices in anticipation of subsequent bills for health care costs. The other reason was that a substantial majority of older persons could not afford out-of-pocket payments for health care—a situation that applies as well today (see Moon, 2011; Reno and Veghte, 2011). Yet the notion of limiting health care resources for older persons has persisted in one form or another for more than three decades and is stronger than ever today.

Informal Ageism in Health Care

Informally, lower priority has been given to the health care of older patients for a long time, both in the United States and abroad. In his Pulitzer Prize–winning book published in the mid-1970s—*Why Survive? Growing Older in America*—Robert Butler (1975) pointed out that ageism in cultural attitudes manifested itself in discrimination against older persons within the health care arena and other societal institutions. Butler's observations regarding ageist attitudes toward older patients in U.S. health care settings were vividly reflected a few years later in an autobiographical novel by a recent medical school graduate who was interning at a first-tier hospital in Boston, Massachusetts (Shem, 1978). Among other things, the novel highlighted the annoyance that physicians expressed toward elderly patients who arrived for service at the emergency room, where effort, time, and other resources were scarce. Such a patient was referred to as a "GOMER," standing for "Get Out of My Emergency Room." Although Medicare and Medicaid matured and financed the care of most older Americans in the succeeding decades, ageism in American health care practices continued (Kane, 2002).

Informal attitudes and practices reflecting ageism are hardly confined to the United States. They have also been manifest, for instance, in the British National Health Service (NHS), which is funded by a fixed governmental budget. As long ago as 1980 cardiologists in the NHS who were frustrated by a high demand for a limited number of hospital beds expressed a complaint similar to that embodied in the term GOMERs by referring to patients aged 65 and older as "bed blockers" (Wilson, 1980). In 2006, a joint report of England's Audit Commission, Healthcare Commission, and Commission for Social Care Inspection reported that standards of care for older people are "unacceptably poor" (Eaton, 2006). And a number of surveys indicate that older age is still a barrier to specialist care within the NHS, including palliative care for dying older persons (Gott, Ibrahim, and Binstock, in press).

Public Discussions of Limiting Care for Older Persons

Suggestions that health care for elderly patients should be formally rationed as a matter of public policy began to emerge in U.S. public discourse in the 1980s. Amid widespread concerns about spiraling U.S. health care costs, attention was redirected, in part, from health care providers, suppliers, administrators, and insurers—the parties responsible for setting the prices of care—to elderly persons for whom health care was provided.

In a major public speech in 1983, noted economist Alan Greenspan stated that 30% of Medicare funds are annually spent on Medicare enrollees who die within the year (Schulte, 1983). Although he was overstating this proportion by a few percentage points (see Lubitz and Riley, 1993), Greenspan pointedly asked his audience "whether it [the money we spend] is worth it" (Schulte, 1983, p. 1). About a year later, the governor of Colorado, Richard Lamm, was widely quoted as stating that "older persons have a duty to die and get out of the way" (Slater, 1984).

These widely disseminated quotes from Greenspan and Lamm were the opening shots in a campaign—by some public figures, economists, and bioethicists—to limit health care for older Americans. That campaign has persisted to this day. Conferences and books explicitly addressed the subject of limiting health care of the elderly, with titles such as *Should Medical Care Be Rationed By Age?* (Smeeding, 1987). Ethicists and philosophers began generating principles of equity to govern "justice between age groups" in the provision of health care, rather than, for instance, justice between rich and poor, or justice among ethnic and racial groups (Daniels, 1988; Menzel, 1990).

The most prominent proponent of old-age-based rationing has been biomedical ethicist Daniel Callahan, whose 1987 book entitled *Setting Limits: Medical Goals in an Aging Society* received substantial popular attention. In it he characterized the older population as "a new social threat" and a "demographic, economic, and medical avalanche . . . one that could ultimately (and perhaps already) do [*sic*] great harm" (Callahan, 1987, p. 20). Arguing that health care spending on the elderly will pose an unsustainable fiscal burden, Callahan urged the use of "age as a specific criterion for the allocation and limitation of healthcare." This would be accomplished by denying life-extending health care—as a matter of public policy—to persons who are aged in their "late 70s or early 80s" and/or have "lived out a natural life span" (Callahan, 1987, p. 171). Specifically, he proposed that the Medicare program not pay for such care and hoped that other private insurers would follow suit.

Although Callahan described "the natural life span" as a matter of biography (the personal details of one's life course experiences) rather than biology, he used chronological age as an arbitrary marker to designate when, from a biographical standpoint, the individual should have reached the end of a natural life. In a subsequent article he expressed the view that the only deaths that are "premature" are those that occur before age 65 (Callahan, 2000).

Callahan's rationing proposal attracted considerable attention. It provoked widespread and ongoing discussion in the media and directly inspired a number of books and scores of articles in national magazines and academic journals (see, e.g., Barry and Bradley, 1991; Binstock and Post, 1991). Although many of these books and articles strongly criticized the idea of old-age-based rationing, the idea has stayed alive and has even been advocated recently by physicians in prestigious forums. For instance, in the spring of 2009, the Institute of Medicine and the National Academy of Science organized and hosted a symposium on "The Grand Challenges of Our Aging Society." In a speech entitled "Judicious Use of Resources," a noted geriatrician argued that health care resources are scarce and that we need to think seriously about principles for rationing some of our health care efforts for elderly patients (Reuben, 2009).

Governmental Efforts to Limit Resources

The contemporary contexts of the Great Recession and political concerns about deficit reduction have focused greater attention than ever on reducing government expenditures for Medicare and Medicaid, the two most important resource streams for supporting health care for older Americans. Although one of the factors that will increase costs in those programs is the aging of the baby boom, little can be done to reduce its impact per se. Moreover, cross-national studies over the years have shown that population aging is a relatively minor factor in the growth of health care costs in the United States and other aging industrialized nations (see, e.g., Binstock, 1993; Reinhardt, 2003). Rather, the percentage of national GDP spent on health care is determined by how it is financed—say, through a fixed budget (such as in the British National Health Service) or open-ended reimbursement for charges (as has been the case with most of Medicare)—and how health care providers and manufacturers respond to the available economic incentives.

Steep increases in U.S. health care expenditures are largely due to expense factors in the overall system, in which costs rise much faster than the general rate of inflation. The major sources of rising costs per patient in the health care sector are a constant stream of new and costly technologies, procedures, and drugs; high rates of utilization; huge administrative costs; and unnecessarily high expenses and utilization in some regions and health centers as compared with others. The consensus among analysts of the growth in U.S. health care costs is that the advance and application of medical technologies and procedures are the single most important factors (see, e.g., Congressional Budget Office, 2007).

Consequently, efforts to contain Medicare and Medicaid costs—without limiting coverage for the health care of older patients—should in principle focus on reforming finances in the health care system generally, not just those two government programs. But as the politics of enacting the Patient Protection and Affordable Health Care Act in 2010 vividly demonstrated, there are substantial barriers to sweeping health care reforms for dealing with the high costs of many new technologies, procedures, and drugs—especially because of the large financial stakes that the politically powerful medical industrial complex has in current arrangements. Moreover, the larger health care arena is highly fragmented, so there is no entity "in charge" of it. In contrast, Medicare and Medicaid policies can be implemented more effectively because they can be centralized and carried out through concerted governmental policy actions. So, for the foreseeable future, attempts to contain health care costs are likely to continue focusing on limiting those government programs.

Explorations for Limiting Costly Health Care

Government agencies have begun examining issues that could be setting the stage for subsequent official decisions to implement old-age-based rationing in publicly financed insurance programs that serve the older population. For instance, in 2010, the Centers for Medicare and Medicaid (which administers the two programs) undertook a formal "national coverage analysis" of Provenge, a vaccine approved for treating prostate cancer, a disease that predominantly affects older men (Stein, 2010). The treatment costs $93,000 per patient and has been shown to extend patients' lives by an average of about 4 months (although many patients live much longer). The fact that this "coverage analysis" is taking place, even though Medicare is not supposed to take cost into consideration, is an indication that this treatment may be excluded from coverage by the program.

Even before the Great Recession and deficit concerns, the nonpartisan Congressional Budget Office (2006) published a report that explored analytical strategies for prospectively identifying which Medicare enrollees are likely to be "future high-cost beneficiaries"—possibly a preliminary step for identifying those whose care might be rationed. As the Congressional Budget Office focuses in on finding ways to forecast which individual patients will be high cost, the possibility of eventual public policy to decide which older individuals are to live and die may seem far less remote than when proposed by bioethicists such as Callahan (1987), philosophers such as Daniels (1988), and politicians such as Lamm (Slater, 1984).

Erosion of Resources for Long-Term Care

Meanwhile, Medicaid has become among the top three items funded by state governments; on average, it accounts for 22% of state budgets (State Budget Solutions, 2010). Because state governments have been experiencing fiscal woes during the Great Recession and are having difficulty fulfilling their constitutional requirements to have balanced budgets, their Medicaid programs have been targets of cutbacks in recent years. In 2009, for example, every state but Arkansas and North Carolina made cuts to some element of their Medicaid programs (Diamond, 2010). Among these cuts have been resources for nursing homes, assisted living facilities, and home care for older and disabled people. And the nursing home industry fears that further cuts are in the offing that will have negative consequences for the quality of care it provides (Pecquet, 2010).

At the same time, individuals who are not very wealthy and wish to finance the enormous expenses of long-term care will find it increasingly difficult to do so. As reported in chapter 3, the national average cost for a private room in a nursing home was $80,000 in 2009. A compounded 5% annual increase in rates (reflecting typical increases historically) suggests that the average cost can be expected to exceed $107,000 in 2015. In 2010, Metlife, one of the major insurers of long-term care, joined a number of other insurers that have withdrawn from the market because their actuarial assumptions regarding the viability of the product had been too optimistic (Holm, 2010). Others sought costly raises in the premium rates paid by its customers. For instance, Genworth Financial was seeking permission from state regulators for an 18% rate increase for 25% of its long-term customers, and John Hancock was trying to get permission for an average rate increase of 40% affecting about 80% of its insurees (Lieber, 2010).

As described in chapter 3, the Patient Protection and Affordable Care Act of 2010 did create a voluntary public mechanism for long-term care insurance, the Community Living and Assistance Services and Supports Program (often referred to as the CLASS Act). It is estimated that when the program implements cash payments for home care, adult day programs, assisted living, or institutional care in 2016, those payments will average from about $50 to $75 a day (see Wiener, 2010). These amounts may be useful in supplementing private resources for purchasing services and make things financially easier for caregivers who are both working and providing care to a family member. However, payments under the CLASS Act program would be far from sufficient to cover the costs of institutional care or round-the-clock care at home.

LOOKING AHEAD: THE POLITICS OF RESOURCE RETRENCHMENT

Will proposals for explicit cuts in or withdrawal of Medicare and Medicaid coverage for selected procedures and services engender political backlash from older voters and old-age interest groups such as the more-than-40-

million-member AARP? Might such a backlash stave off such limitations in health care resources?

Health Reform and the 2010 Election

Harbingers that policies for limiting resources for health care of older persons could energize and solidify older people as a countervailing, oppositional voting constituency emerged in recent years. For instance, the theme of health care rationing for older Americans became especially prominent in the summer of 2009. A health care reform bill in the House of Representatives had in it a provision that expanded Medicare to cover the costs of a voluntary consultation with a physician, every 5 years, concerning end-of-life planning through living wills and health care durable-power-of-attorney documents (see Blumenauer, 2009). Moreover, from the outset of the 2009–10 health care reform effort, an overarching message from President Obama was that the costs of reform would be substantially offset by savings in the Medicare program to be achieved by reducing excess government subsidies to Medicare Advantage programs (see White House, 2009). A number of prominent Republican politicians and conservative broadcasters distorted these two themes—end-of life planning, and savings from Medicare—by transforming them into the specters of "death panels" and efforts to "pull the plug on granny." When members of Congress returned to their districts during the summer recess to hold town hall style meetings, they faced rowdy crowds in which older persons expressed concern about rationing in the Medicare program (Blumenauer, 2009). Subsequently, AARP acknowledged that it faced a challenge in explaining to its members why it had endorsed health care reform (Calmes, 2009); reportedly, about 60,000 members quit the organization (CBS News, 2009).

Advertisements for Republican and Tea Party candidates throughout the nation in the 2010 election campaign consistently hammered on the theme that President Obama and Democratic members of Congress were intent on rationing Medicare (see Steinhauer, 2010). For instance, an ad run by the 60 Plus Association (which billed itself as the conservative alternative to AARP) attacked an incumbent Democratic congressman in the following way: "Boyd voted for Nancy Pelosi's health care bill which will cut $500 billion from Medicare. That will hurt the quality of our care" (Holan, 2010, B1).

Such advertisements, added to the president's message that the savings for health care reform would come from Medicare, apparently had an impact on

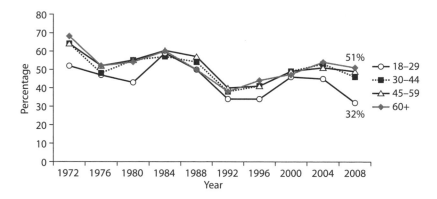

Fig. 18.1. Percent voting for Republican U.S. presidential candidates, by age groups, 1972-2008. *Source*: Binstock, 2010, with permission

older voters in the 2010 election. Until then age-group voting patterns in American elections had shown no discernible sign of older persons voting as a bloc in response to old-age policy issues, regardless of what competing candidates for election had to say about them (Campbell and Binstock, 2011). As figure 18.1 shows, for example, during the preceding four decades older persons had distributed their votes among candidates in very similar patterns to all voters aged in their thirties and above. Only voters in their teens and twenties, least likely to have partisan attachments, tended to show a different pattern. (For a fuller discussion of the reasons behind these patterns see Campbell and Binstock, 2011).

But the age group distributions within the aggregate national vote for congressional candidates in 2010 did show signs of older persons voting as more of a benefits issue bloc than in the past, within the context of repeated campaign portrayals of threats to Medicare coverage, as discussed above. As can be seen in figure 18.2, older voters (whether categorized as aged 60 and older or 65 and older) voted noticeably more in favor of Republican candidates than those aged 45–59 and 30–44. As *New York Times* columnist Frank Rich (2010) put it in a postelection analysis, "[Obama] delayed so long in specifying his own priorities for [health care reform] that his opponents filled the vacuum for him, making fictions like 'death panels' stick."

Because of the age group voting patterns in 2010, politicians (and their consultants) in subsequent years may be wary of supporting policies, both in the governing process and in election campaigns, that might alienate a "sleeping giant" of older voters. These political concerns may serve as a bulwark against major retrenchments in Medicare and Medicaid coverage.

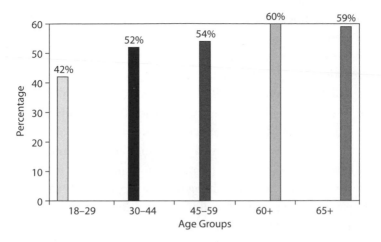

Fig. 18.2. Percent voting for Republican U.S. congressional candidates, 2010, by age groups. *Source*: Connelly, 2010, with permission

Can Our Understanding of the Social Contract Be Reframed?

Ultimately, the likelihood and intensity of maintaining or enhancing governmental resources for the health care of older people will be shaped by the answers to two questions. First, will there be enough national wealth available to redistribute to older people for this purpose? Second, will the prevailing U.S. ideology in the decades ahead support a politics of collectively insuring against the risks of illness and lack of health care in old age? Popular support for Social Security and Medicare has been reasonably strong among all generations up to now (Campbell, 2009). Yet, a strengthening of that collective political will against the vicissitudes of America's national fiscal status and shifting political winds may be needed to mitigate serious cuts in health care resources for the older population.

In his book *Don't Think of an Elephant: Know Your Values and Frame the Debate*, Lakoff (2004) emphasizes the role of metaphors in framing issues and the ongoing influence of rhetorical frameworks in the policy arena. A key challenge for public health in our aging society is to reframe and articulate issues that help the American people appreciate the extent to which our social contract—as expressed through so-called old-age entitlements—actually benefits all generations. Older people are not hermetically sealed from their families, communities, and society. Neither are old-age benefits hermetically sealed from other age groups. The U.S. public needs to understand what significant cutbacks in old-age policies could mean for the nature of family obligations and other familiar social institutions that are integral to the daily life of citizens of all ages.

What are some possible effects of major cuts in old-age benefit programs? Far more elderly persons than today would be financially dependent on their families and local institutions. Because of family financial necessities, we might see the return of three- and four-generation households, instead of preferred independent living arrangements. In the context of the contemporary Great Recession we have already seen an increase in multigenerational families living in one household (Yen, 2010). Many adult children could be financially devastated by policy changes in Medicare and Medicaid that lead them to pay expensive costs of health care and long-term care for their parents. And such responsibilities for health expenses could, in turn, limit the resources available to adult children for raising their own children.

Medicare and Medicaid are not "luxurious" government benefits for a group of Americans that are often depicted in public rhetoric as if they were a separate, selfish tribe of greedy geezers. At the same time, the evidence is clear that older people are among the taxpaying adult generations that support programs for our youth—such as children's health insurance, public education, and many others. Effective dissemination of these broader, intergenerational contexts for perceiving government programs could go a long way toward heading off or moderating potential cuts in health care resources and even enhance the resources essential for public health in our aging society.

ACKNOWLEDGMENTS

The author wishes to acknowledge the intellectual stimulation and support provided by his colleagues in the John D. and Catherine T. MacArthur Foundation Research Network on an Aging Society (John W. Rowe, Director). Portions of this chapter are adapted from Robert H. Binstock, 2010. From compassionate ageism to intergenerational conflict? *Gerontologist* 50:574–85.

REFERENCES

Altman, N. J. 2005. The Battle for Social Security: From FDR's Vision to Bush's Gamble. Hoboken, NJ: John Wiley and Sons.
Barry, R. L., and G. V. Bradley, eds. 1991. Set No Limits: A Rebuttal to Daniel Callahan's Proposal to Limit Health Care for the Elderly. Urbana: University of Illinois Press.
Binstock, R. H. 1983. The aged as scapegoat. Gerontologist 23:136–43.
Binstock, R. H. 1993. Health care costs around the world: Is aging a fiscal "black hole"? Generations 24(4):37–42.

Binstock, R. H. 2010. From compassionate ageism to intergenerational conflict? Gerontologist 50:574–85.

Binstock, R. H., and S. G. Post, eds. 1991. Too Old for Health Care? Controversies in Medicine, Law, Economics, and Ethics. Baltimore: Johns Hopkins University Press.

Blumenauer, E. 2009. My near death panel experience. New York Times, November 15, 12wk.

Board of Trustees of the Federal Hospital Insurance Trust Fund. 2010. 2010 Annual Report of the Board of Trustees of the Federal Hospital Insurance and Federal Supplementary Medical Insurance Trust Funds. Retrieved December 1, 2010, from www.cms.gov/ReportsTrustFunds/downloads/tr2010.pdf.

Butler, R. N. 1975. Why Survive? Being Old in America. New York: Harper and Row.

Callahan, D. 1987. Setting Limits: Medical Goals in an Aging Society. New York: Simon and Schuster.

Callahan, D. 2000. Death and the research imperative. New England Journal of Medicine 342:654–56.

Calmes, J. 2009. AARP says its chore is educating members on bill's benefits. New York Times, October 14. Retrieved October 14, 2009, from http://prescriptions.blogs.nytimes.com/2009/1014/aarp-says-its-chore-is-educating-elderly-on-bills-benefits/.

Campbell, A. L. 2009. Is the economic crisis driving wedges between young and old? Rich and poor? Generations 33(3):47–53.

Campbell, A. L., and R. H. Binstock. 2011. Politics and aging in the United States. In Handbook of Aging and the Social Sciences, 7th ed., ed. R. H. Binstock and L. K. George, pp. 265–79. San Diego: Elsevier.

Carballo, M. 1981. Extra votes for parents? Boston Globe, December 17, 35.

CBS News. 2009. Thousands quit AARP over health reform. Retrieved December 15, 2010, from www.cbsnews.com/stories/2009/08/17/eveningnews/main5247916.shtml?loc=interstitialskip.

Chan, S. 2010. Bernanke says a plan to address the U.S. deficit could keep rates down. New York Times, April 15, B8.

Chan, S., and J. C. Hernandez. 2010. Bernanke says nation must take action soon to shape fiscal future. Retrieved April 8, 2010, from www.nytimes.com/2010/04/08/business/economy/08fed.html.

Committee on the Fiscal Future of the United States. 2010. Choosing the Nation's Fiscal Future. Washington, DC: National Academies Press.

Congressional Budget Office. 2006. High-Cost Medicare Beneficiaries. Retrieved April 12, 2006, from http://cbo.gov/showdoc.cfm?index=6332&sequence=0.

Congressional Budget Office. 2007. The Long-Term Outlook for Health Care Spending. Washington, DC: U.S. Government Printing Office, November.

Congressional Budget Office. 2009. The Budget and Economic Outlook: An Update. Washington, DC: author.

Connelly, M. 2010. Rightward march. New York Times, November 7, wk3.

Daniels, N. 1988. Am I My Parents Keeper? An Essay on Justice between the Young and the Old. New York: Oxford University Press.

Diamond, D. 2010. Rationalizing rationing in Arizona's Medicaid program. California Healthline, December 8. Retrieved December 8, 2010, from www.california healthline.org/road-to-reform/2010/rationalizing-rationing-in-arizonas-medicaid -program.aspx.

Eaton, L. 2006. Care of England's older people still "unacceptably poor." British Medical Journal 332:746.

Esping-Andersen, G. 1999. Social Foundations of Postindustrial Economies. New York: Oxford University Press.

Estes, C. L. 1983. Social Security: The social construction of a crisis. Milbank Memorial Fund Quarterly/Health and Society 61:445–61.

Federal Interagency Forum on Aging-Related Statistics. 2010. Older Americans 2010. Key Indicators of WellBeing. Washington, DC: U.S. Government Printing Office.

Gibbs, N. R. 1980. Grays on the go. Time 131(8):66–75.

Gist, J. 2011. Fiscal implications of population aging. In Handbook of Aging and the Social Sciences, 7th ed., ed. R. H. Binstock and L. K. George, pp. 353–66. San Diego: Elsevier.

Gott, M., A. Ibrahim, and R. H. Binstock. In press. The disadvantaged dying: Ageing, ageism, and palliative care provision for older people in the UK. In Living with Ageing and Dying: End of Life Care for Older People, ed. M. Gott and C. Ingleton. London: Oxford University Press.

Hartz, L. 1955. The Liberal Tradition in America. New York: Harcourt Brace.

Holan, A. D. 2010. Ad intent on attack rather than accuracy. Plain Dealer, September 23, B1–2.

Holm, E. 2010. Update: MetLife discontinues sales of long-term care coverage. Wall Street Journal, November 11. Retrieved May 14, 2011, from www.advfn.com/ news_UPDATE-MetLife-Discontinues-Sales-Of-Long-Term-Care-Coverage_ 45198642.html.

Horney, J. R., P. N. Van de Water, and R. Greenstein. 2010. Rivlin-Domenici deficit reduction plan is superior to Bowles-Simpson in most areas: But health proposal is very troubling. Center on Budget and Policy Priorities, November 30. Retrieved November 30, 2010, from www.Cbpp.org/cms/index.cfm?fa=view&id=3333.

Hudson, R. B. (1978). The "graying" of the federal budget and its consequences for old age policy. Gerontologist 18:428–40.

Institute of Medicine. 2008. Retooling for an Aging America: Building the Healthcare Workforce. Washington, DC: National Academies Press.

Kane, R. L. 2002. The future history of geriatrics: Geriatrics at the crossroads. Journals of Gerontology Series A: Biological Sciences and Medical Sciences 57:M803–5.

Kohli, M., and C. Arza, C. 2011. The political economy of pension reform in Europe. In Handbook of Aging and the Social Sciences, 7th ed., ed. R. H. Binstock and L. K. George, pp. 251–64. San Diego: Elsevier.

Krugman, P. 2010. British fashion victims. New York Times, October 21. Retrieved December 3, 2010, from www.nytimes.com/2010/10/22/opinion/22krugman.html.

Lakoff, G. 2004. Don't Think of an Elephant: Know Your Values and Frame the Debate — the Essential Guide for Progressives. White River Junction, VT: Chelsea Green.

Lieber, R. 2010. When a safety net is yanked away. New York Times, November 12. Retrieved November 15, 2010, from www.nytimes.com/2010/11/13/your-money/13money.html.

Light, P. C. (1985). Artful Work: The Politics of Social Security Reform. New York: Random House.

Locke, J. 1924. Of Civil Government, Two Treatises. London: J. M. Dent and Sons. (Original work published 1690)

Lockett, B. A. 1983. Aging, Politics, and Research: Setting the Federal Agenda for Research on Aging. New York: Springer Publishing Company.

Longman, P. 1989. Elderly, affluent—selfish. New York Times, October 10, p. A27.

Lubitz, J. S., and G. F. Riley. 1993. Trends in Medicare payments in the last year of life. New England Journal of Medicine 328:1092–96.

Medicare Payment Advisory Commission. 2006. Report to the Congress: Medicare Payment Policy. Washington, DC: U.S. Government Printing Office.

Menzel, P. T. 1990. Strong Medicine: The Ethical Rationing of Health Care. New York: Oxford University Press.

Moon, M. 2011. Organization and financing of healthcare. In Handbook of Aging and the Social Sciences, 7th ed., ed. R. H. Binstock and L. K. George, pp. 295–308. San Diego: Elsevier.

The National Commission on Fiscal Responsibility and Reform. 2010. The Moment of Truth: Report of the National Commission on Fiscal Responsibility and Reform. Washington, DC: Author.

Neugarten, B. L., ed. 1982. Age or Need? Public Policies for Older People. Beverly Hills: Sage.

The New Republic. 1988. [The magazine's cover] 198.

Pecquet, J. 2010. Nursing home industry fears pending Medicaid cuts. Healthwatch: The Hills Healthcare Blog, November 8. Retrieved November 9, 2010, from http://thehill.com/blogs/healthwatch/medicaid/128161–nursing-home-industry-fears-pending-medicaid-cuts.

Peterson, P. G. 1987. The morning after. Atlantic Monthly 260(4):43–49.

Preston, S. H. 1984. Children and the elderly in the U.S. Scientific American 51(6): 44–49.

Quinn, B. 2010. UK budget 2010: New era of austerity in Europe? Christian Science Monitor, June 22. Retrieved December 2, 2010, from www.csmonitor.com/layout/set/print/content/view/print/309302.

Reinhardt, U. E. 2003. Does the aging of the population really drive the demand for health care? Health Affairs 22(6):27–39.

Reno, V. R., and B. Veghte. 2011. Economic status of the aged in the United States. In Handbook of Aging and the Social Sciences, 7th ed., ed. R. H. Binstock and L. K. George, pp. 175–92. San Diego: Elsevier.

Reuben, D. B. 2009. Judicious use of resources (a speech delivered at the National Academies on May 28 in Washington, D.C.). Documentation of program retrieved on January 14, 2010, from www.iom.edu/Activities/Workforce/agingamerica/2009–May-28.aspx.

Rich, F. 2010. Barack Obama, phone home. New York Times, October 7. Retrieved

December 14, 2010, from www.nytimes.com/2010/11/07/opinion/07rich.html?_r=1&ref=frankrich.

Rosenzweig, R. M. 1990. Address at the president's opening session, 43rd Annual Meeting of the Gerontological Society of America, Boston, MA (typewritten copy), November 16.

Salholz, E. 1990. Blaming the voters: Hapless budgeteers single out "greedy geezers." Newsweek, October 29, 36.

Samuelson, R. J. 1978. Aging America: Who will shoulder the growing burden? National Journal 10:1712–17.

Sawhill, I., and E. Monea. 2008. Old news. Democracy: A Journal of Ideas 9(Summer):20–31.

Schlesinger, A. M., Jr. 1958. The Coming of the New Deal. Boston: Houghton Mifflin.

Schulte, J. 1983. Terminal patients deplete Medicare, Greenspan says. Dallas Morning News, April 26, 1.

Shem, S. 1978. The House of God: The Classic Novel of Life and Death in an American Hospital. New York: Marek.

Slater, W. 1984. Latest Lamm remark angers the elderly. Arizona Daily Star, March 29, 1.

Smeeding, T. M., ed. 1987. Should Medical Care Be Rationed By Age? Totowa, NJ: Rowman and Littlefield.

Smith, A. 2003. The Wealth of Nations. New York: Bantam Classics. (Original work published 1776)

Smith, L. 1992. The tyranny of America's old. Fortune 125(1):68–72.

State Budget Solutions. 2010. Health Care Reform, Medicaid and State Budget Woes, March 10. Retrieved December 8, 2010, from www.statebudgetsolutions .org/publications/detail/health-care-reform-medicaid-and-state-budget-woes.

Stein, R. 2010. Review of prostate cancer drug Provenge renews medical cost-benefit debate. Washington Post, November 8. Retrieved May 14, 2011, from www.washing tonpost.com/wp-dyn/content/article/2010/11/07/AR2010110705205.html.

Steinhauer, J. 2010. Ads use Medicare cuts as rallying point. New York Times, October 30. Retrieved May 14, 2011, from www.nytimes.com/2010/10/31/us/politics/31 medicare.html.

U.S. Census Bureau. 2009. Income, Poverty, and Health Insurance Coverage in the United States: 2008. Retrieved May 14, 2011, from www.census.gov/prod/2009 pubs/p60–236.pdf.

Vienna Institute of Demography. 2010. European Demographic Data Sheet, 2010. Retrieved September 12, 2010, from www.oeaw.ac.at/vid/datasheet/index.html.

The White House. 2009. America's Seniors and Health Insurance Reform: Protecting Coverage and Strengthening Medicare. Retrieved December 18, 2009, from www.healthreform.gov/reports/seniors/index.html.

The White House. 2010. Executive Order—National Commission on Fiscal Responsibility. Office of the Press Secretary, Feburary 18. Retrieved December 3, 2010, from www.whitehouse.gov/the-press-office/executive-order-national-commission -fiscal-responsibility-and reform.

Wiener, J. M. 2010. What does health reform mean for long-term care? Public Policy and Aging Report 20(2):8–15.

Wilson, L. A. 1980. Blocked beds. Lancet 316:1013.

Yen, H. 2010. More multigenerational families living together. Retrieved May 14, 2011, from www.boston.com/news/nation/articles/2010/03/18/more_multigenera tional_families_living_together.

Index

Page numbers in italics refer to tables

AARP, 59, 405

accountability, 65, 83, 133, 385

accountable care organizations (ACOs), 18

Active Choices (AC), 166–67

Active Living Every Day (ALED), 166–67

activities of daily living (ADL), 105, 125–26, 127, 183, 189, 305, 308, 313

acute care, 54, 60, 66, 67, 189, 269, 383

Administration on Aging (AoA), 83, 304, 318

Advanced Cognitive Training for Independent and Vital Elderly (ACTIVE), 37

AdvantAge Initiative, 46, 83

Advisory Committee on Immunization Practices, 238, 241

Affordable Care Act (ACA). *See* Patient Protection and Affordable Care Act

African Americans, 211, 212, 329, 338; as caregivers, 185, 190; and health disparities, 32, 104, 128

Age Discrimination Act of 1975, 394

Age Discrimination in Employment Act of 1967, 393–94

ageism, 46, 318; compassionate, 393–94; environmental, 345–46; and health care, 108, 399–400

Agency for Healthcare Research and Quality (AHRQ), 4, 240, 315

Agency for Toxic Substances and Disease Registry, 4

Aging and Disability Resource Center (ADRC), 68, 311, 313

Ainsworth, B. E., 336

Albert, Steven M., 353–67

alcohol and alcoholism, 104, 121, 139, 143, 161

Alvarado, V. J., 210

Alzheimer's disease, 36, 354, 356, 361, 362, 363, 364

Alzheimer's Disease Research Centers (ADRCs), 285, 293

American Public Health Association, 123, 281

American Recovery and Reinvestment Act of 2009, 258, 288

American Society of Health-Systems Pharmacists, 283

Americans with Disabilities Act, 121

AmeriCorps, 219
Anderson, Lynda A., 74–92
Area Agencies on Aging (AAAs), 61, 83, 220, 311
Arizona, 67
arthritis, 10, 42, 133–34, 140, 141, 153
Asian Americans, 8, 13, 397
assisted living, 59, 313, 314–15
assistive technologies, 262
Assistive Technology Act of 1998, 261
Association of State and Territorial Health Officials (ASTHO), 277
Atlantic Philanthropies, 284

baby boomers, 70, 268, 397, 402
baby boom generation, 127, 219
Bangladesh, 27
Barbados, 386
Barmada, M. Michael, 353–67
Beacon Community Program, 260
behavior, health: change, 40–41, 112–13, 131–32, 144–46, 382–83; genetic information and, 366; impact of, 17, 36; and socio-economic status, 8, 112–13; and theories, 139, 145, 330
behavioral risk factors: co-occurrence of, 153; and disability, 119, 133; and health outcomes, 138, 139, 161; measurement of, 84; public health interventions to reduce, 144–46, 152–53, 234–36, 384
Behavioral Risk Factor Surveillance System (BRFSS), 90, 124
behavioral therapy, 109
Benson, William F., 53–71
Bernanke, Ben, 398
bicycling, 231–32
Binstock, Robert H., 391–408

bioterrorism, 12–13, 299
Branch, Laurence G., 119–34, 371–88
Breast and Prostate Cancer Cohort Consortium, 360
Brown, Lisa M., 299–319
Buchner, David M., 228–47
Bureau of Health Professions, 280, 281
Bush, George W., 302, 394
Butler, Robert N., 345, 399–400

California, 284
California Geriatric Education Center (CGEC), 280
cancer, 36, 377, 379, 383
Cancer Genetic Markers of Susceptibility (CGEMS), 360
cardiovascular disease, 27, 35–36, 213, 215, 365; as cause of death, 10, 377–78, 379; prevention of, 32, 112–13
Cardiovascular Health Study, 35, 360
Care of Persons with Dementia in their Environments (COPE), 173
Caribbean, 387
cell phones, 263, 264
Center for Home Care Policy and Research, 46–47
Center for Medicare and Medicaid Innovation (CMMI), 270
Center for Substance Abuse Treatment, 143
Centers for Disease Control and Prevention (CDC), 20, 111, 230, 329; BRFSS of, 90–91; definitions by, 78, 84, 101, 346; and disasters, 302, 307, 314, 318, 319; environmental policies recommended by, 339, 340; health promotion efforts of, 16; Healthy

Aging Program, 140; Healthy Aging Research Network of, 77, 328–29; Minority Health and Health Disparities office, 100; Prevention Research Centers (PRC) Program, 285, 292; REACH program of, 89; responsibilities of, 4, 243; on tobacco use, 235–36; training programs of, 285, 292–93

Centers for Medicare and Medicaid Services (CMS), 154, 259, 269, 315, 318, 403

children, 7

China, 27

Choosing the Nation's Fiscal Future, 398

Chronic Care Model (CCM), 386

chronic conditions or diseases, 10, 34, 216; and behavioral change, 382–83; and burden, 240; and disability, 132–33, 140, 141–42; and disasters, 307–8, 310; expense of, 58; and functioning, 77, 188, 216; growing prevalence of, 35, 99, 182; multiple, 53, 305; and prevention efforts, 10, 32, 33, 38, 132–33; and use of technology, 267

Chronic Disease Indicators, 83

Chronic Disease Self-Management Program (CDSMP), 153, 166, 170, 288, 386; and technology, 255, 264

chronic non-communicable diseases (CNCDs), 387

chronic pain, 216, 241

cities: age-friendly, 30, 44, 46, 48, 145, 219–20; urban informatics and, 266

civic engagement, 207, 208, 220

Claude D. Pepper Older Americans Independence Center, 286

clinical trials, 148, 176. *See also* randomized controlled trials

Cochrane Collaboration, 163

cognitive function, 213, 214, 215

cognitive impairment, 37, 173–74, 308. *See also* dementia

cohort effects, 81, 89

Common Disease–Common Variant (CDCV) hypothesis, 355

Commonwealth Fund, 17

"Communities Putting Prevention to Work," 288

community assessment, 82–83

community-based approach, 9, 34, 42, 44

community-based participatory research (CBPR), 19, 150

community-based programs, 37, 42, 163, 165–66, 169–70; development and refinement of, 173–74; dissemination of, 173, 175–76; environmental factors in, 170–71; funding for, 243; participant attrition in, 169; and public health network, 176–77; RE-AIM evaluation of, 167–68; recruitment to, 167, 168–69; stakeholder engagement in, 171–72; sustainability and maintenance of, 167–68, 171, 173

Community First Choice Option, 69

community health promotion, 383

Community Health Status Indicators (CHSI), 91

community health workers, 173

community indicators, 46–47

Community Living Assistance Services and Supports (CLASS), 62–64, 71, 404 comorbidity, 12. *See also* chronic conditions or diseases

Comprehensive Geriatric Education Programs (CGEP), 290

Congressional Budget Office, 403

coping strategies and techniques, 216

copy-number variations (CNVs), 359

Cornell University Environmental Geriatrics Program, 265–66

cost-effectiveness, 36, 67–68, 234, 244, 268, 269–70

costs and financing, 53–54, 154; of family caregiving, 182, 191–93, 198; government efforts to limit, 402–4; and health reform law, 20–21; of long-term care, 58–60, 61–62; of medications, 109; and program sustainability, 171, 173; rising, 70, 108–9, 402; statistics on, 55

cost savings: and family caregiving, 192, 194, 198; from health care reform law, 18, 57, 405; technology and, 256, 258; through prevention, 144, 234, 256

Council on Social Work Education, 283

Crump, C., 377, 379

Data Sources on Older Americans, 84

Declaration of Port of Spain, 387

deCODE/Icelandic Studies, 361

deCODEme, 363

Deficit Reduction Act of 2005, 62

Deficit Reduction Commission, 398

dementia, 190, 192, 214, 308, 362

dental coverage, 107

Department of Health and Human Services (DHHS), 4, 20, 63, 89, 139, 277, 317

Department of Homeland Security, 299, 302, 303, 317

Department of Housing and Urban Development, 329

Department of Veterans Affairs, 58, 61, 66

depression and anxiety, 40, 164, 189, 190

developing countries, 27, 28–29, 371–72

diabetes, 10, 32, 35, 36, 141, 383

Diabetes Prevention Program (DPP), 172

diet, 140–41, 161, 363, 379

Dietary Guidelines for Americans, 140, 229

disability, 68, 131, 228; and built environment, 333–34; causes of, 39–40; characteristics of, 120–21; definitions, 121–22, 126, 134; and disparities, 32, 105, 110, 112, 127–28; future direction around, 133–34; and impairment, 120, 122; measurement of, 122, 123–26, 134; models of, 120; pathology, 122; prevalence and change in, 126–27; prevention efforts, 119, 128–29, 131–33; statistics on, 261

Disability in America: Toward a National Agenda for Prevention, 119

disasters: all-hazards planning for, 301, 315; conceptualization of, 301–2; definition of, 300; evacuations during, 307, 308, 312, 316–17; and housing for elderly, 309–17; informal support during, 311–12; infrastructure for, 299; public health response to, 318–19; public shelters during, 309, 312, 318–19; recovery

phase, 301, 302, 312–13; vulnerability to, 299–300, 305, 307–9, 310,
312, 318. *See also* emergency
preparedness and response
drug addiction, 121
dysregulation, physiologic, 37–38

ecological public health models,
327–28
economy, U.S., 105, 192–93, 402, 403
education, 218; and health, 106, 231;
and socioeconomic position, 102,
106
Edward R. Roybal Centers, 286, 293
Elderhostel, 218
E-learning programs, 265–66
electronic health records (EHRs), 18,
258–61
Emergency Assistance Guide, 304
emergency operations centers (EOCs),
302–3, 318
emergency preparedness and response,
13, 40, 300, 318; structure of in
U.S., 302–5. *See also* disasters
Emergency Support Functions (ESFs),
304–5, 306–7
emerging diseases, 12–13, 237, 302
Employee Retirement Income
Security Act of 1974, 394
ENCODE (Encyclopedia of DNA
Elements), 355
EnhanceFitness, 166–67
environment, built and physical:
adaptation to, 342; definition of,
328–29; development of models for,
343–44; and disability, 333–34; and
genomic studies, 363; and health
behaviors, 329–35; and healthy
aging, 328–29; importance of as

factor, 90, 99, 170–71; individual's
fit to, 120, 342; measurement and
conceptualization, 336–39; modification of, 341–42; and older adult
needs, 30, 44, 123, 245–46; pathways
of, 329–30; and prevention, 234;
public health interventions around,
328, 342, 343, 345, 346, 385;
research studies on, 331–32, 343–44,
345; and social engagement, 211;
and socioeconomic status, 333;
technology and, 263; walking and,
331–33, 335, 339, 341
environmental audits, 337–39
environmental competence press
theory, 123
environmental policies, 231
Environmental Protection Agency,
329, 339, 340
Established Populations for Epidemiologic Studies of the Elderly
(EPESE), 344
EverCare program, 66
evidence, 268, 269–70; for programs,
17, 233–34, 241, 383
excise taxes, 144, 236, 385, 387
Experience Corps, 37, 42
Expert Patients Program (EPP), 170

Fair Housing Act, 244–45
Faith in Action, 166
falls, 170, 210, 261–62, 343
family caregiving, 192, 207; amount
of time providing, 184–85, 197;
caregiver characteristics, 181,
185–86; caregiver involvement in
treatment, 193–94, 197; caregiver
stress in, 189, 192, 194; costs of, 182,
191–93, 198; and demographic

family caregiving (*cont.*)
transitions, 182–83; episodic, 184, 187; ethical questions in, 198; and health disparities, 191, 197; health effects of, 188–89, 197; prevalence of, 182, 183–85, 186, 311; programs to support caregivers, 193–96; and public health, 195–97, 198; research studies on, 190–91, 195; type of care provided, 181–82, 186–88; women and, 183, 190
federal deficit, 398–99, 402
Federal Emergency Management Agency (FEMA), 299, 313
federalism, 302
Federal Poverty Guidelines (FPL), 103–4
fertility rates, 7, 372, 397
fibromyalgia, 216
Fit & Strong!, 153, 166–67
Florida, 220
Florida Health Care Association (FHCA), 304, 317
Food and Drug Administration, 4
Fortune, 395
Foster Grandparents, 218
Framework for Public Health Action, 278
France, 381
Frank, Janet C., 275–96
Fried, Linda P., 26–48
Frieden, T. R., 170, 231, 234–35, 278
functional limitation, 54, 104, 122, 127, 186, 240, 334; as conceptual disability model, 120, 121
Furner, Sylvia E., 74–92
Future of Public Health in the 21st Century, 6

Galway Consensus Statement, 16
gender, 143; and caregiving, 183, 190; and inequality, 31, 102, 103; and life expectancy, 28; and social engagement, 211, 214, 216–17
Genes, Environment, and Health Initiative (GEI), 360
Genetic Association Information Network (GAIN), 360–61
genome, 354, 355
genome-wide association studies (GWAS): about, 354–55; analytic challenges for, 358–60; behavioral and ethical questions in, 363–66; choosing phenotype for, 357–58; study design considerations for, 361–63
genomics, 11, 363; about, 354–57; and aging, 353–54, 356, 360–61, 366–67; clinical utility of, 365–66; functional, 355; population, 355–56, 361, 367; and public health, 353, 356–57; and risk profiles, 360, 363, 364, 366; testing, 363–65
genotype, 354
Genworth Financial, 404
geographic information systems (GIS), 319, 336–37
geographic location, 8
geospatial mapping, 19
Geriatric Education Centers (GECs), 285, 290
geriatric medicine, 48, 282, 288
Geriatric Research Education and Clinical Center (GRECC), 286, 296
Germany, 380, 381
Gerontological Society of America, 394
Gitlin, Laura N., 181–222

Glasgow, Russell E., 161–77
globalization, 382
Global Positioning System (GPS),
    335–36
Great Recession, 402, 403
Greenspan, Alan, 400
Group Health Cooperative (Seattle),
    366
Guide to Community Preventive
    Services, 163, 339
Guralnik, Jack M., 119–34

Hartz, Louis, 392
health-behavior model, 14
health care access, 31, 107–8, 110,
    253, 263, 271, 307, 386–87
health care delivery system, 15, 18,
    64–70; focused on acute care, 383,
    386; fragmented nature of, 10, 64,
    70; integration and coordination in,
    65, 384, 386; and long-term care,
    68–69; primary care, 384, 385–87;
    technology and, 255, 264, 271
Healthcare Effectiveness Data and
    Information Set (HEDIS), 173
health care professionals, 71
health definitions, 4, 78
health disparities, 32, 89, 90, 140; in
    caregiving, 191, 197; definition, 13;
    and disability, 32, 105, 110, 112,
    127–28; global, 374–75; and health
    inequities, 101–2; and health status,
    104–8; models of, 14; and popu-
    lation diversity, 8; and psychological
    stress, 109–10; as public health
    concern, 13–15; race as determinant
    of, 14, 104; in social engagement,
    211; socioeconomic, 8, 14, 31, 105,
    109, 110–11, 112

health impact pyramid, 230–31,
    234–35, 278
health inequities, 100–101, 106,
    111–14. See also health disparities
Health Information Technology (HIT),
    258–61
Health Information Technology for
    Economic and Clinical Health
    (HITECH) Act, 258, 259, 260
health insurance: under health care
    reform law, 20–21, 63, 104; for
    long-term care, 61–62; prior to
    Medicare and Medicaid, 56, 399;
    and public health policy, 108; for
    same-sex couples, 14; supplemental,
    57–58, 69, 112
health intervention trials: duration of,
    150; fidelity in, 151–52, 165; pilot
    tests, 148; program retention, 150;
    recruitment to, 149–50; and
    reinvention, 165; testing
    effectiveness, 148–49, 151
Health Interview Scale (HIS), 125
health maintenance organizations
    (HMOs), 18, 66
health promotion, 15–17, 221, 383,
    387; community- and home-
    based, 34, 162; evidence, 146–47;
    health care reform law and, 154;
    population-based, 384, 386, 387;
    programs, 166–67, 170, 177
health-related quality of life
    (HRQOL), 78
Health Resources and Services
    Administration (HRSA), 4, 280,
    285, 290–91
healthy aging concept, 47–48, 77–78,
    286, 328–29, 346
Healthy Aging Program, 140

Healthy Aging Research Network (HAN), 77, 292, 328–29, 338. *See also* Centers for Disease Control and Prevention

Healthy Caribbean Coalition, 387

Healthy IDEAS, 166–67

Healthy People, 89, 90, 129, *130*, 152–53, 195; about, 239–40

hearing care, 107

Henry Ford Health System (Detroit), 366

herpes zoster (shingles), 241

Hispanics, 8, 101, 104, 128, 185, 190

HIV/AIDS, 11, 12, 374

Home and Community Based Services (HCBS), 68

Home-Based Primary Care (HBPC), 66

home health services, 34, 66, 68, 318; annual cost of, 59; federal funding for, 60; home health aides, 59; for long-term care, 68–69

hospitalization, 66, 186, 237, 262, 316; risks of, 38, 40

housing: assisted living, 59, 313, 314–15; community housing with services, 313–14; design of, 40, 44; nursing homes, 58–59, 60, 68, 183, 188, 315–17, 404; older adults living in community, 311–13; patient-centered medical homes, 10; retirement communities, 244–45; smart homes, 263

HuGE Navigator, 365

Hughes, Susan L., 138–54

Human Ageing Genomic Resources project, 355

Hurricane and Disaster Preparedness for Long-Term Care Facilities, 317

Hurricane Katrina, 303, 304, 305, 307, 310, 314; mortality from, 299–300, 316

Hyer, Kathryn, 299–319

hypertension, 32, 104, 131, 140, 235, 360, 378

hypothalamic-pituitary-adrenal (HPA) functioning, 215

Iceland, 374

Illinois, 219

Improving Access to Assistive Technology for Individuals with Disabilities Act of 2004, 261

Incident Command System (ICS), 303–4

incontinence, 109, 316

Independence at Home Demonstration, 66

Index of Independence in Activities of Daily Living, 122

India, 27

Indian Health Service, 4, 58, 61

infant mortality, 376–77, 378–79

infectious disease, 11, 99, 377

influenza, 12, 237–39, 302

informal caregivers, 64, 311. *See also* family caregiving

Institute of Medicine (IOM), 63, 197; on disability, 119, 121, 129; on disaster preparedness and response, 315; on public health policy, 3, 5–6, 12, 401; on public health professionals, 9, 276–77, 288–89; works: *Disability in America: Toward a National Agenda for Prevention*, 119; *Research Priorities Report*, 315; "Retooling for an Aging America,"

276, 288–89; *Unequal Treatment,*
    107
instrumental activities of daily living
    (IADL), 183, 313
insurance companies, 61, 399, 404.
    See also health insurance
Integrated Dynamic Research-Practice
    Partnership, 177
intergenerational inequity, 396
International Classification of Func-
    tioning, Disability and Health
    (ICF), 122, 123
International HapMap Project, 354,
    358, 359
International Network on Public
    Health and Aging, 8
Internet, 91, 174, 220, 258, 267
Ireland, 184
Italy, 27

Japan, 27, 373
Japanese Americans, 214
John A. Hartford Foundation (JAHF),
    284, 288, 317
John Hancock, 404

Kaiser Permanente, 260

Lamm, Richard, 400, 403
Latinos. *See* Hispanics
Lee, Chanam, 327–46
leisure-time physical activity (LTPA),
    140
liberalism, 392, 393
Liberal Tradition in America, The
    (Hartz), 392
life course approach, 29, 31–33, 89,
    110–11

life expectancy, 79, 105, 142, 212,
    380–81; active, 33, 79, 382–83;
    global variation in, 372–73, 376;
    health disparities and, 14, 109; and
    population aging, 7, 27, 228, 372
Lifespan Respite Care Act of 2006,
    195
Lindeman, David, 253–71
location-tracking technologies, 262
Long-Life Family Study, 361
long-term care (LTC), 53, 54, 67,
    260; CLASS program and, 62–64;
    consumer direction in, 69–70; costs
    and financing, 58–60, 61–62; and
    health care delivery system, 68–69;
    PACE program and, 65

Maasticht Social Participation Profile,
    208
MacArthur Foundation, 76
Madrid International Plan of Action
    on Ageing, 29
malaria, 11
Mather's More than a Café, 218
Matter of Balance, 166–67
meals programs, 61, 308, 311, 312
measurement, 90–91, 387; of age
    effects, 81; of built environment,
    336–39; community indicators as,
    46–47; of disability, 122, 123–26,
    134; performance-based, 124, 126;
    and public accounting, 75–76;
    of quality of life, 79, 80, 85–88;
    of social engagement, 208–9; of
    socioeconomic status, 112; types,
    45–47; of walking and physical
    activity, 335–36. *See also* research;
    surveys

Measuring Health: A Guide to Rating Scales and Questionnaires (McDowell), 122

Medicaid, 20, 58, 64, 70, 408; and CLASS program, 63; cuts to, 398–99, 403–4; establishment of, 393, 399; and home and family care, 192, 314; and long-term care, 54, 59–60; and PACE program, 65; transformational impact of, 31

Medicare, 54, 64, 132, 154, 408; cost and financing, 17, 70, 192, 397–98, 400; cuts to, 398–99; establishment of, 56, 393, 399; gaps in coverage of, 57–58, 107; and health care reform law, 20, 66; and long-term care, 60; and PACE program, 65; popular support for, 407; and prevention, 107, 238, 241–42, 246; structure of, 56–57; transformational impact of, 31

Medicare Modernization Act of 2003, 57, 67

Medicare Savings Program (MSP), 58

medications: and disasters, 310; rising costs of, 109; technology and, 257

Meng, Hongdao, 119–34, 371–88

Metlife, 404

Mexico, 27

migration, 30

Minnesota, 67, 220

mobile health technologies, 263–64

morbidity, 38, 110, 142; compression of, 33, 45, 234

mortality, 316, 375, 382; premature and preventable, 377, 379; and socioeconomic status, 14, 104–6, 107, 110

Multiplex Initiative, 366

National Academy of Public Administration, 398

National Academy of Sciences, 329, 401

"National Agenda for Geriatric Education, A: White Papers," 280, *281*

National Association of County and City Health Officials (NACCHO), 277

National Cancer Institute, 366

National Center for Health Statistics, 121, 125

National Center on Minority and Health Disparities, 15

National Council on Aging, 16, 164

National Expert Panel on Community Health Promotion, 16–17

National Family Caregiver Support Program (NFCSP), 195

National Health and Nutrition Examination Surveys (NHANES), 127

National Healthcare Disparities Report, 100–101

National Health Interview Survey, 142

National Human Genome Research Institute (NHGRI), 355, 359, 366

National Incident Management System (NIMS), 303

National Institute on Aging (NIA), 344, 372, 394; training programs of, 285–86, 293–95

National Institute on Alcohol Abuse and Alcoholism, 143

National Institutes of Health (NIH), 4, 15, 100

National Long-Term Care Survey, 64, 142, 183, 194

National Registry of Evidence-based Programs and Practices (NREPP), 164

National Research Council, 398

National Response Framework, 303

National Social Life, Health, and Aging Project, 143

Nationwide Health Information Network (NHIN), 260

Native Americans, 58, 61

Navigenics, 363

Neighborhood Environment Walkability Survey (NEWS), 336

neighborhoods: and social participation, 211; and socioeconomic status, 106–8, 110, 113; walkable, 331, 332, 341

neoliberalism, 394–95

Netherlands, 231

New Deal, 393

New England Centenarians Study, 361

New England Healthcare Institute (NEHI), 256, 257

New Freedom Initiative, 68

New York Times, 395, 406

nongovernmental organizations (NGOs), 4

Nummela, O., 212

nurses, 264, 282–83, 386

Nursing Home Emergency Preparedness and Response during Recent Hurricanes, 315

nursing homes, 183, 188; cost and financing, 58–59, 60, 68, 404; during disasters, 315–17

OASIS Institute, 218

Obama, Barack, 398, 405

obesity and overweight, 379; health impact of, 5, 10, 133, 141–42; and public health policy, 10, 32, 113, 379, 385

Office of Management and Budget (OMB), 83

Office of Personnel Management (OPM), 62

Office of Public Health Genomics (OPHG), 353

Office of the Surgeon General, 121, 128–29

older adults: ageism toward, 108–9, 345–46, 393–94, 399–400; devalued status of, 109; health status continuum of, 36, 41–42; heterogeneity of, 38; public perceptions of, 76; rationing care for, 400–402, 403; scapegoating of, 108–9, 394–96, 408; as social category, 101; societal benefits from, 29–30, 34, 41, 48; special needs of, 30, 34, 44, 47–48, 123, 245–46; vulnerabilities of, 286, 299–300, 305, 307–9, 310, 312, 318

Older Americans Act, 61, 218, 393

Olmstead v. L.C., 68

Ory, Marcia G., 138–54, 327–46

Partnership for Prevention, 244

Patient-Centered Medical Home (PCMH), 10, 384

Patient Protection and Affordable Care Act (PPACA), 18, 69, 230, 275; CLASS program under, 63, 404; financing care under, 20–21; health promotion efforts of, 154; and Medicare, 57, 144, 241–42; political debate over, 21, 402, 404–6; prevention efforts under, 21, 144,

Patient Protection and Affordable Care Act (PPACA) (cont.) 241–42, 246–47; service integration under, 65, 66–67; and SNP program, 68

Patient-Reported Outcomes Measurement Information System (PROMIS), 77, 90–91

patient-safety monitoring, 261–62

Pension Benefit Guaranty Corporation, 394

pensions, employment-linked, 102

personal emergency response systems (PERS), 262

pharmacists, 283

phenotype, 354, 355, 357–58, 359, 361

physical activity: guidelines for, 139–40; health benefits of, 36; need to enhance, 40; social engagement and, 215–16. See also walking

physical inactivity: as health risk, 139–40, 161, 330; as public health question, 379

physical therapy, 132

physicians, 5, 276, 282

Pillars for the Care of Older Persons in the Caribbean: A Comprehensive Community-Based Framework, 383–85

point-of-care monitoring devices, 256

pollution, 113

population aging: causes of, 7, 27, 372, 397; as global phenomenon, 27–28, 371–72, 397; impact on society of, 29–30; need to expand study of, 344–45; and public health, 27, 28–29, 48, 182, 318, 372–73, 382, 383–85; statistics on, 7, 27–28, 182, 319, 371–72, 373, 397

Population Association of America, 396

population perspective model, 4

poverty, 31, 102–4, 396; and health, 8, 104–5, 108

Press-Competence model, 330

prevention, 40, 107, 245, 386; of cardiovascular disease, 35, 112–13; and chronic conditions, 10, 32, 33, 36, 38, 132–33; cost-effectiveness of, 234; directed toward older adults, 34–36; of disability, 119, 128–29, 131–33; genomics and, 364; health care reform law and, 21, 144, 241–42, 246–47; life course approach to, 31–33; Medicare and, 107, 241–42, 246; and personal responsibility, 234; primary, secondary, and tertiary, 33–34, 35, 131–33, 231; public health and, 26–27, 32, 228, 229, 242–43, 246–47, 286, 387; and screening, 39, 143–44; vaccination, 143–44, 228, 237–39, 241, 403

Prevention Research Centers (PRC), 285. See also Centers for Disease Control and Prevention

primary care, 18, 54, 60, 383; by family caregivers, 182, 192; under health care reform law, 66; integrated, 66, 385–87; low compensation for, 243; and prevention, 243, 384

privacy and confidentiality, 18, 267

Program of All-Inclusive Care for the Elderly (PACE), 65–66

Program to Encourage Active Rewarding Lives for Seniors (PEARLS), 164

Prohaska, Thomas R., 161–77

Prostate, Lung, Colorectal, and Ovary (PLCO) study, 360

Provenge, 403
proxies, 124–25, 187
psychiatric disorders, 121, 309
psychological first aid, 308–9
psychosocial stress model, 14
public health: community-based approach to, 9, 34, 42, 44, 243–46; coordination and oversight of, 6; definitions, 3, 230; and disability prevention, 132–33; and disaster response, 318–19; dispersed responsibility for, 3–4; environmental interventions, 342; evidence-based policy in, 17, 146–47, 163–64, 166–67, 170, 177, 233–34, 241, 383; and family caregiving, 195–97, 198; functions of, 5–7; future approaches to, 40–41; and genomics, 353, 356–57; goals of, 33–34, 74; and health behavior, 37, 40–41, 146–47, 152–54; and health equity, 100–101; and healthy aging, 47–48; history of, 26, 99, 229, 230; and infant mortality, 377, 378–79; intervention design and evaluation, 9, 19–20, 146–47, 246; and mortality rate, 377, 378–79; need for improved infrastructure of, 6, 12–13, 32–33, 382; and obesity and overweight, 10, 32, 113, 379, 385; and population aging, 27, 28–29, 48, 182, 318, 372–73, 382, 383–85; prevention focus in, 26–27, 32, 239–41; reframing of issues in, 407–8; and risk factors, 144–46, 152–54, 161–62, 376–77; social benefits of, 38–39, 48; and social-ecological aging model, 4–5, 77, 91, 228–29, 232, 242–43; and social

engagement, 217–20, 221; and technology, 254; and tobacco use, 20, 113–14, 144, 235–36, 237, 385, 387; vaccinations, 237–39, 241. See also health intervention trials
Public Health Genomics, 353
public health movements, 113–14
Public Health Prevention Service (PHPS), 292
public health professionals, 5, 19–20, 287, 290; aging of, 8, 277, 288; competencies of, 276, 288–89; definition of, 276–77; and emergency preparedness, 13; medical licensing of, 265; number of, 276; and older person's self-management skills, 287–88; roles and functions of, 278–79; shortages of, 183; and succession planning, 277–78; and technology, 71, 255–56, 264–66, 267, 268, 271; training of, 8–9, 13, 197, 264–66, 267, 275, 282–86, 287, 308–9, 318
Public Health Training Center (PHTC), 285
Public Health Workforce Enumeration 2000 report, 278
public-private partnerships, 9, 268–69

quality of life, 90, 132; defining, 78; measurement of, 79, 80, 85–88

race, 14, 101, 104
Racial and Ethnic Approaches to Community Health across the U.S. (REACH U.S.), 89–90, 111. See also Centers for Disease Control and Prevention
racial-genetic model, 14

racism, 14, 15, 111

randomized controlled trials (RCT), 148–49, 162, 164, 176, 193, 268

rationing of health care, 400–402, 403

Reagan, Ronald, 394

RE-AIM framework, 147, 167–68, 171, 172, 177

regional extension centers (RECs), 259

rehabilitation, 54, 60, 123

remote patient monitoring (RPM), 255–56

research: cross-sectional studies, 331; data collection, 74–75, 81–84, 85–88, 91–92, 387; demographic, 81; and evaluation models, 144; future directions for, 89–91; longitudinal studies, 331, 332, 334, 339, 344; and practice, 16, 339, 341–42; social-ecological model, 91; strategies, 19–20; translational, 163–66, 171–72, 174, 175, 176–77; during twentieth century, 138. *See also* measurement; surveys

Research on Aging Act, 394

Research Priorities Report, 315

Resource Centers for Minority Aging Research (RCMAR), 286

retail clinics, 18

retirement age, 29, 112, 380–81

retirement communities, 244–45

Risk Evaluation and Education for Alzheimer's disease study, 365

risk factors: attention to, 99, 376–77; complexity of, 39; genetics and, 360, 363, 364, 366; and prevention, 31, 32; social activity as, 217. *See also* behavioral risk factors

Robert T. Stafford Disaster Relief and Emergency Assistance Act, 302

Robert Wood Johnson Foundation, 171, 239

Roosevelt, Franklin, 393

Rosalynn Carter Institute for Caregiving, 265

Satariano, William A., 327–46

schools of medicine and health science, 275, 280–82, 283–84

Schulz, Richard, 181–222

screening, 39, 42, 143–44

seatbelt laws, 229

self-assessments and reports, 79, 111, 123–24, 126, 212–13

Senior Companions, 218

Senior Walking Environment Assessment Tool, 338

Service Corps of Retired Executives (SCORE), 218

Setting Limits: Medical Goals in an Aging Society (Callahan), 401

sexual orientation, 14

Seymour, Rachel B., 138–54

Shepherd's Centers of America, 218

Sherwin, Angela, 3–21

Should Medical Care Be Rationed By Age?, 401

Sickness Prevention Achieved through Regional Collaboration (SPARC), 243

single nucleotide polymorphism (SNP), 354–55, 357, 358–59

smart homes, 263

smartphones, 263

Smith-Ray, Renae, 161–77

smoking. *See* tobacco use

social capital, 207–8, 221

social determinants, 4–5, 90, 99, 208, 328; ageism as, 108–9; and health disparities, 99–100, 104–8; impact on medical care, 100, 109–10; and life course, 110–11; public health and, 113, 230–31; social institutions and, 111–12

social engagement, 205, 206, 385; decreases with age, 211–12; definitions and characteristics, 206–9; epidemiology of, 209–12; and gender, 216–17; health impact of, 36, 41, 42, 212–14, 215–17, 221; and life satisfaction, 213, 214; measurement of, 208–9; and mental health, 210, 213; and public health, 217–20, 221; research studies on, 206–7, 209–10, 221; types of, 216, 217; unique role of, 205–6

social isolation, 213, 215, 216–17

social networking and media, 19–20, 266, 319

social networks, 207, 215, 311–12

Social Security, 121, 314, 393; cash flow problem in, 395; and disparities, 102, 112; popular support for, 407; and retirement age, 29, 112, 380–81; transformative role of, 31, 396

social workers, 283–84

socioecological model, 4–5, 77, 91, 228–29, 242–43

socioeconomic status, 101; and environment, 333; and health, 8, 14, 31, 105, 109, 110–11, 112; income equality, 112; income

inequity, 104; by race, class, and gender, 102–4; and social engagement, 211, 216

Special Needs Plans (SNPs), 67–68

STAMPEED (SNP Typing for Association with Multiple Phenotypes from Existing Epidemiologic Data), 360

Stanford Diabetes Self-Management Program, 154

State Health Information Exchange Cooperative Agreement Program, 260

St. Louis Environment and Physical Activity Instrument, 336

Stone, Robyn I., 53–71

Strategic Health IT Advanced Research Projects (SHARP), 260

stress, 214; caregivers', 189, 192, 194; in disasters, 309, 313; from social isolation, 216–17

Strong for Life, 166, 169

structural constructivist model, 14

Substance Abuse and Mental Health Services, 4

successful aging, 45, 76

support-dependency ratio, 45

Supreme Court, 68

"Surgeon General's Call to Action to Improve the Health and Wellness of Persons with Disabilities, The," 128–29

surveillance, health, 3–4, 84, 90, 133, 195, 239, 385

Survey of Health, Ageing and Retirement in Europe (SHARE), 213

Survey of Income and Program Participation (SIPP), 127

surveys, *80*, 89–90; as data collection tools, 75, 83–84
syndemics, 12

Task Force on Community Preventive Services, 164, 233, 235, 243–46
teams, 385–87
technology, 11, 256; assistive, 262; barriers to adoption of, 266–69; comparative effectiveness research on, 269–70; and cost, 267, 268–69, 271; and family caregiving, 182–83; and health care delivery system, 169, 255; and health care workforce, 71, 255–56, 264–66, 271; Health Information Technology, 258–61; mobile health, 263–64; monitoring, 255–56, 261–62; older adults and, 220, 254–55, 261, 266, 267, 268, 270, 271; and public health, 254; and public health system, 253–54, 271; and quality of care, 271; reimbursement for, 270–71; scalability and sustainability of, 269; smart homes, 263; telehealth, 257–58; as transformative agent, 271
telehealth, 257–58
Texas, 67
text messaging, 264
Time, 395
tobacco use, 106; impact on health, 142–43, 161; public health policy toward, 20, 113–14, 144, 235–36, 237, 385, 387
trans fats, 113, 385
transportation, 40, 231
Transportation Research Board, 329
TRUTH, 20
tuberculosis, 11, 12

Unequal Treatment, 107
United Healthcare, 66
United Kingdom, 170, 386, 400
Upshur, R. E. G., 17
urban informatics, 266
urbanization, 30
U.S. Preventive Services Task Force (USPSTF), 240–41

vaccination, 143–44, 228, 241, 403; for influenza, 237–39
Veterans Administration (VA), 260, 286, 296. *See also* Department of Veterans Affairs
Veterans Health Administration (VHA), 256, 257, 265
videoconferencing, 258, 265
vision coverage, 107
Visiting Nurse Service of New York (VNSNY), 264
volunteering, 212, 218–19, 220; health benefits of, 205–6, 207, 214, 215, 216

walking: and built environment, 331–33, 335, 339, 341; disabled people and, 334; health effects of, 330–31, 344, 379; measurement and conceptualization, 335–36
Wallace, Steven P., 99–114
Weiss, Joan, 275–96
Welcome Trust Case Control Consortium (WTCCC), 361
Wetle, Terrie, 3–21
Why Survive? Growing Older in America (Butler), 399–400
World Health Organization (WHO), 17, 195, 197, 380; on cities and

urbanization, 30, 44; on community
health promotion, 383; definition of
health by, 4, 75; on disability, 122;
on disasters, 300, 301; environmental recommendations of, 339,
340; health inequity concept of, 101;
on social determinants of health, 90,
110; on social engagement, 210

YMCA, 218

About the Editors

THOMAS R. PROHASKA is Professor in the Division of Community Health Sciences at the University of Illinois at Chicago (UIC) School of Public Health and Co-Director of the Center for Research on Health and Aging at UIC's Institute for Health Research and Policy. He has over 100 publications in gerontological health and behavioral health risk factors in older populations. He previously edited (along with Tom Hickey and Marjorie Speers) *Public Health and Aging* (1997), a predecessor to the present volume. During his more than 30 years of experience in gerontological research, Dr. Prohaska has been the principal investigator of several federally funded research studies and co-investigator on many others. His recent research funding sources include the National Institute on Aging, the U.S. Administration on Aging, the Retirement Research Foundation, and Easter Seals. His research interests focus on gerontological public health including health behavior, illness behavior in older adults, self-care and chronic disease management in older populations, doctor–older patient interaction studies, and the translation and dissemination of evidence-based research and health innovations in older populations. He serves on the editorial boards of the *Gerontologist*, the *Journal of Gerontology Social Sciences*, and the *Journal of Aging and Health*. He has also served on advisory and review panels for the National Institutes of Health, the Robert Wood Johnson Foundation, and several other research foundations. Dr. Prohaska received his PhD in Experimental Psychology at Virginia Commonwealth University, Medical College of Virginia and his postdoctoral training in Health Psychology and Gerontology at the University of Wisconsin–Madison.

LYNDA A. ANDERSON is the Director of the Healthy Aging Program, Division of Adult and Community Health in the National Center for Chronic Disease Prevention and Health Promotion at the Centers for Disease Control and Prevention (CDC), U.S. Department of Health and Human Services. She is also Adjunct Associate Professor at the Rollins School of Public Health at Emory University, Atlanta, Georgia. Dr. Anderson is responsible for leading innovative CDC projects to facilitate the translation of research to practice to improve the lives of older adults. She has over 100 publications, including peer-reviewed manuscripts, book chapters, and invited articles. She is a current member of the advisory boards of the Health and Aging Policy Fellows Program and the Healthy Aging Regional Collaborative Leadership Council. She served as a guest editor for several special journal issues, including the *American Journal of Preventive Medicine* and *Health Behavior and Health Education*. She is the recipient of numerous U.S. Department of Health and Human Services Public Health Services honor awards and the Eunice Tyler Practice Award from the University of North Carolina. Dr. Anderson received her doctorate from the School of Public Health at the University of North Carolina at Chapel Hill. She completed a 2-year NIA Postdoctoral Fellowship in aging at the Duke University Center for the Study of Aging and Human Development.

ROBERT H. BINSTOCK was, until his death in November 2011, Professor of Aging, Health, and Society at Case Western Reserve University. A former President of the Gerontological Society of America, and former Chair of the Gerontological Health Section of the American Public Health Association, he served as director of a White House Task Force on Older Americans and frequently testified before the U.S. Congress. He was a member of the MacArthur Foundation's Research Network on an Aging Society. Dr. Binstock authored about 300 articles, book chapters, and monographs, most of them dealing with politics and policies related to aging. His 26 authored and edited books include seven editions of the *Handbook of Aging and the Social Sciences* (the latest published in 2011 and coedited with Linda K. George) and *Aging Nation: The Economics and Politics of Growing Older in America* (2008, coauthored with James Schulz). Among the honors he received for contributions to gerontology and the well-being of older persons are the Kent and Brookdale awards from the Gerontological Society of America, the Lifetime Achievement and Key awards from the Gerontological Health Section of the American Public Health Association, the American Society on Aging Award, the American Society on Aging's Hall of Fame Award, and the Ollie A. Randall Award from the National Council on Aging.